Praise for *Breas*

Dr Frank Reeves's memoir is an account of living with cancer, hi̱ cancer in men and the process invol ...̱ ̱ ̱ this rare cancer. Dr Reeves's book will encourage a whole host of important conversations.

- Jo Judges, Head of Service for the Midlands, Macmillan Cancer Support UK

This most useful and thoroughly interesting book provides, perhaps for the first time, a brutally honest account of the experience of a man diagnosed with breast cancer, and the extensive treatment he received, revealing in graphic detail his ongoing bodily and emotional reactions. While breast cancer is rare in men, those men who are diagnosed with it will find much here of value, as will cancer patients generally, regardless of their gender. But the book has a much greater relevance. It transcends the personal by vividly depicting the sheer disruptive force of cancer on an active life and the renewed pleasure in the everyday and relationships that a reminder of mortality brings. Just as importantly, Frank Reeves balances the personal and intimate with a wider social perspective, depicting an NHS hospital from a patient's point of view, while simultaneously demonstrating a profound political and historical appreciation of the NHS as an institution.

- Diana Holmes, Professor of French at the University of Leeds and former breast cancer patient

Men account annually for only 0.6 per cent of the cases of breast cancer. Yet Frank Reeves, an academic and political campaigner, in this detailed account of his illness and treatment, never makes the despairing plea, "why me?". Instead, from the moment of diagnosis, he sets out to record the course of his treatment, the impact it has had on him, his outlook on life and his relationships. It offers reasons both to celebrate and be critical of the management of his treatment pathway through cancer. It also opens up a gradual exploration of male identity faced with the consequences of serious illness and turbulent emotions. Anyone will find this account engrossing and thought-provoking. Patients, medical professionals, and NHS managers should mine it for the rich seams of analysis and insight it contains. This is the story of cancer born of a lived experience, allied to a forensic examination of the realities of treatment in one Midlands hospital.

- Professor Geoff Hurd, Deputy Vice-Chancellor at the University of Wolverhampton, now retired

A moving description and analysis of the diagnosis and treatment of cancer in one man. I was gripped emotionally and intellectually as the scene shifted between home and hospital in the ten months of Frank's illness.

- Dr Anna Frankel, former manager, Heart of Birmingham Primary Care Trust

BREAST CANCER MAN

by Frank Reeves,

with the assistance of his wife, Mel Chevannes,

his children, other family members, and friends.

A 72-year old grandfather's story of his diagnosis,

operations and treatment for breast cancer

at an NHS hospital in the West Midlands,

including an account of his chemotherapy,

radiotherapy, and hormone therapy,

together with reflections on the social, cultural

and institutional context in which treatment took place.

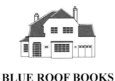

BLUE ROOF BOOKS

First published in Great Britain in 2018 by Blue Roof Books, 53 Woodthorne Road, Tettenhall, Wolverhampton , WV6 8TU

ISBN 978-0-9570042-2-1

Printed and bound by Heathcotes Print and Design, Unit C1, Hilton Trading Estate, Hilton Road, Lanesfield, Wolverhampton, WV6 8TU. To be released as a Kindle ebook in 2019.

Individual copies of the first edition of *Breast Cancer Man* may be obtained free on request by emailing blueroofbooks@yahoo.com, or by writing to Blue Roof Books, 53 Woodthorne Road, Tettenhall, Wolverhampton WV6 8TU. Please supply your name, and postal address and provide a reason for your interest, eg., you have been diagnosed with breast cancer, or are employed in the NHS, etc. Appreciative readers are encouraged as a quid pro quo to make a donation to Supporter Donations, Macmillan Cancer Support, FREEPOST LON15851, 89 Albert Embankment, London SE1 7UQ. Also available on Amazon.

BREAST CANCER MAN

CONTENTS

Dedicated

to all those, like me, who have been diagnosed with breast cancer and are undergoing, or have undergone, treatment.

to my wife, children and grandchildren, who brightened my life during the ten months of my cancer treatment.

to my grandson, Ulysses Equiano Hubbard, who came into the world on the 6th October 2018, as *Breast Cancer Man* went to press.

to other family members and friends, whose kindness and concern for my health and wellbeing were incomparable and overwhelming.

to the memory of Dennis Turner, a dear friend, former MP for Wolverhampton South East, and then peer of the realm, who campaigned ceaselessly for the National Health Service and social care for the elderly and infirm, until he developed terminal cancer. He was attended at home in his final hours by Macmillan cancer nurses.

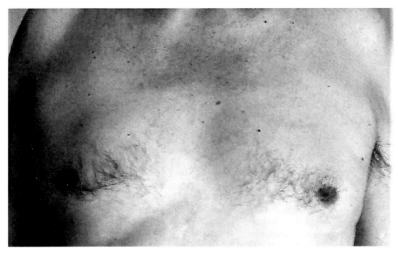

Frank's chest prior to the mastectomy

Preface: why I came to write this book

Aware of my habit of keeping a written record of the significant events in my life, my wife, Mel, and daughter, Toussaint, suggested that I write a diary about my breast cancer diagnosis, operations and treatment. They conceived the project, quite spontaneously, as a therapy for helping me come to terms with my cancer, or for distracting me from the discomfort of its treatment. It was only later that I read in a Macmillan Cancer Care practical guide that 'some people find it helpful to keep a diary, journal, or on-line blog, where they can write down all their thoughts, feelings and frustrations'.[1] I saw the diary as a useful opportunity to record my experiences and improve my understanding at first hand of modern scientifically-based medical procedures and my own and others' responses to them. As my treatment progressed, I learned that making a record on a systematic daily basis helped me to digest the information I was given about my cancer, the operations I underwent, and the medication I was prescribed, and to accept and come to anticipate the side effects of the chemotherapy,

1

radiotherapy and hormone therapy I was given. Likewise, I found myself obliged to contextualise and compare my individual experiences with those of fellow patients, and gained comfort from knowing that I was merely one among many, and there were always some far worse off than myself.

As treatment continued and my diary grew in length, I recognised the limitations of describing my daily experiences in chronological order. I decided to edit out unnecessary repetition and self-consciously to adopt a more thematic and explanatory approach. I realised from the start that my experience of being a patient was occurring along with those of thousands of other people in the context of a large National Health Service hospital, and that what I felt and thought and came to accept in the process of treatment was a result of a complex interplay between my 70-or-so years of personal history, current 21st-century medical practice in relation to breast cancer, and the all-prevailing UK social, political and institutional environment in which I, my family and my fellow patients lived out our lives. The most atypical aspect of all this, and possibly its only noteworthy feature, was the fact that I, as a man, had been diagnosed with breast cancer, and that there were only 350 instances of men with breast cancer per year in the UK[2] and that just two or three of these anomalies occurred in the Wolverhampton area annually.

Over the ten months of hospital treatment, my personal account of 'the patient experience' grew, like Topsy, into an 80,000-word manuscript. When I informed doctors and nurses that I was keeping a record of the treatment I was receiving, they invariably encouraged me in my endeavour, pointing out that it was important for them and the NHS as a whole to listen to those they were treating, learn from them, and take action. Feedback of this kind, they said, was essential for improving the quality of hospital care. Some of the staff asked whether I would send them a copy of the finished account, to which I readily acceded, provided that they gave me an email address.

The essence of the manuscript was indeed an account of a patient's personal experience of being diagnosed and treated for breast cancer at an NHS hospital. But to provide such an account in any meaningful way, I had not only to describe my mental and physical reactions to the diagnosis, surgery, and adjuvant therapy, but to explain my thoughts and feelings in the full context of my daily domestic routines, my visits to the GP and hospital, the hospital's physical and social environment, the technical apparatus used on me, the medical protocols, the relationships I established with hospital staff in the course of my treatment, the empathy generated in my contact with fellow patients on wards and in waiting rooms, and much more besides. And coming from a philosophical, sociological and anthropological background, I could not help but reveal my interest in the ethnography of the moment. My patient experience was self-evidently socially mediated.

At the start of my second cycle of chemotherapy, it was put to me by family and friends that the account of my personal experiences and feelings might provide information, reassurance, and a male perspective to other men newly diagnosed with breast cancer, as well as to breast cancer patients more generally. Perhaps I could work up my account of one man's experience of breast cancer into a publication aimed primarily at newly-diagnosed male breast cancer patients to prepare them for what to expect from their treatment. The prospect of producing a book appealed to me as I had written and published before. I was also attracted by the idea of helping others to cope with what I had had to endure, although I was conscious that they might well be alarmed by my more graphic accounts of the various side effects. Nevertheless, it occurred to me that I might publish a book, entitled *Breast Cancer Man*, at my own expense, which I could then make freely available to men diagnosed with breast cancer in the UK. There were, after all, only 350 men each year!

Once the project had been conceived formally in this way, I came to recognise that the project I had embarked upon required the input, assistance and scrutiny of all those involved in my treatment and care. The cooperation of hospital staff, my local GPs, family and friends was essential, not only for sustaining my ongoing physical and mental health, but to provide the dramatis personae, scenes, settings, and twists and turns of my story, and to ensure my mention of medical procedures and medications was accurate.

From then on, I worked hard to involve family members, friends, acquaintances and the doctors, nurses and radiographers who had treated me, in commenting, contributing, correcting, amending, and improving on the content of chapters, which were circulated electronically to those who expressed, or might be considered to have an interest in the project and were prepared to provide me with their email address. In the course of my treatment I must have had contact with 70 or more health service staff at my local GP surgery (the Castlecroft Medical Practice) and at the hospital (New Cross, run by the NHS Wolverhampton Royal Hospital Trust). I learned the names of at least 55 of those people and conversed, often at length, with doctors, nurses, radiographers and ancillary staff, my memory of them assisted by the names displayed on calling letters, appointment cards, notice boards, treatment rooms, security tags, and lapel badges. In short, I was positively encouraged or invited to refer by first or second name to those treating my condition and, in reciprocal fashion, they used the name on my medical record to address me as 'Francis' (but rarely as 'Frank', which I would have preferred).

Over the ten-month period of hospital attendance, my familiarity and friendly exchanges with hospital staff developed. I told them about my diary and project of publishing a book about my experience of being a patient. Many expressed interest and asked me to send them an electronic copy of my manuscript once it was nearing completion. Encouraged in this way, I built up a list of 25 staff and their email addresses and sent them a copy of either the completed manuscript or, in accordance with their contribution, the chapter in which the services they rendered were mentioned. A covering note invited them to respond, with comments, corrections, or suggestions for improvement by a suitably distant deadline. Apart from a few friendly acknowledgments of receipt of the covering letter and attachment, I received only one response. It was from a nurse who had befriended us but who had recently retired from a senior position at the hospital. Her comment was that she wouldn't change a word of my account! I received no further communication or comment in response to the circulation of the manuscript to the 24 others at the hospital. I attributed this ominous electronic silence to the pressure of work on exhausted staff and gave no further thought to the matter. At this stage, I believed the accuracy, immediacy and honesty of my account would be appreciated and well received. I had sought only to describe as truthfully and vividly as I could, the series of events that had occupied my ten months of treatment.

Surgery, other medical procedures and adjuvant therapies are never pleasant, but can be made more tolerable by the quality of the care provided by the staff who administer them. For me, the social environment of the hospital was overwhelmingly supportive. Only on rare occasions did I find the attitude of staff disrespectful and upsetting. In telling the story of my treatment, I sought to credit the people who helped me by giving them a presence and personality, of which describing their actions and naming them constituted an essential element. In my view, a significant part of the patient experience - at least as significant as the physical sensations and side effects - is the social context of sympathetic consideration, understanding, compassion, respect and kindness in which the treatment takes place. To emphasise its overwhelming importance, I chose to omit the names of staff who had been brusque, unhelpful, or caused me distress. I assumed that this would deny them the opportunity to respond defensively with accusations that I had damaged or defamed their professional reputation. Conversely, staff who received positive mention and accolades would be pleased by my acknowledging the quality of their contribution.

I first became aware of the alarm that the receipt of my manuscript had caused at the hospital when one of the doctors requested politely that I remove his name from it, in order, he said, to protect his privacy. He hinted that other staff who had dealt with me felt the same way as he did, but were reluctant to say. Despite the fact that they were employed in public positions in the National Health Service and providing treatment to all who needed it, I was led to believe that the medical staff, with whom I had such amicable contact, assumed that they had a right to privacy and were unhappy that I had so freely made use of their names. If that were true, then clearly, in their eyes, an account of the patient experience was all well and good, as long as the persons involved in providing that experience were not identified by name.

Not wanting to offend anyone unnecessarily, or jeopardise the publication of *Breast Cancer Man*, I readily agreed to replace all actual names of doctors, nurses, radiographers and ancillary staff with pseudonyms in the hope that that would satisfy the desire for privacy, while at the same time retaining the integrity and accuracy of the narrative relating to my multiple social encounters with the essential providers of my course of treatment. (In the text, I denote pseudonyms with italics.) This decision also entailed anonymising the greater proportion of the directory of named persons which I had compiled to assist readers' understanding of the course of events, and of the degree to which hospital arrangements resulted in contact with the same staff, and a semblance of continuity in care.

In addition, I sought the informal advice of friends who were trained and qualified in legal matters, one a solicitor. They reasoned, as all legal advisors do, that it was best to err on the side of caution, but were of the opinion that privacy law applied to people's private and family lives and not to their roles in the public domain. To be on the safe side, however, they thought it best to obtain the written consent of everyone who was named in the book. Even if I could have accessed the contact details of hospital personnel (which I could not), this would have proved an almost impossible task. As I had already agreed to remove the actual names of all NHS staff, I proceeded no further along that path. But I became curious to discover how others who had written about the patient experience had handled the privacy issue.

I noticed that in her book, *Dear Cancer, love Victoria*[3], Victoria Derbyshire, the journalist and television presenter, sometimes referred to medical staff by their actual names, and sometimes by their role, for example, nurse, or radiographer, perhaps because she had gained permission from some to use their names, while for others she had never learned their names, or had forgotten to ask whether they minded her using them. What was most apparent, however, were the book's photographs of the (named) team of nurses who attended to her in the infusion suite, the (named) surgeon who 'saved her life', and one of the nurses she liked, together with selfies of her with her extended family, children, and actor friends, Julie Walters and Robbie Coltrane.[4] There was little evidence of a desire for anonymity here. On the contrary, Victoria Derbyshire's use of her celebrity status to demystify breast cancer treatment for women was widely appreciated, leading those around her to join her campaign and abandon any preference they might have for privacy. Breast cancer in men awaits its celebrity advocate.

The hospital staff's preference for privacy also led me to abandon my plan to illustrate my narrative systematically with pictures of the medical teams or the various stages of my treatment, for example, of my having my blood taken, being given an infusion of chemo drugs, or lying beneath a Linac machine. Staff did not object to Mel taking the occasional snap of me in the course of my treatment, but they would have become perturbed at the suggestion that the photographs were to feature in a published book - with the attendant risk of breaching the confidentiality of other patients, or the privacy of staff. I suspected that the ever-present laudable preoccupation with safeguarding patient confidentiality had led to a similar expectation regarding staff privacy. In due course, an official request to take photographs to the hospital authority might have been granted, but with stringent conditions attached. Better not to alert the sleeping giant!

I chose the photograph that forms part of the book's cover design, not because it was a selfie and I didn't need permission to use it, or to frighten away or shock potential readers, but to emphasise an obvious and socially-significant difference between men's breasts and women's breasts. I can use an image of my chest in this way precisely because men's breasts are not regarded as private and intimate organs. In appropriate context - a beach, building site, hospital ward, while scything a Cornish meadow, or on the cover of a book about breast-cancer - men can expose their breasts to the public without risk of censure.

In stark contrast, in the United Kingdom, women's breasts are invariably considered to be private and intimate parts of their bodies. They are expected to shield their breasts from the public gaze and, on occasion, have even been condemned for exposing themselves in order to breast feed their babies in public places. The contrasting social attitude to men and women's breasts helps to explain the difference between the sexes in their experiences of, responses to, and treatment for breast cancer, including the variation in the provision made for them in the hospital setting, one of the themes that I touch on in the chapters that follow. (There is, of course, another issue here, relating to the presentation or representation of bodily deformity in public, in this instance, of scar tissue arising from a mastectomy, but it would be inappropriate to explore it further at this point.)

When my breast cancer was first diagnosed, the breast cancer nurse gave me a copy of *Understanding Breast Cancer in Men*,[5] one of the excellent Macmillan Cancer Care practical guides, carefully and simply written to inform patients with cancer about their condition. During my treatment I had cause to peruse many of those Macmillan guides and found them very helpful in preparing me for what to expect. They also provided me with reassurance that my condition was run-of-the-mill and that I was one among many. Useful, too, were Breast Cancer Care's booklets, *Radiotherapy for Primary Breast Cancer*, and *Tamoxifen*.

Convinced of the quality and efficacy of the available literature for cancer patients, I contacted Macmillan to explore how my project might best be targetted at men diagnosed with breast cancer, explaining that I would like to make copies of my story freely available to them. Would Macmillan help to publicise *Breast Cancer Man*? Would it be able to provide me with a recommendatory quote for the dust cover? Could it play any part in helping me distribute it free to other men diagnosed with breast cancer?

I am grateful to Sophie Beresford, Macmillan's Communications Officer for the West Midlands Region, and to Sue Hawkins, Macmillan's Information Materials Researcher in Cancer Information Development, for their courtesy, encouragement and advice on publicising my book. They promised to add details of my book to the Macmillan web directory of resources for people affected by cancer. Sophie contacted Jo Judges, Head of Services for the Midlands, who, after perusing the manuscript, provided me most generously with a suitable quote of praise for the book. Sophie also promised to assist me in publicising my breast cancer story by producing press releases for the local media. While Macmillan Cancer Support has encouraged me to make public my story (in line with its ubiquitous advice on the therapeutic value of talking about and recording experiences), I should make clear that the publication of *Breast Cancer Man* is an entirely independent private initiative and the opinions expressed herein are my own.

Macmillan was unable to assist me in the distribution of *Breast Cancer Man* to the 350 men diagnosed every year in the UK with breast cancer, and I am still looking into ways of contacting them. But while considering the issue of the target readership, I became convinced that the book should be made freely available, not only to men with breast cancer, but to women as well and, indeed, to all who were willing to read it. I realised that just as importantly as sharing my story with fellow cancer patients was the business of informing health service providers of the impact of their treatment regimes in the hope that they might initiate ways of improving the patient experience. My efforts could only bring that about if they, too, read the book.

If errors remain in *Breast Cancer Man*, as surely they must, it is not for want of seeking, receiving and acting on help and advice. I am particularly indebted to academic friends, Professor Mel Chevannes (my wife), Dr Anna Frankel, Professor Diana Holmes, and Professor Geoff Hurd, who went to great lengths to appraise the manuscript, as if it were a student's assignment or thesis, making incisive observations and proposing amendments accordingly. They were unwavering in their support for my project which, I trust, was due to an assessment of its merit, and not out of sympathy for my condition. To improve access to and understanding of the information embedded in the book, they variously recommended the addition of references and footnotes, a glossary of medical terms, a directory of named individuals, and a general index. I took up their suggestions and, as I went on writing, compiled the requisite lists.

I am profoundly grateful to Philip Lopez, a longstanding friend, who, as on previous occasions, worked closely with me on the laborious task of formatting and paginating the manuscript in preparation for printing. I also wish to thank Ted Heathcote and Matt Dunne of Heathcotes Print and Design, Lanesfield, Wolverhampton, for their friendship, advice, encouragement, and technical know-how, which helped to turn my rudimentary text into a very presentable book. Their efforts on my behalf seemed to me like a labour of love - a personal commitment - extending well beyond mere commercial considerations.

Other friends and family members gave support and encouragement in different ways. For example, I was told that I had brought tears to their eyes with the vivid accounts of my pain and suffering, They complimented me on the concision and clarity of some of the chapters. In particular, they liked the chapters on hair loss, therapy, and New Cross Hospital. They inquired about the state of my health, my recovery, and the progress I was making on the manuscript. They tried to place orders for autographed copies of the book following its publication, offering to pay me in advance of its appearance to speed up the process.

I have explained how I came to produce the book and the social and psychological benefits I personally gained from keeping a detailed account of my treatment from start to finish, and the encouragement I was given by family and friends, the NHS staff who treated me, and persons at Macmillan Cancer Support. But why go further and publish what is, in effect, a very private and intimate insight into my experiences, bodily functions and emotions, as well as my social life and political views?

I am bold enough to believe that an honest and accurate description of my experience of being treated for breast cancer may help to inform other newly-diagnosed patients - especially men - of what they can expect, and to reassure them that their reactions, both physical and psychological, to surgery and adjuvant therapies, are perfectly normal and commonplace. If I, a very ordinary chap, along with hundreds of other men annually, could cope with the treatment and survive it, then so can they. Like me, they will be able to discover and make use of their own ways of dealing with the side effects - for example, the therapies that suit them. Expressed in more popular lyrical mode, you, the reader, can walk with me, holding your head high, no longer afraid of the dark uncertainty of cancer, but with hope in your heart:

'And you'll never walk alone
You'll never walk alone.'

If, in addition, the health service can be improved by listening carefully to, and acting on patient opinion, as hospital administrators, doctors and nurses are keen to claim, then my story is surely worth publishing.

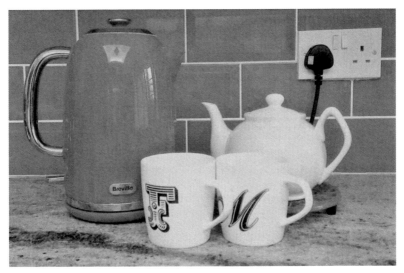

The kettle that led to Frank's diagnosis

Chapter 1

A lump in the breast

I first experienced a twinge in my breast late in July 2017. I was trying to lift the lid on an electric kettle to fill it with water to make our early morning cup of tea. The next day, while repeating the tea-making routine, I experienced the same tension. After my shower, I examined the spot on my chest where I had felt the tweak, and was surprised to discover a small hard lump, below the skin, situated near to my left nipple. It was not very obvious or pronounced, but I asked my wife, Mel, to look at it. She quickly detected the same lump and pointed out that the nipple next to it was slightly inverted, a further feature that I had failed to notice. I had never looked closely at that part of my anatomy before, let alone examined or felt it deliberately. I had no idea whether my diminutive nipples were turned out or turned in. I could best be termed totally male breast-blind, rather than being 'breast aware', as urged in breast health education campaigns directed at women.

Mel impressed on me the urgency of having the lump checked out and insisted I make an appointment at our medical practice. On the 9th August, I was examined by *Dr Tasleema Ahmed*, a GP at the Castlecroft Medical Centre. She made me lie on the couch and raise my hands above my head before carefully palpating both left and right breasts. She confirmed that I had a lump that was worthy of further investigation and, without more ado, referred me for an urgent appointment to Wolverhampton's New Cross Hospital.

I was not at this stage unduly concerned. A former personal assistant and friend had recently been referred to the hospital after finding lumps in her breasts. Despite her fears, they turned out to be cysts and were drained with a syringe there and then. I knew even at that stage that men could have breast cancer, but that instances in men were extremely rare. I thought of myself as an average bloke, one most likely to be among the statistical majority. I believed the lump would turn out to be non-cancerous and be easily and painlessly removed, just as my friend's had been.

Hospital appointments

I received an afternoon appointment for Wednesday 23rd August 2017 at New Cross Hospital to attend the breast clinic in the outpatients' department. I was weighed, my height was measured, and a blood sample was taken by a nurse. I was examined by a kindly registrar who, when I questioned him, affirmed that my lump could well be cancerous.

I was then seen by *Mr Suri Venkatramanan*, the NHS consultant oncoplastic breast surgeon, with expertise in the management of breast conditions, breast cancer and reconstruction.[1] My first impression was of a handsome younger man, well spoken and with a friendly smiling demeanour. He was seated next to *Sister Carys Jevons*, the designated senior breast-cancer nurse

Mr Venkatramanan inquired about my general state of health and how long I had become aware of my lump. Was there a family history of breast cancer and did I have any close relatives who had developed the disease? I told him that, as far as I was aware, no-one, male or female, on either side of my family had been diagnosed with breast cancer. My three sisters were healthy and well into their sixties. My parents and many of my uncles and aunts had lived into their eighties or nineties.

I read later that 1 in 5 of men with breast cancer (20 per cent) had a close relative who also had breast cancer, indicating an inherited form of the disease linked to the so-called BRCA 1 or BRCA 2 genes.[2] My family history showed that my cancer was more likely to be related to the presence of the hormone oestrogen (American spelling 'estrogen'), known as 'oestrogen-receptor positive breast cancer', abbreviated to ER-positive. Around 90 per cent of male breast cancers turned out not to be genetic (in the BRCA sense), but ER-positive.[3]

Mammogram, ultra-sound scan and biopsy

Mr Venkatramanan explained that he would need to confirm the diagnosis. He sent me to the imaging department for a breast x-ray, ultra-sound scan, and breast biopsy. The breast x-ray, known as a mammogram, was done on both breasts by pressing plates tightly against my chest. The ultra-sound scan examination took longer. A friendly sonographer scanned both breasts, the area of the lump, and the locations of the lymph nodes under my arms. She told me that she had found no sign of further lumps or swollen nodes.

I was then subjected to a breast biopsy, which extracted four samples of subcutaneous tissue in the vicinity of my lump, by means of a hollow needle attached to a spring, which sounded and felt as if I were being shot with a staple gun, but was not particularly painful. Each needle was extracted replete with a core of tissue, a little like an auger extracting a core of soil. Once those procedures had been completed, I returned to the Outpatients' Department and was given an appointment a week later to discuss the results with *Mr Venkatramanan.*

Cancer diagnosis

At 4.45 pm on 29th August 2017 (accompanied by my wife, Mel, who had been helping with grandchildren in London at the time of my initial hospital appointment), I returned to the breast clinic to learn the outcome of the tests. *Mr Venkatramanan* explained simply, painstakingly, compassionately, and in considerable detail, what had been discovered and what he proposed to do about it.

He sat me facing him across the desk, with Mel, and *Sister Carys Jevons* from the breast cancer nursing team, seated further back. He told me that I had cancer in my left breast, but that it had been detected early and there was no evidence that it had spread. Pre-operative histology showed that the lump measured 12mm x 11mm and was graded as a 2.[4]

He proposed treating it by performing a left mastectomy, as well as a sentinel node biopsy to discover whether the cancer had spread any further.[5] A form consenting to the operation was filled out there and then, with the provisional date for the procedure set for the 22nd September 2017. I signed the form immediately, knowing full well that the cancerous cells needed to be removed as soon as possible. I paid scant attention to *Mr Venkatramanan's* meticulous encapsulation of the risks attendant on the procedure. It was only later on my carbon copy of the consent form that I studied the list: 'infection, bleeding, seroma, lymphoedema, arm pain/stiffness, reaction to blue dye, deep vein thrombosis, pulmonary embolism, need for further surgery'. And at that stage, I did not know what 'seroma', or 'lymphoedema', meant.

Throughout our meeting, *Mr Venkatramanan* encouraged me to ask questions about my diagnosis and treatment. My immediate reaction was to quiz him on why I had developed the cancer. Why me and in that part of my body? What was its cause? Was it related in any way to my lifestyle? Had I been eating too much red meat, or quaffing too many glasses of wine?

He explained simply and clearly that breast cancer could occur in males at any age, but it was most frequently diagnosed in 71-year-old men[5] and, at 72, I was a typical case. It was not a common diagnosis, with an incidence in Europe of only 1 in 100,000 men.[7] Various risk factors had been identified. Breast cancer was associated with cirrhosis of the liver which resulted in increased oestrogen levels, but he could see no sign that I was an excessive alcohol drinker. I would need more than a few glasses of wine! Obesity was another factor, but I was not fat and had never smoked.[8] Revealingly, evidence gathered from large-scale studies showed that most people of either gender who developed breast cancer had no apparent risk factor for the disease, and the majority of male patients had no detectable hormone imbalance.[9] Neither he, nor medical science, could answer my questions with any authority.

With my interest in ethnic relations, migration and family history, I was curious to learn more about my surgeon's name,

'*Venkatramanan*'. Having spent time in Tamil Nadu supporting the development of community colleges in Chennai and Madurái, I inferred that '*Venkatramanan*' was a Tamil name, and could not resist asking whether my assumption was right. Mr *Venkatramanan* confirmed that his surname was Tamil, but that his family origins lay in Sri Lanka. Mel thought my inquiry intrusive, unnecessary and contrary to customary protocol on practitioner/patient relations, especially at a first meeting. He was a highly-skilled surgeon and I had no business asking personal questions like that. I should have focussed my attention entirely on his professional competence!

Confirmation that I had cancer and, furthermore, that it was breast cancer which would require a mastectomy, came as a shock to me, as well as to my wife, Mel. When the consultation with the surgeon concluded, *Sister Jevons* took us to another room, where she explained in more detail what would happen next, and reassured me that her dedicated breast cancer nursing team were there to give me any support that I might need. She was kindly and reassuring, and managed to convince me that I was in capable hands, and that the procedures were entirely routine.

She had come well prepared for the occasion by bringing along a Macmillan Cancer Support Information booklet entitled *Understanding Breast Cancer in Men*, published in 2015. She acknowledged apologetically that much of the literature on the subject was targeted at women. I told her that her apology was unnecessary and the discrepancy was understandable, given the vast difference between men and women's breast cancer rates. In the United Kingdom, there are approximately 55,000 cases annually of women with breast cancer, as compared with 350 cases of men.[10] Put another way, 1 in 8 women are diagnosed with breast cancer during their lifetime, but a mere 1 in 870 men.[11] I learned later that I was only the third case of male breast cancer to be treated at New Cross Hospital in 2017.

The condition's statistical oddity did not make it any less worrying for me. While googling 'male breast cancer', I came across an article written in July 2008 by Dr Christian Rudlowski at the University Hospital in Bonn (Germany), summarising much of the research on breast cancer in men, and acknowledging just how rare a disease it was, representing less than 1 per cent of total breast cancer cases worldwide. Because of its low incidence rates, there were no randomised clinical studies providing information on the optimal diagnostics and therapy for male breast cancer patients. The treatment recommendations were derived entirely from the established guidelines for breast cancer in women.[12] Because of the rarity of male breast cancer, the scant information available in 2008 about the disease derived from retrospective or small-scale studies conducted in single institutions.

In subsequent meetings with members of the New Cross Hospital Breast Cancer Nursing Team, it was suggested that, as a man, I should exercise caution when informing people about my diagnosis, the news of which was, in their experience, sometimes met with incredulity or derision. They implied that male colleagues at the workplace or pub might find an instance of a man with breast cancer extraordinary, bizarre, or funny, in the mistaken belief that only women had proper breasts and that breast cancer was an exclusively female condition.

In hindsight, my personal experience led me to conclude that their cautionary advice was misdirected. Without exception, the men in whom I confided responded to my news with sympathy, being as surprised and shocked by the 'c' word as I was, irrespective of whether it applied to the breast, or any other part of the human anatomy. They all had a friend or colleague who was diagnosed or living with cancer - more often than not, prostate cancer, whose proximity to the urethra or penis they considered with trepidation. Breast cancer, above the waist and some distance away, disturbed them far less.

Most of the women I told also reacted with sensitivity and kindness, and respected the privacy of my confidence. It was my misfortune, however, to be acquainted with a handful of significant exceptions, exemplified by the following conversation.

When I told one woman friend my news, she smiled wryly and said that I should always remember that breast cancer was a women's disease. Being aware of the statistics in relation to both breast and prostate cancer, I nodded in agreement.

"It won't have the same impact on you," she continued, "You don't have proper breasts."

"Women's breasts," she added, "define their beauty and sexual attractiveness, and removing them is an assault on their womanhood."

At a cerebral level, I respected all that she said, but sensed she betrayed an inability to empathise with me as a man. In hindsight, I was struck by her failure to mention the impact of cancer treatment on women's fertility - the ability to have children - which, from my point of view, would be a far worse blow than the removal of breast tissue, or the loss of hair. Some chemotherapy drugs affected men's fertility, too, stopping them, but usually only temporarily, from producing sperm.[13] Side effects of the various breast cancer therapies listed loss of sex drive (libido) and the inability to get an erection (impotence), which, at my age, I found more worrying than my ability to father a child.[14]

After the initial diagnosis, my immediate inclination was to keep news of the breast cancer secret, to tell no-one other than my wife and children, and to forbid them from telling anyone else. But it was the diagnosis of any form of cancer – not breast cancer specifically – that I was reluctant to share, mainly because I believed at that point that the use of the 'c' word was likely to cause unnecessary distress, fear and anxiety among those who knew me. Many people assumed that a diagnosis of cancer resulted inevitably in serious debility, rapid decline, and death. At the current stage of diagnosis, investigation and treatment, I was not in a position to reassure them to the contrary. Henceforth, I divulged the news of my cancer slowly and gradually to extended family, close friends and colleagues on the principle of 'need to know.' It was only later during chemotherapy, that I began to tell anyone who I thought might be interested.

I was numbed at the news that I had cancer - not of breast cancer, but of any form of cancer - but remained convinced that such a small lump could easily be removed by a simple and relatively minor surgical intervention. I resigned myself dispassionately to the operation in the knowledge that I was in the hands of a capable surgeon, fully versed in the practice of scientific medicine, and equipped with up-to-date machinery and carefully-developed drugs. I believed myself to be physically robust. The operation would take place soon, and I would go on to make a full and rapid recovery.

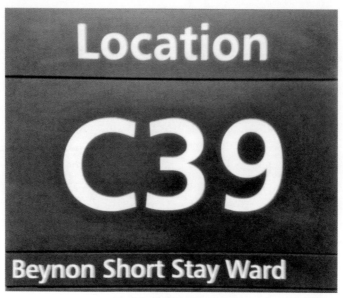

The Beynon Short Stay Ward

Chapter 2

Mastectomy, lymph node biopsy and clearance

Following a pre-operative assessment earlier in the week to check my general health and fitness, I was admitted for day surgery to the Appleby Suite at New Cross Hospital at 7.00 am on Friday 22nd September 2017. I bade goodbye to Mel when a male nurse came to collect me from the waiting room and to conduct me to a ward.. I was told to take off my clothes and dress in a flimsy hospital gown, open at the back. I was given no guidance as to whether to retain my underpants to assist in maintaining my dignity and hiding my naked bottom. I kept on my underwear, put on my slippers, and wrapped my dressing gown around me, before sitting on the chair next to my hospital bed and submersing myself in my book, entitled *King of Kings, the Triumph and Tragedy of Emperor Haile Selassie I of Ethiopia,* by Asfa-Wossen Asserate.

The nurse asked me various questions, checking that I was the Francis Reeves born on the 7th of the 2nd 1945 and living at Blue Roof, 53 Woodthorne Road, before fastening an identity tag to my wrist. He sought assurance that I had taken nil by mouth. I had had no food since 7.00 pm the night before. White surgical stockings were distributed on the ward to everyone awaiting surgery. I pulled mine over my instep and up my calves, in the knowledge that they were meant to stop blood clots from forming in my legs during the time I spent on the operating table. (I had worn them before on long-distance air flights.)

A physiotherapist paid me a visit and handed me a fold-out leaflet with pictures of the exercises I would be expected to do after my operation[1]. An hour or so later, *Mr Venkatramanan* arrived on the ward with another doctor. He drew black lines with a marker pen on my left breast and armpit, where he planned to make incisions.

I went on reading my book until around 1.00 pm, when a porter collected me on a wheel chair and pushed me along corridors to a room adjacent to an operating theatre. I volunteered to walk, but he made it clear he preferred me to sit in the chair. When we arrived, I was told by theatre attendants to climb onto a gurney. I was asked further questions to establish my identity and given another consent form to sign. My slippers, dressing gown, dentures and spectacles were taken back to the Appleby Suite. The anaesthetist questioned me, I recall, about my previous operations, breathing problems and allergies, before inserting a cannula into the back of my right hand. Other staff dressed in tabards and trousers engaged me in small talk in an effort to distract and relax me. Various substances were then injected into me before I eventually passed out.

I must have lain unconscious for two or three hours. I woke on Appleby ward later that afternoon in a relaxed state and not in any pain, the only sign of surgical intervention being a large waterproof dressing on the left of my chest and a cannula and plaster on the back of my right hand. When fully awake and once more experiencing the tedium of my hospitalisation, I turned once more to my book.

Post-operative complication

The nurse brought me a glass and a large plastic jug of water, and explained that I needed to drink plenty of fluids following my nil-by-mouth regime and operation. I would have to stay on the ward and could not be discharged from the hospital until I passed urine. Desperate to go home, I went on drinking – at least two-and-a-half litres of water and three cups of tea. I went to the lavatory on a number of occasions but, however hard I tried, I was unable to produce a single drop. The nurse told me that, while I had been in the lavatory, *Mr Venkatramanan* had come to the ward to tell me how the operation had gone but, after waiting ten minutes for me to return, had left. By 9.30 pm, there was still no sign of micturition.

Increasingly concerned for my wellbeing, and phoning the hospital for news of my discharge, Mel had come to the hospital and had been waiting in the corridor for nearly two hours to take me home. Conscious that I was the only patient left on the day ward, I approached the nursing station and pleaded to be discharged. A nurse phoned a doctor on another ward and secured my release, on the condition that I called a hospital number if my bladder filled and I was still unable to urinate.

As I felt ravenously hungry, Mel took me to Nando's at Bentley Bridge and ordered chicken and rice and a large mango juice. We consumed our meals and dinner on the premises, but still I felt no urge or ability to urinate. Only when we arrived home around 11 pm that evening did I succeed in passing urine. Thereafter, I was unable to stop.

Frequency

Every ten minutes, throughout the night, I was obliged to rise from my bed and make my way to the lavatory. By Saturday morning, I was exhausted, but the frequency continued for the whole of Saturday and Sunday, too.

On Sunday, I was so tired that I fell asleep and woke up on Monday, having wet the bed. On Monday 25th September, I made an emergency appointment with *Dr Agrasen* at the Castlecroft Medical Centre. He suggested that my complaint was a consequence of the anaesthetic and that, if it continued, I should contact the hospital. He believed I had developed a urinary infection and prescribed the antibiotic, trimethoprim.

The frequency persisted and I took to wearing absorbent pants. By Thursday, six days after the operation, I was still suffering from frequency and soreness. The antibiotics appeared to have had little effect.

Mel phoned the hospital (as advised) in the hope of speaking to someone knowledgeable or responsible for my case, and was variously referred to the Appleby Suite and a surgical ward, but could get no one to help. She was told to take me to the New Cross Walk-In Clinic on the hospital site, but organised and independent of the NHS Trust.

We made our way there and waited for nearly four hours among crowds of women with children and babies in prams, who seemed to take precedence following the triaging process. I felt tired and ill, regularly visiting the lavatory in the clinic as the frequency persisted.

At last we saw a *Dr Rukhsana Iqbal*, who listened to my story sympathetically, requested a urine sample (which tested positive for an infection), and prescribed the antibiotic, nitrofurantoin. She confirmed that the sequence of post-operative events had most likely been triggered by the anaesthetic.

Two days later, the antibiotics began to take effect and my micturition became less frequent. One consequence of my frequency and urinary infection was that I had given no thought or attention to my mastectomy operation for over a week, although Mel had made sure I regularly undertook my prescribed physiotherapy exercises.

In terms of anxiety, unremitting discomfort, prolonged sleep deprivation, failure to access much-needed medical care, and feelings of utter despair, I shall remember this period as one of the most miserable in my life. Paradoxically, my complaints were only tangentially related to my breast cancer operation which, to my great relief, had been painless.

The physiotherapy regime

After two previous operations on my hands, I had been given physiotherapy homework and was aware of the contribution of physio to ensuring a full recovery. The day after the mastectomy, until the completion of chemotherapy and radiotherapy, I undertook the recommended exercises three times a day – morning, afternoon and evening – in accordance with the excellent illustrated set of instructions produced by the Breast Cancer Care charity[2] and issued by the hospital Therapy Services Department. The aim was to regain full arm movement after breast or lymph node surgery or radiotherapy, and to reduce the occurrence of lymphoedema (a build-up of lymph fluid under the skin),

While the exercises seemed to improve movement in stiff or numb muscles and limbs, and reduce and eliminate the sensation of cording running down my left arm to my fingers, they had little effect on the repeated formation of a substantial lymphoedema near to the scar tissue.

In the first week, I memorised and repeated the basic exercises – at least three times a day – shoulder shrugs, shoulder circling, arm bending, back scratching and making wings behind my head. In the second week, I added the advanced exercises: wall climbing, arm lifting and lifting my head by pushing up with my arms. Thereafter, I began to increase the number of movements and to add exercises of my own, such as backward arm circling and trunk curls. The movement I found most beneficial was the wall climbing, high on the wall as far as I could reach. I was convinced that it eased the cording sensation I experienced and was responsible for its eventual disappearance. (Cording is a feeling that a rope is being stretched along the inner arm from the shoulder to the finger tips, thus causing pain and restricting movement, but see the glossary of medical terms.)

Post-operative examination of breast tissue

On the 3rd October 2017, Mel and I returned to *Mr Vennkatramanan*'s Breast Cancer Clinic in the Outpatients' Department for a post-operative examination of my breast tissue.

When the dressing was removed, my wound was found to have healed well. A seroma (an accumulation of fluid under the skin, see medical glossary) had collected on the side but, at that stage, it was not causing discomfort and *Mr Venkatramanan* advised that it be left alone.

Mel and I told him of the negative aftermath of the surgery, the urinary symptoms I had experienced following my discharge, and our difficulty in obtaining help from the hospital. *Mr Venkatramanan* apologised and said he would look into the circumstances that had let me down. A further sample of my urine was sent off for microscopy and he decided, there and then, to refer me to the urology department for my urinary tract to be checked. Despite his timely referral, almost four months elapsed before I was offered an appointment.

Lymph node biopsy and clearance

A week later on the 10th October, we returned to *Mr Venkatramanan's* clinic to learn the results of the sentinel lymph node biopsy. I was apprehensive, but fatalistic in my attitude, resolving to act on whatever scientifically-grounded findings and medical advice I was given. *Mr Venkatramanan* explained at some length, and with great sympathy, the lab results. The lump measured 13.5mm and was grade 2, but of no special type, with a surrounding high grade DCIS (ductal carcinoma in situ).[3]

In regard to the lymph node biopsy, one of the two nodes had been ER (estrogen receptor) positive but HER 2 (human epidermal growth factor) negative. Because the cancer had been detected in my lymph nodes, *Mr Venkatramanan* recommended a further operation – a left completion axillary node clearance, to remove the remaining lymph nodes in my left armpit –to be performed as soon as possible.[4]

He filled in the consent form for me to sign and booked me in for day surgery on the 20th October 2017. As before, he detailed the unavoidable risks of the operation which, with the shock of the news that the cancer had spread, I scarcely took in. The list was almost identical to the risks of the mastectomy, with the addition of 'damage to nerves and vessels'.

I was disappointed to learn that my cancer had spread and that a further operation was necessary. I consoled myself that *Mr Venkatramanan* had taken immediate action to deal with the problem and was quietly confident that his further intervention would be effective. In view of my previous experience, he arranged that I be kept in for monitoring and observation overnight after the operation.

The prospect of the lymph node clearance left me with an additional anxiety about the impact of the possible after-effects on me personally. My nerves might be injured during the operation, which could leave me with numbness and tingling in my upper arm that in some cases could be permanent, resulting in a debilitating loss of strength and dexterity. In my case, the incision would be made under my left arm pit, on the same side as the mastectomy that had removed my left breast and nipple. My concern was that I was one of the 10 per cent of the population who was left-handed, relying heavily on the left side of my body for all operations involving strength and dexterity. If the operation went wrong, my ability to chisel, cut, draw, drill, hammer, paint, pour tea, punch, screw, write, etc, might be impaired, thus radically limiting my daily role and activities.

Removing the lymph nodes in my breast under my left arm could also cause lymphoedema, which I read about in the Macmillan practical guide, *Understanding Lymphoedema*. I read that the lymphadenectomy (the technical name for the surgical removal of my lymph nodes) could cause chronic swelling, changes to sensation, skin stretching and flaking, and pain, as a result of the build-up of fluid following damage and disruption to the normal working of the lymphatic system and, furthermore, that the damage was irreparable, and that lymphoedema symptoms might develop a few months, or even years, after surgery.[5]

This was also the first time that it dawned on me that my condition could be serious and potentially life-threatening. If the cancer had spread to the lymph nodes, could it have already metastasised elsewhere in my body? I had only recently learned the word – 'metastasised' – the spread of disease, especially cancer – but unlike other newly-acquired vocabulary, I dreaded the mention of it. I thought for a while about my mortality: 'he cometh forth like a flower, and is cut down', and consoled myself that, at 72, I had had a good innings, a loving wife, three children, and a growing number of grandchildren. I recognised at once the futility of indulging in this kind of introspection and rededicated my mind to logic and reason. Was I going to die? Yes. How long had I left? Only medical science could give me an answer. And that meant waiting stoically for the results of biopsies and scans, and acting on medical advice.

Lymph gland clearance operation

Mel drove me to the hospital on Friday 20th October for the 7 am admission to the Appleby Suite for the lymph gland clearance operation. This time, I was familiar with the procedure and knew what to expect. I put on my surgical gown and stockings and retained my underpants. *Mr Venkatramanan*, accompanied by a colleague, came to the ward and, as before, marked the point of incision with a black line. He told me that I would be first on his list, which would give me time on the ward for observation prior to spending the night in the Beynon Short-Stay Suite.

Around 10.30 am, I was taken to the operating theatre, where an anaesthetist showed interest in my case and seemed to be familiar with my previous post-operative problem. The anaesthetics were administered. I lost consciousness. The operation occurred.

I woke up on the ward, read my book, ate a sandwich on offer, and drank moderately. This time, a few hours after the surgery, I was able to pass urine. *Mr Venkatramanan* came to the ward to say hello, tell me the surgery had gone to plan, and ask how I felt. Nevertheless, in the late afternoon, I was taken by a porter along lengthy corridors to the Beynon Suite for an overnight stay and monitoring.

Night on the Beynon Short-Stay Suite

The Beynon short stay facility consisted of a lobby with nurse station and toilets and three small wards each containing eight to ten beds. I was allocated to a room with three other occupants – three elderly men, two of whom wore back-tying-hospital gowns and appeared to be confused, wandering at intervals into the lobby to inadvertently reveal their naked white bottoms, and having to be steered back to their beds or chairs by the patient nursing staff.

Mel came in the evening to visit, by which time I had eaten a meal, drunk tea, and was passing urine regularly. The nurse allocated to look after me measured my urine output after each micturition and made a note of the quantity. Once visiting time was over, Mel departed, and I read my book until a nurse came to draw the curtains around my bed. The lights were dimmed and I eventually drifted off to sleep.

It must have been about two o'clock in the morning when I was woken by loud banging, men's raised voices and the rattling of chains, sounding like Marley's ghost in *A Christmas Carol*. With the bed curtains drawn, I was unable to work out what was happening, but the racket gradually reduced until all that I could hear were two gruff male voices conducting an indistinct but endless conversation in the corner of the room, which kept me awake until morning.

When my curtains were drawn back, I looked across and could see a man lying in the bed with two other men wearing prison-officer uniforms seated on either side of him. The patient on the bed was attached by a chain to one of the prison officers, who would periodically lead him to the lavatory in the corridor, to the sound of clanking metal.

From observation and the snatches of conversation overheard on the ward, I was able to piece together that, during the night, the man's jaw had been broken in a fight at the prison and that he now had to be fed through a straw. Predictably, he remained silent while, over his head, the prison officers carried on talking and joking with each other.

Waiting for my discharge

I had passed urine regularly since my operation on Friday morning and had almost finished my book. I wanted to know when I would be discharged and could phone Mel to take me home. The nurse told me that only a doctor could discharge me and that I would have to wait on his round. By now it was lunch time and I was becoming increasingly bored. The nurse estimated that, as it was Saturday, it would be around 4 00 pm before the doctor arrived. I decided to leave the ward in my dressing gown and walk to the hospital shop to buy *The Guardian.*

When I returned, another patient had been admitted and was lying in the bed next to mine. We exchanged pleasantries. He told me that he had a nasty infection between his shoulder blades and had been admitted for an emergency operation to remove pus and prevent septicaemia.

He expressed strong support for the NHS. I learned that he had been in the army and had served in Iraq and Afghanistan, but was vehemently opposed to Western military intervention in either country. Sensing that we might have something in common, I asked if he were involved in politics.

"Yes", he said, "I'm a socialist –a national socialist", and went on to tell me that Hitler was not as bad as he had been painted. He added that what was needed was strong leadership to take Britain out of the European Union, make it great again, and to kick all of the immigrants out.

At this point, a Mauritian nurse came round to do some tests on him and I was able to retreat behind my newspaper. Mel came at visiting time, but we had to wait until 4.30 pm before I was finally discharged from Beynon.

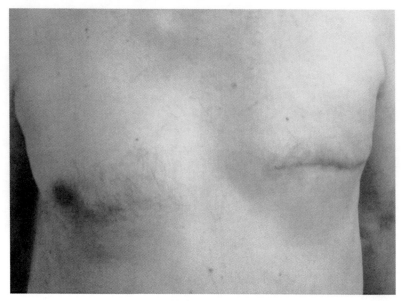

Frank's chest after the mastectomy

Chapter 3

Biopsies, scans and adjuvant therapies

Seroma and aspiration

After the lymph gland clearance operation, I continued with physiotherapy exercises, but found them to be coming more painful because of swelling in the area of my left breast[1], near to where my mastectomy and lymphadenectomy had occurred. Mel said she thought it was a seroma, a build-up of serum under the skin – a fluid accumulation made up of blood plasma from injured cells – which can occur after surgery.

Despite Mel's reassuring diagnosis, I was worried, nevertheless, that it might be the first sign of a lymphoedema that would never go away. I googled 'seroma', and discovered it to be a relatively common side effect of breast cancer surgery. The swelling was usually located near to the site of the incision and was short-term, clearing up of its own accord, or requiring draining with a needle, until the wound fully healed. A seroma that persisted over a prolonged period, say of two months , could turn into a lymphoedema, but most lymphoedemas emerged in any area of the upper body (but on the same side as the original breast cancer), such as arm, breast, chest, hand and trunk, long after the completion of breast cancer treatment. Lymphoedema was a consequence, not of the breast surgery, but of the damage inflicted on the lymphatic system. Yet people who had a seroma were at increased risk of developing a lymphoedema.

On the 26th October, I returned with Mel to the Breast Cancer Clinic to have my dressing and wound inspected by *Sister Carys Jevons*. Diagnosing a seroma and recognising that the swelling was causing me discomfort, *Carys* inserted a cannula and drew off 255ml of clear orange serum. We joked that it resembled a quality lager or lucozade. Thereafter, I returned on a regular basis to have my breast drained.

On the 31st October, *Nurse Donna Dobson* withdrew 305ml. On the 7th November, 225ml were aspirated, by the 15th, 195ml, by the 21st, 165ml, and by the 28th, 45ml but, by the 6th December, after a thorough examination, *Nurse Margery Catterall* thought the problem had resolved itself and that regular aspiration was no longer needed. Not a lymphoedema after all!

Biopsy result

Mr Venkatramanan saw me and Mel on the 7th November to tell us the results of the biopsy performed on the removed axillary nodes. He told us that 3 of the 20 nodes had turned out to be cancerous, that my left breast was most likely to have been the primary site, but that there was still a possibility that the cancer had spread beyond the axilla[2], although the chance was low. This meant that, in medical jargon, my breast cancer was referred to as 'node positive' (it had spread to the nodes) – as opposed to 'node negative' (when biopsy results showed the nodes to be non-cancerous).

With my node-positive status, *Mr Venkatramanan*'s aim now was to reduce the risk of the cancer spreading or returning. He proposed that I undertake various adjuvant therapies ('adjuvant' meaning treatment to suppress secondary tumour formation) in the form of a course of chemotherapy, chest-wall radiotherapy, and tamoxifen (an oestrogen receptor modulator).[3]

He must have seen my look of dismay at the mention of chemotherapy, and sought to reassure me. All the treatments he was proposing were aimed at reducing the risk of the cancer returning.

"Frank", he said, "we're going to beat this. I have every confidence that with these treatments you can outlive this cancer."

To make sure that the cancer had not spread and 'to exclude any distant disease', he would also arrange appointments for CT scans of my chest, abdomen, pelvis and bones. (I was soon to learn that CT or CAT stands for 'computerised axial tomography, a procedure in which I would be expected to lie on a table that slides into a barrel-like scanning machine, which then rotates to allow an x-ray beam to create a 3d image of my bodily tissues and organs). These procedures were not his specialism and he would refer me on to the imaging department and the oncologist.[4]

The prospect of chemotherapy

The prospect of chemotherapy filled me with dread. I, in common with the rest of the population, had talked to family members and friends at various stages of their treatment for cancer, and was fully aware of the unpleasant effects of the anti-cancer drugs, and the usually prolonged duration of the treatment.

For a couple of days after the consultation, I remained in a morose, dejected, and pessimistic mood, but soon came to realise that I was making those nearest to me – Mel and my children – more miserable than myself. I resolved in future to avoid that pointless and gratuitous form of self-indulgence – a kind of sulky irrational cowardice – and face up to the scientific reality. These advanced and expensive adjuvant therapies were being made freely available to me under the NHS with the sole aim of reducing the risk of my cancer returning. (I read somewhere that a course of FEC-T cost around £70,000.) Unpleasant they might be, but their purpose was preventive and they were being provided entirely for my benefit.

To convince and reassure myself beyond all reasonable doubt, I began to explore the medical research. An article in *The Lancet* (14th-20th May 2005) reviewing randomised trials, described the effects of chemotherapy (including FEC) and hormonal therapy (tamoxifen) on the recurrence of breast cancer and 15-year survival rate among women who had had breast cancer.[5] However, all the randomised trials that the authors examined were undertaken on women. There was no comparative study of men.[6]

Chemotherapy was found to reduce the annual breast cancer death rate by about 38 per cent for women younger than 50 years of age, and by 20 per cent for those aged 50 to 69, from the time they were first diagnosed. (Very few women aged 70 plus were entered for the chemotherapy trials.) Hormone therapy in the form of five years of treatment with tamoxifen reduced women's annual death rate for ER-positive forms of breast cancer by 31 per cent, irrespective of their age (under 50, between 50 to 69, or 70 plus).[7]

For middle-aged women diagnosed with ER-positive disease (the commonest type of breast cancer, and what I had been diagnosed with), chemotherapy, in the form of FEC followed by five years of tamoxifen, reduced the breast cancer mortality rate after fifteen years by half.[8] Despite the fact that I was a man aged 70-plus years and did not belong to the target group, any sensible reading of this article convinced me that *Mr Venkatramanan*'s post-operative prescription for me of chemotherapy and hormone therapy was entirely correct and in my best interests.

The isotope bone scan

Appointment letters arrived regularly throughout November, the first on the 14th, for an isotope bone scan of my whole body at the nuclear imaging section of the Radiology Department. Before the scan, a radioactive isotope tracer was injected into my right arm. (The isotopes gave off gamma rays which were then detected by a gamma camera and used to build up a computer image of the bone structure, aimed at revealing malignant tumours that might have developed away from the primary site of my breast cancer.) After a wait of approximately two hours, I was asked to lie on a couch which was projected forward into a barrel to which a special camera was attached. The camera rotated from side to side, first scanning my head and then my body, as the couch transported me slowly into and out of the barrel.

The scan itself must have lasted about 40 minutes. Afterwards I was expected to drink two litres of liquid during the day to wash the isotopic material out of my body. I was also advised to avoid close contact with children or pregnant women. After the procedure, Mel drove me to the Royal Oak, where we dealt with the requisite fluid intake by drinking beer.

Scans of bone, thorax, abdomen and pelvis

On the 21st November, Mel accompanied me once more to the Radiology Department for what was termed a 'CT Thorax Abdo Pelvis Contrast'. This time I was given a jug of water to drink and was expected to undress and put on a hospital gown. I came prepared with my dressing gown and slippers. After a short wait in which I drank the water, I was taken into the x-ray room and asked to lie down on the couch. A strap and padding were applied to keep me in position. An injection was administered through a cannula on the back of my right hand, the radiologist warning me that I might feel a hot glow around my waist and a strong taste in my mouth. The couch then slid into the barrel-like structure, or 'doughnut', housing the x-ray cameras.

The radiographer retreated to the control room and the machine began rotating around me and whining. I felt warm around my waist and a bitter taste in my mouth. Now and again, a recorded voice would tell me to breathe out and hold my breath and then to breathe in again. Around 20 minutes elapsed before the couch was withdrawn from beneath the cameras, after which I had to wait in a little waiting room with other patients in dressing gowns before the cannula was extracted.

My elderly men and women companions were discussing and joking about their health and treatment. One jolly old lady remarked that she had recently signed an organ donor form. "I was happy to sign", she said, "but I haven't got many organs left. They've already taken my gall bladder, a kidney, fallopian tubes and womb."

First appointment with *Dr Grigoryev*, the oncologist

On the 27th November, Mel accompanied me to the Oncology Clinic at the Deanesly Outpatients' Department to see *Dr Grozdan Grigoryev*, the oncology consultant. *Dr Hetu Charitha Gupta*, one of his registrars, and an attendant nurse were also present. *Dr Grigoryev* explained the course of treatment he was proposing. With a pre-assessment scheduled for the 27th December, my chemotherapy would begin in early January and consist of a series of six cycles, each lasting 21 days, or three weeks. The chemotherapy would be followed by 15 days of radiotherapy, when I would be expected to attend the hospital on successive days (bar Saturdays and Sundays).

Given my node-positive status, *Dr Grigoryev* proposed a course of chemotherapy known as FEC-T, named after the initials of the drugs used in the treatment: fluorouracil, epirubicin, cyclophosphamide and docetaxel (or Taxatere).[9] These would be administered by means of a thin tube inserted through a cannula in the back of the hand. At this point, the nurse examined the back of my hand for prominent veins and expressed her satisfaction with their visibility.

Dr Grigoryev impressed us with his compassionate manner, patience and self-evident kindness and concern for his patients' welfare. He spent time explaining the possible side effects of the chemotherapy before getting me to sign the consent form. The list of side effects was lengthy, but it was most unlikely that I would experience all of them, as the drugs affected everyone differently. The main side effects were: risk of infection, loss of appetite, changes in the taste of food, sore mouth, skin dryness, rashes and bruising, soreness or tingling of hand palms and soles of feet, sore eyes, headaches, feelings of nausea, fatigue, diarrhoea, and hair loss, etc.[10]

On this occasion, the mention of nausea and hair loss concerned me most. *Dr Grigoryev* explained that feelings of nausea and vomiting were controlled by an area of the brain known as the vomiting centre or, in medical parlance, the chemo-receptor-trigger zone. Depending on their kind and dose, the chemotherapy drugs injected into the veins would circulate to the brain and stimulate the vomiting centre. He reassured me that special anti-emetic and steroid drugs would be given during and after the chemotherapy to counteract and prevent any feelings of sickness or nausea, thus enabling me to go on eating and drinking normally.

In regard to the hair loss, I had read: 'You usually lose all the hair on your head. Your eyelashes, eyebrows and other body hair may also thin or fall out.'[11] I wanted to know whether the treatment was likely to affect my beard. *Dr Grigoryev* told me that it might, but he was unable to say with certainty, as each person reacted differently; some individuals managed to retain all their hair, but this was rare. He took the trouble to explain that cancer cells and hair follicle cells shared in common the attribute of dividing rapidly. In the process of attacking the cancer cells, the chemotherapy drugs also affected the hair follicle cells, interfering with the hair growth cycle and causing hairs to fall out. He was keen to tell me that, unlike the cancer cells, my hair follicle cells would recover and my hair would grow back.

I was reassured that my responses would be monitored very closely throughout the course. If there were serious side-effects, I was instructed to phone either of the telephone numbers given (the nursing team at the oncology clinic, or A & E) and make my way to the hospital without delay.

As the meeting concluded, I couldn't resist inquiring about *Dr Grigoryev's* surname. "Is it Eastern European?" I asked. "Yes," he said with a smile, "It's Bulgarian." Mel frowned from her seat in the corner, believing that the inquiry could have waited for a subsequent visit.

Cardiac investigation at the Heart and Lung Centre

A few days after meeting the oncologist, I received an appointment for a cardiac investigation at the Heart and Lung Centre at New Cross. On the 5th December, Mel accompanied me to the hospital for an ECG (an electro-cardiogram) and an ultra sound examination. A cardiac physiologist took me to a room, got me to take off my shirt and lie on a couch. The aim was to detect and measure the electrical impulses produced by my beating heart. The sensors or electrodes were connected by wires to a recording machine. The procedure lasted for about five minutes.

For the ultra-sound examination, the physiologist put gel on my chest and held a sensor over my heart , moving it systematically to and fro to build up a sonic picture on a screen above my head. He told me that he was experiencing difficulty in obtaining a clear image of my heart. After a good half hour, he called in his supervisor to assess progress. In the meantime, I began to feel discomfort as the sensor was rubbed repeatedly against the scar tissue left by my mastectomy.

Eventually, the two operatives decided that their investigation was complete, the gel was wiped off my chest, and I was allowed to rejoin Mel who was sitting patiently in the waiting room with her sudoku book. I gathered that the ECG and ultrasound scan of my heart had been commissioned by *Dr Grigoryev* to establish my fitness for chemotherapy.

A week or so later, Mel thought it was about time I was told the results of my scans and insisted I phone up *Mr Venkatramanan*'s secretary. His secretary said she would ask Mr *V*. She phoned back later on the 8th December to confirm that both the bone scan and the chest, abdomen and pelvis scan had come back clear – that is, with no sign of secondaries – good news, which I happily relayed to my children. Shortly afterwards, a letter arrived in the post to confirm that the results showed no evidence of metastatic disease.[12]

Pre-assessment meeting with the palliative care nurse

Immediately after the Christmas festivities spent at Blue Roof with Toussaint, Luc and Caio, Mel and I went to ward A24 at New Cross Hospital on the 27th December 2017 for an assessment meeting prior to the chemotherapy treatment. The waiting room was crowded but, half an hour after the time scheduled, Mel and I were seen by *Sister Natalie Edmunds*, the lead palliative care nurse, a very genial. approachable and fun-loving person, who took a sample of my blood, talked me through the procedures that I would be receiving, how the FEC-T drugs would be given and in what cycles, and the side effects I was likely to experience at the time the drugs were administered and then afterwards at home. *Sister*

Edmunds was very patient and took time to explain, making sure we understood matters of significance, and answering in detail all the questions we asked her.

We were told that one common side effect in the days after chemotherapy was a feeling of nausea, or vomiting. To prevent or reduce sickness, I would be given anti-emetic drugs prior to the treatment. Because the FEC-T drugs would reduce my white blood cells, I would be at an increased risk of infection, but the cells were likely to recover to normal levels before the next bout of treatment. It was important to avoid possible sources of infection, such as people with chicken pox or shingles. We remembered that our friend, Bob Major, had had shingles for almost a year, and thought how unfortunate it was that, henceforth, we would have to avoid him. *Sister Edmunds* said that it was 90 per cent likely that I would lose all my hair, including my beard, after the second round of treatment. I was also likely to experience a sore mouth, loss of appetite and taste, dry skin, and fatigue.

The side effects were many and varied but, if I felt any of the following:

- chest pain,
- a temperature of 37.5^0c or above,
- a fever, or flu-like symptoms,
- an obvious infection,
- shortness of breath,
- diarrhoea,
- nausea and vomiting,
- weakness, or loss of function,
- swollen arms or chest,
- felt very unwell,

I had to contact the oncology patient 24-hour emergency helpline[13]. We were told to acquire a thermometer to record my temperature twice daily, aqueous cream to moisten my skin, Corsodyl mouth wash to reduce the risk of mouth infection, and a note book to write down questions for the nurse or doctor and any information they gave us. We must have spent about 90 minutes with *Sister Natalie Edmunds*. She was unstinting with her time and very thorough.

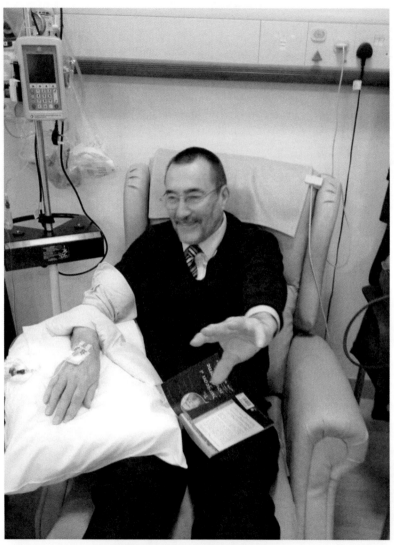

Frank concluding his first course of FEC chemotherapy
in the Snowdrop Suite

Chapter 4

Beginning chemotherapy with FEC

Day 1 (Wednesday 3rd January 2018)

First session of chemotherapy at the Snowdrop Millennial Suite

On Wednesday 3rd January 2018, Mel and I turned up for my 10 am appointment at the Snowdrop Millennium Suite at the Deanesly Centre at New Cross Hospital, where we waited for 25 minutes. I noticed that most of the other patients and their companions seated in the waiting room were of our age or older, perhaps an indicative sample of the modal age of those diagnosed with cancer. A senior nurse, *Sister Jemima Holyoak*, took me to be weighed and measured, and then directed us to a u-shaped ward divided into seventeen curtained units, each equipped with a reclining chair for a patient, a chair for a patient's companion, a drip stand, a blood-pressure monitor, and a table.

After taking off my coat and jacket, I was told to sit on the vacant patient's chair, while Mel sat on the companion's chair next to me. I was given a capsule of aprepitant, an anti-emetic, to swallow. The nurse then placed my right hand on a pillow rested on the arm of the chair and put a hot compress on the back of my hand to bring up the veins. After a while, a cannula was inserted and attached to a transparent plastic tube through which saline and anti-emetic liquids fed down from bags hung from the drip stand. Two nurses checked the drugs that were prepared in the pharmacy and sent over for me. I was asked for my name, date of birth and first line of my address. The procedure took approximately half an hour.

47

Once completed, the nurse inserted a syringe into the cannula and began slowly to inject a red fluid, the E, epirubicin (the clue to its colour lies in the name) into my vein. I think there were three full syringes of this fluid – a total of 150ml – and I was told that the colour of the fluid would reveal itself afterwards in my urine. Syringes full of clear fluids, the C, cyclophosphamide, and the F, flurouracil, followed. The total of the three drugs amounted to 1,000 ml. This cocktail of drugs, referred to by the acronym, FEC (fluorouracil, epirubicin, cyclophosphamide), was to be injected into me three times in all, and constituted the first , second, and third cycles of my chemotherapy.[1]

Sister Holyoak concentrated on her task, while I tried to ignore the process by reading. The book I had brought with me, *The Surgeon of Crowthorne*, given to me at Christmas by my sister, Maggie, served as an admirable distraction and I was scarcely aware of the FEC treatment until the nurse told me she had finished at 12.10 pm, after which I was reattached to the bag of sodium chloride fluid on the drip stand.

Sister Holyoak then assembled the medicines from the hospital pharmacy for me to take home – the anti-emetics, steroid tablets, and syringes full of drugs to counter any fall in my blood count. She also scheduled an appointment for the next round of chemotherapy in twenty-one days' time on the 24th January 2018 – on the assumption that the blood count test to be taken on the 22nd January would show I had recovered sufficiently to undergo a further cycle.

After a short rest to allow for any adverse reaction, I left the ward with Mel and we made our way back to the car. I felt perfectly normal, but asked Mel to drive just in case. The chemotherapy had been administered painlessly in a relaxed and friendly manner on a busy ward, fully occupied with other patients receiving treatment for a variety of cancers. The man seated opposite me had gesticulated to point out my chair's reclining button, at which point I realised that he had a laryngectomy vent in his throat which prevented him using his voice-box. I derived fortitude and solace from the knowledge that I was surrounded by fellow patients, all calmly submitting to chemotherapy, many for cancers more advanced or serious than mine. I was further assured by the fact that already I had completed one sixth or 16.6 per cent of my chemotherapy course, and more than half of day one of the first three-week cycle.

The first signs of the chemotherapy injections came in the form of blood orange urine on the first two occasions that I went to the lavatory, but the colour thereafter returned to normal. As instructed, I took an 8 mg ondansetron anti-emetic tablet that evening, and managed to drink 1.8 litres of fluid in the form of tea but mostly tap water. I took a light lunch at 12.30 pm and a normal supper at 7.30 pm with no accompanying feeling of nausea, but perhaps a little indigestion. We retired to bed around 11 pm, and I fell into a deep sleep for about two hours, before entering a state of manic dreaming or semi-conscious thinking in which my head swirled with life-changing ideas for new projects. Unable to relax, I went downstairs at around 3.30 am to make a cup of tea, before returning to sleep for perhaps an hour before those exciting thoughts woke me up again.

Day 2 (Thursday 4th January)

Mel cooked me oats porridge with nutmeg mace for breakfast, which I ate with honey and a date. Twice daily, she took my temperature, which turned out to be normal – 36.9^{0}c in the morning and 36.5^{0}c in the evening. At 7.00 am, I took one 8 mg anti-emetic ondansetron tablet, at 9.00 am, two 2 mg dexamethasone soluble steroid tablets and, at 10.25 am, one 80 mg anti-emetic aprepitant capsule. My urination was normal and my bowel movements were regular, but I noticed the stools were firmer than yesterday.

Mel took me into town to do some shopping and bought me a cappuccino and cake in Costas, where we met Margaret Dasent, a friend and nurse, for a chat, which included an account of my recent chemotherapy. Returning home, Mel and I had a lunch of bread and soup and, after working for a while on the PC, I went for an afternoon nap for an hour.

Mel prepared a delicious supper of boiled potatoes, salmon and broccoli, which I ate hungrily, but noticed that it did not taste as good as it looked, one of the side effects of the chemotherapy that *Sister Natalie Edmunds* had mentioned. My fluid intake amounted to approximately 1.6 litres, consisting of tea, coffee and water. I would have felt ill if I'd forced myself to drink more. As the evening progressed, I experienced a bout of hiccups, followed by burping and belching, which continued on and off to bedtime at 11 pm. As on the previous night, I fell asleep for about two hours but then was woken by the need to sit up and belch, followed by more hiccups, which disturbed my night's rest – and Mel's – until morning.

Day 3 (Friday 5th January)

The belching continued, and, at 6.30 am, I went to make tea, taking the final anti-emetic Ondansetron tablet. Mel cooked cornmeal porridge with nutmeg mace for breakfast, which I took with honey and a date, along with the two 2 mg steroid dexamethasone tablets.

At 10.25 am, I downed the 80 mg anti-emetic aprepitant capsule. The belching reduced, but I still felt mildly indigested. My bowels were regular, but the stools were firmer. My temperature remained steady: 36.5^0c in the morning and 36.4^0c in the evening.

I did various jobs around the house but spent much of the day on the PC amending a document. Lunch was the normal bread, cheese and soup. Supper at 8.30 pm consisted of a tasty paella made of rice, black pudding, bacon , onion, ginger, garlic and mushrooms but, as before, I was unable to appreciate its full flavour. At 11 pm bedtime, I slept for two hours but was woken once more by the need to sit up and belch, which I did on at least three occasions. Dreaming was vivid and thought-flow abnormally active, and at 3.30 am I went downstairs to make a cup of tea. Sleep thereafter was better but intermittent.

Day 4 (Saturday 6ᵗʰ January)

I arose, showered and dressed by 8.30 am, feeling mildly agitated, slightly light-headed and giddy. Thinking my blood sugar was low, I added muscovado sugar, lashings of honey and a date to the plate of oats porridge Mel had prepared for me. I also took the dissolved 2 mg tablet of dexamethasone steroid. Mel took my temperature, which remained stable at 36.8^0c.

After breakfast, I still felt light-headed and giddy, but decided to go shopping with Mel to get out of the house for a breadth of fresh air. Nevertheless, I staggered down the drive and was relieved to sit in the car passenger seat. We drove to the B & M supermarket on the Bilston Road, where I wandered around the aisles very slowly. The feelings of faintness gradually subsided. In Dunelm, I began to function normally and was able to stand at the checkout for a 7-minute wait. We then drove to Sainsbury's to buy provisions – a tub of soap and a pizza – which we ate for lunch later. Returning home, I became conscious of my severe burping and dyspepsia, and took one of the 10 mg domperidone tablets. Shortly afterwards, I ate some chicken soup and a couple of slices of pizza. The burping and indigestion continued all afternoon. I took another domperidone tablet in the evening and had paella for supper.

The burping and belching continued until 11 pm bed time. I was tired and fell asleep easily but was woken up around 3.00 am, feeling most uncomfortable and needing to sit up and belch, a routine repeated until 5.30 am, when I eventually fell into a deep sleep until 9.00 am on the Sunday morning. It was as if my chest was an over-inflated plastic bag, or bubble-rap that needed to be popped!

Day 5 (Sunday 7th January)

I took a 10 mg anti-emetic domperidone tablet, drank a cup of tea, and then had a bowl of cornmeal porridge with nutmeg mace, honey, muscovado sugar, a date and a large prune, the last added to my diet in the knowledge that I was beginning to feel constipated. I dissolved and drank the remaining 2mg dexamethasone steroid tablet. After breakfast, Mel and I walked to the shop to buy Sunday papers.

As soon as I started the journey, I became aware that the heel and sole of my left foot felt sore and bruised, but I limped on in pain, determined I would not be halted. Was this a side effect of the treatment? I was weaker and more breathless than usual and had to slacken my pace. Taking it slowly, stopping occasionally to breathe and burp, I made it to the shop and back – a distance of approximately two miles. On our return, Mel made me a cup of ginger tea from fresh ginger to help settle my stomach It was refreshing and gave me temporary relief.

Home injection

It was now around 12.30 pm, and I plucked up the courage to administer the remainder of my day 5 medication – a syringe full of 300 micrograms (5 ml) of filgrastim, a drug used to treat neutropenia following chemotherapy by stimulating the bone marrow to increase the production of neutrophils. (I looked up filgrastim on Google and discovered that it cost the NHS about £50.15 per 300 ug dose). Never before in my life had I given myself an injection and, despite Mel's reassurance, I became very anxious.

Eventually, I unbuttoned my shirt and, in accordance with the guidance given at the pre-assessment, pinched a pouch of flesh on my midriff, cleaned the skin with a wipe, and stuck in the needle, pushing the plunger slowly down into the barrel. I completed the task in a jiffy. It was painless at the time, but the spot stung for a little while afterwards. Mel took the syringe pump away to dispose of it in the sharps box given by the hospital for that purpose.

An hour or so later, still troubled by indigestion and burping, I took a further 10 mg domperidone tablet, then waited for a while before eating lunch. We had chicken mulligatawny soup, cold pizza slices, and artichoke hearts. After lunch, Mel made a tea of real ginger with the intention of easing my indigestion.

In the afternoon, I read the Sunday papers and did a little writing, interrupted occasionally by bouts of belching. I began to feel distinctly constipated which, I had been told, was a common side effect of the treatment, and spent some time on the lavatory attempting to extrude a very firm stool. Even after I succeeded, I remained uncomfortably blocked, resolving to take more prunes with my breakfast. In preparation for supper, I took a domperidone tablet with water. The meal was a lamb stew with potatoes and leeks, most appetising, and I was comforted by the fact that my sense of taste had returned. Throughout day 5, my temperature remained normal at 36.8^0c.

We went to bed earlier than usual at 10.00 pm and I slept until 2.00 am but after that, as on previous nights, I was obliged to sit up at regular intervals to express wind. I must have dropped off again between the burping, but my sleep pattern remained disturbed and fitful.

Day 6 (Monday 8th January)

I took a 10 mg domperidone anti-emetic tablet and made morning tea. We rose early to await the arrival of the fitters, who were scheduled to install smart meters to our energy supply. Mel cooked oats porridge with nutmeg mace and cinnamon. I added muscovado sugar, honey, a date, and a large prune. Despite wanting to evacuate my bowels, I was unable to do so. My temperature stood at 37.0^oc.

I drove to the dentist to keep my appointment for my six-monthly check-up, informing him, as I sat down, that I was undergoing chemotherapy, in which he showed interest and sympathy. He was aware, of course, of the danger of infection from cuts and abrasions and, after examining my teeth, told me that I had no build-up of plaque or tartar, and that there really was no need for the follow-on appointment with the hygienist.

On returning home, I was now able to empty my bowels and felt much relieved, a success which I attributed to the previous days' diet of vegetables, oranges and prunes. Scheduled to arrive between 8.00 am and 12 noon, the smart meter fitters cancelled in late morning for a second time, thus disrupting our arrangements. I was already becoming anxious at the prospect of injecting myself with the second syringe of filgrastim due at 12.30 pm. Seeing my concern, Mel offered to help. I pinched the flesh on my belly, while she rapidly administered the shot, remarking that I was fortunate I wasn't a diabetic.

I took a domperidone anti-emetic tablet, we had lunch, and went shopping for groceries but, as on the previous day, my heel felt bruised and I found walking painful. It was a cold day, and I soon became exhausted, pleased to return to the comfort of the car and conscious of the impact the chemotherapy had had on my previous fitness. Once back at home with a hot cup of tea, I felt much better, convincing myself that I was over the worst and one step nearer recovery.

Mel cooked a supper of smoked haddock with ginger, potato, and sprouts, which I ate without preparing myself with a 10 mg domperidone anti-emetic tablet. I had no feeling of nausea, before or afterwards, and experienced no burping or bloating. We watched *East Enders* and the first in a new series of *Silent Witness* on television before retiring to bed early at 10.00 pm. After recording my temperature at 36.8°c, I went to sleep easily enough, but kept waking up regularly during the night to sip water and visit the lavatory.

Day 7 (Tuesday 9th January)

After my shower and physiotherapy exercises, Mel took my temperature and massaged my bruised left heel. I decided once more to do without the domperidone anti-emetic tablet and hungrily polished off my cornmeal porridge with nutmeg mace and cinnamon, muscovado sugar, honey, date and prune. My daughter, Toussaint, texted me to find out how I was doing and whether I was still feeling 'high'. I texted back to tell her I was coping: "My main complaints are constant burping which I have tried to counter by reducing my intake of anti-emetics, and what appears to be bruising on the heels of my feet, which make it painful to walk. I am also a little constipated but have managed a firm stool everyday so far". She said she hadn't meant me to go into detail.

Later that morning while I wrote my diary, Mel made me a mug of real ginger tea to ensure my stomach remained settled. The prunes and vegetables consumed on previous days had the desired effect and I vacated my bowels with ease, but the stools were still well-formed. I noticed that I was experiencing a certain stiffness and cramping in my arms, shoulders and leg joints.

As the time of my third injection of filgrastim approached, I became anxious again but, this time, resolved to administer the dose myself, although I readily accepted Mel's offer to supervise. I wiped and pinched the skin on my abdomen and then stuck in the needle and pushed the plunger, thus proving I was not a wimp.

Visit of Mel's brother and sister-in-law

Lloyd and Bernadette, Mel's brother and sister-in-law, drove from Sutton Coldfield to visit us and learn about my health. They were curious to know how I had discovered my breast cancer and to receive a blow-by-blow account of my treatment – particularly the chemotherapy. Of course, they knew others who had been treated for cancer and had subsequently survived, as well as others, no doubt, who had died, whom they refrained from mentioning.

Aware that they were genuinely concerned and interested in my condition, I became suddenly conscious that I was gaining satisfaction from demonstrating an expert personal knowledge of my diagnosis and treatment. The four of us ate lunch of soup and pizza. Before Lloyd and Bernadette left, I began to feel very tired and went up to bed for a nap. I got up later and did some writing, before Mel cooked supper – another stew that I liked – and more ginger tea. After watching television, we went to bed. I slept much better that night without being made uncomfortable by the burping, but still had to rise a few times during the night to cope with the amount of fluid I had drunk. My temperature remained steady, morning and evening, at around 36.8^0c.

Day 8 (Wednesday 10th January)

I woke feeling hungry and eagerly consumed my porridge. Noticing I had a sore throat and a few abrasions in my mouth, I cleaned my teeth and gargled with Corsodyl mouthwash. The previous days' prunes had done their work, and I had a full loose evacuation of the bowels. Mel massaged my heels, but I was still sore when I walked, and my joints were stiff and cramped.

As it was Wednesday – Diamond Club discount day – I drove Mel to B & Q in Bilston to buy some seeds for the greenhouse and vegetable patch – broad bean, onion, swede, kale, kohl rabi and courgette. When we returned home, I felt hungry again, and prepared and ate lunch. Soon afterwards, I felt unusually tired, lay on the bed and immediately went to sleep, not waking up until 5.00

pm. When I came to, I found a cup of cold ginger tea on the bedside table that Mel had brought up for me. I drank it cold.

Our friend, Bob, phoned from Wales to inquire after my health and to ask when we were coming to stay. I knew he had been suffering from shingles for over a year and had to explain that, even if we came down, we would only be able to converse on the phone because of the chemotherapy and my compromised immune system.

Day 9 (Thursday 11ᵗʰ January)

My temperature remained steady at around 37.0^0c. My bowel movements were regular and normal for me. Nevertheless, I woke with a sore throat and, after breakfast of cornmeal porridge, date and prunes, felt slightly nauseous, a sensation that led me to take a 10 mg anti-emetic domperidone tablet before lunch, when I ate chicken soup and slices of pizza. When I complained once more of the bruising sensation in my left heel, Mel massaged my feet, and we took a gentle afternoon walk to Tettenhall Upper Green. By the time I got back to the house, I felt very tired and went to bed at around 4.00 pm for an hour-long nap. I dropped off to sleep once more at 10.30 pm, but woke up early in a restless state, before making tea at 7.00 am.

Day 10 (Friday 12ᵗʰ January)

My temperature rose to 37.5^0c, what proved to be its highest point in the cycle. My bowel movements were regular and soft, if not loose. In regard to my general health, I experienced a sore throat, as well as a burning sensation between my buttocks and when wiping my anus. In the afternoon, I felt very tired and retired for an afternoon nap from 3.30 pm to 5.30 pm. This did not prevent me from going to bed again at 10.30 pm and sleeping well until 6.00 am, when I got up to make tea.

Days 11 to 21 (Saturday 13th – Tuesday 23rd January)

The remaining ten days of the first cycle followed the same routine. At first, the mild indigestion continued and I went on experiencing a bruising sensation in the heels and soles of my feet, but this gradually went away. Instead, on Friday 12th January, I unexpectedly developed another complaint: soreness in the trough between my buttocks and around my anus, the latter causing me intense discomfort after defecation, especially when wiping myself.

On examination, Mel told me the skin was now raw and red, and showed signs of deteriorating still further. When we googled the symptoms, the term 'intertrigo' appeared (see medical glossary). By Sunday 14th January, Mel noticed that additional areas of soreness had appeared between my buttocks. On Monday the 15th January, I made an emergency appointment to see *Dr Bidemi Oyawale* at the Castlecroft Medical Practice. She listened sympathetically to my complaint, got me to lie on the couch, with a chaperone present, as well as Mel, and examined the area, before writing a prescription for Fucibet cream (consisting of fusidic acid, a kind of antibiotic, and betamethasone valerate, a steroid) used on the skin to kill germs and reduce soreness. I was told to apply the cream to the infected area two times a day in the expectation that the area would heal in about seven days. The intertrigo responded to treatment and, by the time I saw *Dr Grigoryev* for an assessment of my health on the 22nd January, it had disappeared, although I continued to use the Fucibet cream as a precaution until the last day of the cycle.

As the first cycle of chemotherapy came to an end, I took the opportunity to review my state of health and wellbeing. My temperature had remained normal. I had not experienced nausea, diarrhoea, vomiting, shortness of breath, hair loss, or a serious infection. But I had suffered from sleeplessness, severe burping, minor constipation, mouth ulcers, painful joints, soreness on the heels of my feet, sores on my buttocks and anus, reduced energy levels, weakness, fatigue and exhaustion. Nevertheless, I judged my glass to be half full, and that my strength had returned in time for the next cycle of treatment on the 24th January. After all, I was being looked after by a caring wife, concerned children, family and friends, and a scientifically-grounded National Health Service of professional doctors and nurses.

On day 20 (Monday the 22nd January) of the first chemotherapy cycle, and two days before the second set of injections were due on Wednesday the 24th, Mel and I returned to the Deanesly Outpatients Department for my second appointment with *Dr Grigoryev*, the consultant oncologist.

We turned up early to allow Tracy, the phlebotomist, to take a sample of my blood. She attended to me as soon as I presented the form. As she took the blood from my right arm, I asked her how many syringes of blood she drew off in a day – around 150, she reckoned. Given that I must have been at least the hundredth patient she had dealt with on her shift, I was impressed with her smile and friendly demeanour.

Chance meeting

Having time to kill before my second appointment at Deanesly, and feeling restless and bored, I left Mel doing sudoku in the waiting room and went for a walk around the hospital site. While heading north on the long eastern corridor, I scarcely noticed a porter pushing a trolley in the opposite direction and was startled to hear a voice call out my name. It came from the trolley. The porter drew up and I turned round to see the face of a frail pale-skinned grey-haired old man peering up at me from under a blanket. It took me a few moments to recognise Norman Davis, a former councillor and friend of ours, whom Mel and I had not seen for several years. He told me that he was suffering from cancer and was being taken for a scan. Why was I at the hospital? I told him that I, too, had cancer and was there for an oncology appointment. He seemed very surprised.

I reported this chance meeting to Mel, who telephoned Norman's wife, by which time Norman had been discharged and was at home, attended by Macmillan nurses. (Norman died aged 84 on the 28th March 2018. He had been leader of Wolverhampton's Labour Group and leader of the council from 1973 to 1984 and, again, from 1986 to 2002.) I think I was more dismayed by the news of Norman's terminal cancer and death because I had seen him that day on the trolley and, like him, I, too, was a cancer patient, with the same intimation of impending mortality.

Reflecting on the encounter, I realised that cancer was widespread, especially among the elderly. In 2015, there were an estimated 2.5 million people living with cancer in the United Kingdom.[2] Almost 40 per cent of the population of the United Kingdom were diagnosed with some form of cancer during their lifetime[3], and more than half of cancer deaths occurred in people aged 75 or over (2012-2014)[4]. In regard to cancer, I was not in any way unique, different or special – just run of the mill. It was salutary to remember that.

Second appointment with *Dr Grigoryev*, the oncologist

On returning to the waiting room and half an hour before my scheduled appointment time, a nurse called out my name to see *Dr Grigoryev*. With his registrar in attendance, *Dr Grigoryev* inquired in a most mild and attentive manner about my experience and response to the first bout of chemotherapy, questioning me closely about its side effects.

I told him of the belching and hiccups, the mouth ulcers, my racing brain but tired body, the feeling of bruising on my heels, and the more recent sores between my buttocks and around my anus. I told him that this last complaint had since responded to the Fucibet cream prescribed by my GP. He asked whether I had become constipated around the third day of the cycle. For me, the constipation occurred around the fifth day, but I had managed to ease it by taking prunes with my breakfast and increasing my intake of vegetables and fruit at supper. *Dr Grigoryev* wrote out prescriptions for capsules to control future belching, and mouth drops to deal with any recurrence of mouth ulcers.

He seemed pleased with my progress and asked whether I had any questions for him. I wanted to know whether the chemotherapy drugs would permanently compromise my immune response and reduce my capacity to resist all the illnesses for which I had been vaccinated, for example shingles, hepatitis, tetanus, or for typhoid, paratyphoid and cholera, or indeed yellow fever. He reassured me that my immune responses would return to normal after the chemotherapy, but pointed out that most immunisations needed repeating or boosting over a lifetime.

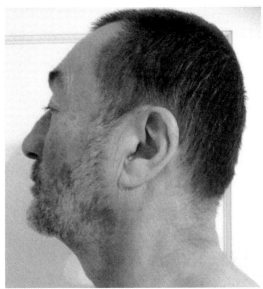

Frank's hair prior to a second cycle
of chemotherapy

Chapter 5

Second chemotherapy cycle

Day 1 (Wednesday 29th January 2018)

Second session of chemotherapy at the Snowdrop Millennium Suite

My second cycle of chemotherapy started on Wednesday 24th January 2018, on the 22nd day after the first dose. The same procedure was followed, with saline, anti-emetic and steroid drugs, and successive injections of epirubicin, cyclophosphamide and fluorouracil administered on the day ward of the Snowdrop Millennium Suite. On this occasion, I was treated by *Nurse Michelle McLean*, who dealt calmly and systematically with the business, commencing by giving me a 125 mg capsule of the anti-emetic aprepitant to swallow.

After my first cycle, I knew what to expect, but did not foresee that, on this occasion, my response would be different. Quite unexpectedly, I found it difficult to relax on the ward, and began to feel anxious. As the treatment commenced, I did my best to submerse myself in the same book that had gripped my attention on the first occasion, but was unable to concentrate.

As the fluids went in, my bladder filled up and I became desperate to urinate. *Nurse McLean* halted the procedure and allowed me to wheel the drip stand along the ward to the lavatory to relieve myself. My bladder filled up again rapidly and I was forced to make the same journey three times in all.

In the course of injecting the FEC drugs into my right arm, *Nurse McLean* noticed that I had become agitated and could not keep still. I was unable to explain either to her, or to Mel, the reason for my distress, nor comprehend to my own satisfaction why I was shaking. When the nurse suggested we pause the process to give me time to recover, I urged her to continue, even more perturbed that my behaviour might result in further delay. The moment soon passed, but I still have no idea why I reacted in this way and so differently from the first cycle of chemotherapy. A friend later suggested that I might have been experiencing a panic attack but, apart from the shaking, I had none of the commonly-listed symptoms of a pounding heart, sweating, nausea, faintness, nervous asthma, or pains in the chest.[1]

As on the previous occasion, I left the ward with an assortment of medicines, in the form of tablets, capsules and syringes, to help me to cope with the side-effects. While walking past other patients in the course of their treatment, I heard someone calling my name and went over to a man in the midst of his chemotherapy, sitting next to his wife. Neither Mel nor I recognised them although their faces looked familiar, but they knew who we were. We had met and drunk together in the Yew Tree Pub some forty years previously. John told me he was on a two-week cycle for bowel cancer, and we rapidly established a communion of cancer camaraderie.

After my treatment, we drove back home for pizza and olives. By the time I got home, I had already passed urine a number of times, removing all trace of the blood-orange coloration from the epirubicin. Later that evening, I took the 8 mg ondansetron (anti-emetic) tablet as prescribed. Mel prepared a tasty supper of spiced chicken, potatoes and sprouts, with which I drank plenty of water, in a vain attempt to reach the recommended 1.8-litre intake of fluid. We relaxed watching television before going to bed at 11.00 pm, but I had an over-active brain and found it impossible to sleep. I dropped off eventually around 3.30 am, waking up around 6.30 am to make tea.

As I tossed and turned, I realised that my scalp felt unduly sore against the pillow, leaving me with the odd sensation that I was lying on a pin cushion. My hairs felt like pins being pushed backwards into their follicles on the scalp. Was that a dream?

Day 2 (Thursday 25th January)

On waking, I noticed a sprinkling of hairs on my pillow, signalling that I was starting to lose my hair. This was the chemotherapy-induced alopecia - the sinisterly-named CIA - that I had been warned to expect.[2]

During the previous cycle, I had learned the importance of organising the day's timetable of my prescribed drug-taking. As before, it included the morning and lunchtime soluble tablets of the steroid, dexamethasone, and the capsule of anti-emetic aprepitant, with the addition, this time round, of a 30 mg tablet of lansoprazole to control my burping, and a pipette-full of nystatin to keep my mouth free of ulcers. I found it quite testing to remember the type, timing, and order of my medicines, and wondered how others coped.

I ate well that day, with cereals for breakfast, Mulligatawny chicken soup for lunch, and smoked haddock with ginger, garlic and chives, potatoes, sprouts and parsnips for supper. I noticed, however, that my stools were very solid, and resolved to increase my intake of fibre. Despite the previous night's lack of sleep, I felt reasonably alert and went out shopping with Mel in the afternoon to Ryman for stationery, to the Works and Waterstones for books, and to Sainsbury and Lidl for groceries.

We went to bed around 11.00 pm, and I fell asleep almost immediately, but woke at 3.00 am, feeling bloated and uncomfortable. I was obliged to sit up at half-hourly intervals to belch, rub my belly, and express wind. Meanwhile, my head stayed in racing mode, and I went over again and again the experience of the previous day's chemotherapy, during which I had become agitated without being able to give a reason. I still could not explain why I found the second set of injections so much more taxing than the first.

Day 3 (Friday 26th January)

The dyspepsia lasted until morning, when I belched when drinking tea at 7.00 am. I inspected my pillow but did not find any further hairs but, as I looked in the mirror, I noticed a distinct thinning and recession of my hair on either side of my forehead. Again, as I placed my dirty clothes in the washing basket, I saw that a significant sprinkling of dead grey skin flakes from my ankles and legs had formed a crusty deposit on my navy-blue socks. A similar powdering was beginning to accumulate on my navy-blue pullover. Skin flaking – desquamation – is highlighted by men's dark winter clothing, but I had no intention so early in the year of wearing my grey summer suit and socks.

Forty-five minutes before breakfast, I took one 30 mg of lansoprazole with water to tackle burping. During breakfast, I dissolved the two soluble 2 mg tablets of dexamethasone and swallowed them, and then took one 8 mg ondansetron tablet. Afterwards I cleaned my teeth and rinsed my mouth with one ml of the nystatin suspension. My course of medication was completed at 10.15 am with an 80 mg capsule of aprepitant.

I took morning coffee and worked on my computer for a while, before deciding to escape from the house for a little retail therapy. Conscious of my changing appearance, I chose to wear my light-blue beanie to disguise my thinning hair. My beard, so far, seemed unaffected. After a visit to Dunelm, where no-one, including the sales assistant, gave me a second glance, I drove to McDonald's for a much-welcomed quarter-pounder meal. Returning home, I confessed to Mel what I had done and was duly scolded for eating out, in the knowledge that my immune system was compromised. Mel directed me to busy myself by tidying up for the weekend visit of our son and daughter-in-law and our two grand children. I decided to go on wearing my light-blue beanie indoors, but to change to a bright orange one as a night cap, reminding Mel, so she said, of sleeping with a detainee of the US camp at Guantanamo Bay.

Visit of my son, daughter-in-law and grand children

At 9.30pm, Robeson, Tasha and grand children arrived from London for the weekend, but with the additional mission of visiting me and asking about my health. It was wonderful to see them and to catch up on their lives, and we did not retire to bed until after midnight. By then feeling very tired, I slept well until 3.00 pm but, thereafter, woke up feeling indigested and bloated, which I was only able to relieve by sitting up straight for a burp. The side effects and their timing were a repetition of the first cycle of the treatment.

Day 4 (Saturday 27th January)

At 7.30 am I went down to make tea and take a capsule of the lansoprazole prescribed to control my burping (and described in the information leaflet as a 'gastro-resistant' used to reduce the amount of acid in the stomach). About an hour later, Mel cooked me oats porridge which I had with prunes in the hope it would prevent me becoming constipated. At the same time, I drank one dissolved 2 mg tablet of dexamethasone which should be taken with food, thus completing my prescribed medicines for the day.

Noticing and coming to terms with hair loss

After breakfast, I showered, noticing as I stepped out of the basin a substantial accumulation of my hair around the sump. On looking more closely, I realised that many of the hairs had come from my body, particularly from my chest and from under my arms. The hair on my head had also thinned, making me decidedly mangy and alopecic, a sight I quickly concealed with my light-blue beanie. My beard and moustache may have thinned, too, but not so noticeably.

In the morning, Robeson drove me and Maxi, my three-year-old grandson, into Wolverhampton to buy a children's football for a kick-around in the garden. Afterwards, I asked Robeson to come shopping with me to Boots for a hair trimmer and shaver, as a precaution against further extreme or uneven hair loss.

I asked a saleswoman for advice on the purchase, mentioning in passing why I needed the trimmer and shaver in one – I was having chemo. She led me to a shelf and took the time and trouble to talk me through the various models and prices, showing me courtesy and concern. I opted for a Philips cordless rechargeable battery-driven trimmer, reduced in price by £20. The saleswoman wished me good luck as I left the till, helping me to appreciate the immense pool of public sympathy and goodwill towards people with cancer. Inexplicably, the compassion she showed almost reduced me to tears.

I had soup with a slice of olive bread for lunch and, feeling fatigued, went upstairs for an afternoon nap. Not having slept well the night before, I quickly dropped off for an hour or so. When I woke, I was conscious of indigestion which I relieved on an hourly basis with a bout of belching. To ensure I would be able to eat my supper without further discomfort, Tasha made me ginger tea and I took a 10 mg domperidone tablet half an hour before the meal.

After the family supper, we played with the children, watched as they splashed in the bath, and conversed for a while. Mel and Tasha went to their beds, while Robeson and I talked about his business ventures, as we watched *Match of the Day*. I eventually went to bed about 12.30 am and slept until 3.00 am. I was disturbed by indigestion and the need to sit up to belch, action repeated at roughly 90-minute intervals.

Day 5 (Sunday 28th January)

Woken by the radio at 7.00 am, I went to make tea, taking my early morning capsule of lansoprazole with water, to control further burping. Around 8.00 am, I joined Robeson and the children in the kitchen and had breakfast of cereals with prunes and dates to avoid constipation, and also took the last of the soluble dexamethasone. Sure enough, I managed to evacuate my bowels, despite the hardness of the stools.

After taking a shower, I noticed more hair in the shower basin, and a further recession of the hair on my forehead and pate. Nevertheless, I had lost far less than on Saturday, and it had fallen away evenly. My beard may have been thinner, but it was still in place. I dressed, put on my beanie, and walked to the shop for the Sunday newspapers.

Around 12 noon, before Robeson, Tasha and the grandchildren departed for London, I went with Mel to the bedroom, where she jabbed in the 5 ml syringe full of filgrastim to assist me in producing the necessary neutrophils. Irrationally, I dreaded the injection and was much relieved when Mel had finished. This time round, I was quite prepared to wimp out of injecting myself.

For lunch, I ate some of the left-overs from last night's supper. Tasha made me a mug of root ginger tea. I felt distinctly fatigued and went for a short afternoon nap.

Later, concerned as to whether I would experience another night's burping, I considered taking a domperidone before supper, but decided against it in the hope that I might be recovering naturally from the gastritis.

Mel cooked a tasty supper of rice and peas and diced chicken, with plenty of sprouts to ease constipation. I drank Ribena, followed by a hot cup of root ginger tea. We watched *Call the Midwife* and *McMafia* on television and went to bed at around 11.00 pm.

I managed to sleep until 3.00 am, when I woke feeling constipated and needing to sit up and burp. Feeling restless and with a head buzzing with ideas, I went downstairs to make myself tea. In an attempt to ease my constipation, I went to the lavatory and, with some effort, managed to evacuate a small stool, thus breaking the bottle neck, so to speak. Returning to bed, I rested, perhaps falling asleep occasionally, but having to sit up at hourly intervals to burp and belch.

Day 6 (Monday 29th January)

At 7.00 am, I went to the kitchen to take a 30 mg capsule of lansoprazole and to make tea. Soon afterwards, I managed a further evacuation of more stubborn stools. An hour or so later, I had a further looser and adequate evacuation, and felt much relieved.

Serious hair loss

While taking my shower, I noticed a build-up of water in the shower tray. Once I had dried myself, I took out the sump cover to investigate and found it clogged with facial and body hairs, which I must have shed while washing myself. When I looked in the mirror, I noticed my hair had receded still further and the little that remained had thinned quite markedly. My beard was grizzlier and greyer and my chest and underarm hair much shorter, although my pubic hair appeared as plentiful and tangled as before. Later that morning, I felt a sharp pain against my retina and realised that one of my eye lashes had fallen into my eye.

After coffee, Mel gave me my filgrastim jab. Invariably, as the time for the injection approached, I became increasingly worried and agitated, despite the fact that, whenever the reality occurred, it was never a prolonged or painful experience, and I was fully aware that diabetic patients routinely took insulin in the same way. After lunch, I went to help Mel with some gardening, but was surprised at how arduous I found the work and how quickly I became fatigued. I went indoors to sit down and fretted about my lack of strength. The rest of the day passed uneventfully and we retired to bed around 10.30 pm.

I slept soundly until 4.00 am, when I got up to empty my bladder and to burp, but then fell asleep easily enough until the alarm went off at 7.00 am. It was the best night's rest I had had since the second cycle began.

Day 7 (Tuesday 30th January)

In the morning, I managed to achieve a small evacuation, but felt bloated and constipated for most of the day, before expressing a meagre but solid stool around 8.00 pm. I glimpsed my steadily increasing baldness in the mirror as I was about to shower, leading me to check the shower basin and sump as soon as I had finished. Hairs had fallen again, but Mel assessed them to be shorter and finer than on the previous day. I took a capsule of lansoprazole before a welcome breakfast of oats porridge, prunes, dates and honey.

Our friend, Philip, came round to assist me on the computer with the design work on my book. After he left, Mel gave me my third and final 300 mg filgrastim jab. She did it in a flash, but once more I reacted irrationally by starting to shake. Never in the past had I bothered one jot about injections, inoculations, or the extraction of blood. What was now different? I couldn't explain, but noted that current jabs were meant to be self-administered at home and into the midriff. But why should I be troubled by that?

Attending a meeting at Citizens Advice

On checking my diary, I noticed that I was scheduled to attend a 5.00 pm meeting of the Wolverhampton Citizens Advice Trustee Board of which I had long been a member, but wondered whether I would be sufficiently fit to participate. Should I offer my apology? I had already made known to the chair and chief officer my current health status and I knew they would not expect me to attend. Nevertheless, I had adopted two guiding principles to help me on my road to recovery: to retain the routines of my life – what might be referred to as 'normalisation' – and to make every effort to sustain my network of friends and social contacts.

I asked Gem Lopez, a friend and fellow trustee, to give me a lift to the meeting, familiarised myself with the agenda and reports, and put on my suit and smartest beanie in readiness. My attendance and appearance passed without comment. A few of the trustees who were my friends and confidants, inquired discreetly about my health and progress but, despite wearing the beanie throughout the meeting, my cancer and I went unnoticed. As usual, several agenda items triggered discussion. I left the meeting feeling happier and more in touch with local concerns than when I arrived.

Day 8 (Wednesday 31st January)

In the morning, I was still slightly indigested, but this settled after breakfast. I remained a little constipated but, after initial straining, I managed to produce a couple of hard stools. The hair loss continued, but there was no repeat of Monday's sump blocking. My hair line had receded still further towards the back of my head and the short grey bristles of my beard were thinning and falling out. Touching my chin was painful, leaving me with a prickling sensation, as if I had splinters. At lunchtime, the top of my head began to hurt, as if the tuft of hair that remained on my pate was being ground by my beanie into my scalp. The stinging continued for half an hour, even after I removed the beanie.

Before lunch, I began to feel nauseous but relieved myself somewhat by belching. I swallowed a 10 mg domperidone tablet as a precaution. This allowed me to consume a cup of spicy jerk chicken soup, a piece of pork pie, and a slice of baguette.

Mel was alarmed by the dead skin she saw on my face, arms, legs and ankles, and massaged those parts of my body with aqueous cream. When working on my ankles, she noticed that they were swollen and insisted I rest them in a raised position on the poof. She became upset when she learned that I planned to walk to Tettenhall Green and back for fresh air and exercise. It was a bitterly cold day, and I was glad to return to the house. After my walk, I felt very tired and went for a short nap on the bed.

The evening took the usual course: supper followed by television (when we watched the final episode of *Kiri* on Channel Four) and bed. I slept comparatively well, only waking twice to belch and relieve myself.

Day 9 (Thursday 1st February)

I noticed a further diminution of hair on the dome of my head, my cheeks, chin, torso and thighs, although my pubic hair seemed unaffected. In assessing my appearance, Mel remarked that my eyebrows and eyelashes remained in place as a recognisable and distinctive facial characteristic. The skin on my face looked dry and flaky. As before, Mel massaged my face, legs and ankles with aqueous cream.

In the late afternoon, Mel and I went to the hospital for my appointment with *Mr Hiyam Shome*, the consultant urological surgeon (see Chapter 6). When we got home, I felt very tired and inexplicably anxious. Following supper, Mel and I watched television, but I fell asleep during the Thursday evening episode of *Death in Paradise*, never to discover 'who done it'. As soon as the programme had finished and still half asleep, I stumbled upstairs, got into bed and did not wake up until 3.00 am. Thereafter, I had a restless few hours, with Thursday's events in the urology department swirling around in my mind. I lay there fitfully until the radio alarm went off at 7.00 am.

Day 10 (Friday 2nd February)

The day started well for me with a normal bowel movement, followed by a further evacuation around 11.00 am. There had been further hair loss, but it was not obvious from looking in the mirror or the shower tray, indicating that the process must have slowed down. Mel thought my face and the skin on my body remained very dry and insisted on massaging them with aqueous cream.

When Mel went out for coffee with her women friends, I received a phone call from Dunelm to tell me our new kitchen curtains were ready to collect.   Freed from Mel's surveillance, I seized the opportunity to fetch the curtains and go to McDonald's for the quarter-pounder meal I yearned for.

Feeling vulnerable and helpless after a boiler breakdown

Later that afternoon, I noticed that the radiators were cold and the temperature in the house was falling.   Mel and I fiddled with the knobs on the combi-boiler.   We knew the break-down of the central heating system was serious, given the cold weather forecast for the weekend, Mel's impending departure to spend time with our grandchildren, and my current health status.   Yet I realised that I felt very tired, if not utterly exhausted, from my morning's activity, and found it difficult to summon the energy to make the necessary arrangements to get the boiler fixed.

I felt vulnerable and helpless.   I could deal with the routines of everyday life, but had not the resilience to respond to emergencies. I took the least stressful option: I phoned a friend.   Philip Lopez responded immediately, turning up on the doorstep with his son-in-law, Lucan Spittle, a boiler engineer, who proceeded to strip down and service the combi.   Lucan concluded that the fault lay with the extractor fan and promised to return the next morning with a friend who was skilled in diagnostics.

In the meanwhile, Mel and I had to live with the cold.   We were left with the gas fire to heat the living room, a portable electric radiator for our bedroom, and a hot shower unit downstairs on a different system.   We would cope.   When we went up to bed at 10.00 pm, I dropped off to sleep immediately and did not wake up until 4.00 am.   I slept again until 6.30 am, when I went to make tea.

Despite or because of the day 10 boiler crisis, I had an excellent night's sleep.

Days 11 to 21 (Saturday 3rd – Tuesday 13th February)

With the boiler out of operation, we had to shower downstairs and eat our porridge in a chilly kitchen. My bowels seemed now to be functioning normally – if still a little loose – from a surfeit of prunes, oranges and vegetables. I drove Mel to the station to catch her train to London, where she was due to help with our grandchildren while Robeson and Tasha moved house. Returning home, I realised how cold the rooms were. Given the state of my immune system, I wondered whether the temperature was putting my health at risk, but realised that there was little I could do but keep my coat on and wait.

Later that morning, Philip, Lucan and a diagnostic boiler engineer came round, Philip to drink coffee and to help me on the computer, Lucan and the other engineer to work on the boiler. Sure enough, the extractor fan was faulty and the part had to be ordered. It would not be in stock until Monday. Lucan would fit it on Monday evening in time for the house to warm up, before the arrival of Mel, Toussaint, our daughter, Luc, our son-in-law, and baby Caio. They were coming up specially from London to visit the sick me and celebrate my birthday.

My main grumble on day 11 was that my mouth and gums had become bruised and sore. I went on regularly brushing my teeth after every meal and washing my mouth with the nystatin suspension. That evening, I noticed my temperature had risen to 37.5^0c, the highest of the second cycle so far, but in line with the pattern of the first cycle.

Selective perception of cancer news

On day 12 (Sunday 4th February) I went to collect my papers, *The Observer* and *The Sunday Times*. After my breast cancer diagnosis, I seemed to have acquired an uncanny ability to spot news items and articles about cancer – a very noticeable selective perception. *The Sunday Times Magazine* (4.2.2018) carried an inspiring story about Nicola Mendelsohn, a Facebook executive, who was diagnosed with follicular lymphoma, a slow-growing, rare and incurable form of cancer. She responded by contacting on Facebook other follicular lymphoma patients across the globe and linking up with an organisation called ' Living with Follicular Lymphoma', helping to build it to a membership of 3,500. Members communicated with one another on a daily basis, shared information about their condition, liaised with doctors and researchers, raised funds for research, and organised conferences and symposia. I found Nicola Mendelsohn's story inspiring. For me, it posed the question of what contribution I should be making to cancer relief.

Emotional outburst on birthday

My 73rd birthday coincided with day 15 of the second cycle, prompting my family and friends to make a special effort to mark the occasion and demonstrate their affection for me. Robeson, our son, and Tasha, our daughter-in-law, sent me a card with the message: 'Always be aware that we, your family, love and care, and will always be there for you'. Toussaint, our daughter, and Luc, our son-in-law, along with baby Caio, had come up from London to spend the weekend with us, and to cook me a gourmet three-course birthday dinner, featuring a large beef fillet slowly and tenderly prepared by using the sous vide method. This birthday present took into account the advice I had been given to avoid eating out during chemotherapy, and the soreness I experienced under my dentures when attempting to chew hard on unyielding morsels.

My children, sisters and my friends showered me with birthday cards through the post, often followed on the day with emails and texts. My sisters, Annie and Maggie, phoned to wish me happy returns and inquire about the progress and side effects of my chemotherapy. Robeson and Tasha, phoned to express their love and affection. I received presents from Philip and Gem – a bottle of Cuban rum to share with Philip once I had completed my treatment, and a bundle of stationery for use in writing my cancer diary. Essie brought round a potted anthurium plant, crowned with hood-like bright red spikes and erect yellow spadices. Was the gift an attempt to revive my flagging virility in the face of the chemo?

Early that evening, Spartaca, our daughter in Kenya, and Patrick, our son-in-law, called me on Facetime to talk about the state of the world, particularly East Africa, and to inquire about the progress of my chemotherapy and its side effects. Patrick signed up to a celebratory drink once the treatment was over. He was unaware, I suspect, that I had not touched a drop of wine or spirits, least of all, my favourite tipple of rum, since the September diagnosis, and no alcohol whatsoever since the chemotherapy began.

When the conversation was over, emotion welled up inside of me, and I started to sob, doing my best to hide it at first, but then weeping openly and uncontrollably. Mel, Toussaint and Luc sprang up to console me but, feeling distraught and embarrassed, I pushed them away, and fled to the living room. For a few minutes, I sat there quietly to collect my feelings, before Mel came in to comfort me.

"What is happening to me?, I asked her. "This is totally out of character. I have never behaved in this way before. I don't deserve this endless profession of love and kindness. Why do I keep bursting into tears? It's so unlike me."

"I agree," Mel said. "As a man, you've always been taught to keep a stiff upper lip. You should listen to your feelings and let them out."

"I don't think that's what it's about, at all," I replied. "There is nothing in there to come out. I can't explain that shameful display of emotion to myself, let alone to you. How could any normal person respond to his birthday greetings in such a strange way?"

"Of course," Mel said. "We are all aware that it's a side effect of the drugs you're taking. If you weren't on chemo, it wouldn't have happened."

Over dinner that night, I apologised to Toussaint and Luc for my emotional outburst.

"Don't be absurd," they said, "it was quite unlike you. We put it down to the chemo."

Even were my behaviour to have been a consequence of the chemotherapy or steroids, I found it to be the most disturbing side effect so far. However temporarily, it had caused me to relinquish my grip on my emotions and reasoning, and to lose control of what I considered to be the essence of my personality. At first in the sitting room, I imagined that I might indeed be exposing my feminine side and demonstrating features originally revealed by the oestrogen-receptor breast cancer itself. Yet despite my vulnerable emotional state of the moment, I was still sufficiently rational and in charge to dispel such fantasies for the psycho-babble I knew them to be.

When I tried to discover more about the impact of chemotherapy on the emotions and personality, for example, in the Macmillan practical guide, *How are you feeling?*, I noticed that the feelings identified were shock and denial, fear and anxiety, guilt, sadness and depression, and anger.[3] I did not think I had experienced any of those, apart possibly from anxiety (which more accurately, from my point of view, I would have called 'agitation'). Furthermore, those feelings were attributed to being frightened and challenged by the diagnosis of cancer and the possibility that the knowledge of the diagnosis might lead to depression, manifested in weeping, irritability, and difficulty in sleeping. But the emotions that had recently overwhelmed me had occurred not when I learned I had cancer, but after I was given chemotherapy drugs.

Included in the many side effects listed in the Macmillan practical guide, *Understanding Chemotherapy*, is the subheading 'effects on the nerves', telling the reader that 'some drugs can make you feel anxious, restless, dizzy, sleepy or have headaches. Some people find that chemotherapy makes them forgetful or unable to concentrate during their treatment'[4]. Elsewhere, there is mention of the steroids given alongside the chemotherapy drugs: 'Their side effects include indigestion, increased appetite, feeling more energetic or restless, or having difficulty sleeping'.[5] I recognised the indigestion, restlessness and insomnia, but not the anxiety, depression, or forgetfulness. But my own peculiar symptom of uncontrollable and heightened emotional sensitivity was nowhere specifically mentioned.

Towards the end of the second cycle, I woke up on a couple of occasions with amorous feelings towards Mel and an erection but, perhaps because of my age and the weakening effects of the chemotherapy, we never got round to making love. I interpreted my spontaneous arousal as a reassuring sign of recovery, like the green olive leaf that the dove brought to Noah in the story of the flood and, therefore, further good news.

Research on alternatives to chemotherapy

On day 16 of the second cycle (the 8th February), while listening to the *Today Programme* on BBC Radio 4, my ears pricked up at the mention of the immune system and cancer. John Humphrys, the veteran broadcaster, was interviewing Sir John Bell, the Regius Professor of Medicine, at Oxford University. Traditionally, drugs had been given when the human immune system failed. Professor Bell highlighted the increasing recognition of the natural role that the body's immune system played in curing a majority of illnesses, including cancer. A new approach was to focus on the immune system, reviving it when it showed signs of flagging, by turning off signals telling it that it was tired, and boosting and reviving its response towards the cancer cells. So far, results for directing the immune system towards a whole range of cancers had been very positive and had led to prolonged periods of remission. The research promised to improve standards of care for most cancers within the coming decade[6]. I was delighted by the news, interpreting it optimistically to mean that today's forms of chemotherapy and their unpleasant side effects would soon be a thing of the past.

In the months that followed, the press carried various stories of a 'groundbreaking therapy' that harnessed the power of the immune system to fight cancerous tumours. For example, *The Guardian* (5 June 2018) reported how Judy Perkins, aged 49, an engineer from Florida, with late-stage breast cancer, had been successfully treated with her own immune cells. The immune cells had found out and destroyed her metastasised cancer cells, leaving her free from the disease after two years. Her cancer had been at an advanced stage and had already spread to her liver and other areas.

Doctors at the US National Cancer Institute in Maryland had taken tissue from Perkins's tumours, studied its DNA to find mutations specific to her cancer, focusing on those that disrupted genes to produce abnormal proteins. They had then extracted immune cells from the patient's immune system and selected those that could effectively find and destroy her cancer cells by attacking their abnormal proteins. They cultured many millions of the effective immune cells in the laboratory and injected them into her body along with another drug. After 42 weeks, tests showed the cancer had disappeared. It had not returned since.[7]

Appointment at the oncology department prior to the third chemotherapy cycle

On Monday 12th February (day 20), I had two hospital appointments – one in the morning and one in the late afternoon. Mel accompanied me to both. In the morning, I had my blood taken to check my white cell and red cell count were sufficient for the third chemotherapy to go ahead. The phlebotomist was *Elsie Montagu*, the very affable phlebotomy team leader, who saw me immediately and managed to distract me with such effect that I scarcely noticed the procedure until it was over. In the afternoon, we returned to the Deanesly Centre for my appointment with *Dr Grigoryev*, prior to the third chemotherapy cycle.

The electronic message board informed us that *Dr Grigoryev* was running an hour late, but we were seen very quickly by his registrar, *Dr Tahir Raja*, who asked whether we minded dealing with him instead. *Dr Raja* inquired about the second cycle and my experience of side effects. I mentioned the burping, soreness of gums, occasional agitation, and irregular sleep patterns. He listened to me very attentively, seeking clarification on several points. I went on to ask him about my strange emotional sensitivity and outbursts of weeping. I said that I did not believe I was depressed or anxious about the cancer. I thought it was directly related to the chemotherapy.

He suggested it might be the result of hormone imbalance brought about by the drugs. He felt that this was unusual at such an early stage in the treatment, but warned that the docetaxel (Taxotere) of the 4th, 5th and 6th cycles might affect me in much the same way. In regard to the burping and indigestion, he advised me to double up on the lansoprazole capsules, taking one in the morning and one in the afternoon. He wrote out a prescription for further supplies of lansoprazole to reduce stomach acid, and nystatin oral suspension to prevent mouth infections, as well as one half-tablet of lorazepam (a benzodiazepine given as a therapy for anxiety) to swallow with water on the night before chemotherapy, in order to calm the agitation I experienced before.

Second cycle in summary

The distinguishing features of the second chemotherapy cycle were my hair loss and my intense emotional sensitivity. The indigestion, belching and irregular sleep patterns had stayed much the same.

Unlike in the first cycle, I continued throughout the twenty-one days to shed hair, rapidly at first, but then at a slower rate, like the fall of leaves in the Autumn. It dropped out from most parts of the body, but not to the same degree. Some areas lost everything, while others retained a thinner but discernable covering. I judged myself to have lost more hair from my head than elsewhere, but it had fallen out relatively evenly and did not look mangy. A slight showing of hair remained on the scalp to the front of my ears as an ethereal coif, and as a shadowy nap to the rear of my ears on the back and high sides of the dome. The overall effect was to make me appear as if my hair had been trimmed much shorter than usual. As mentioned previously, I retained my eyebrows, eye lashes and beard, but in an attenuated form. When I looked in the mirror, I was reminded of a home-slaughtered chicken, recently plucked and stuffed, with hairs on its skin demanding to be singed, before being put in the oven to roast.

As to my emotional sensitivity, I have described how it manifested itself, with a particularly troubling outburst on my birthday. My family reassured me that they knew it was the effect of the chemo drugs, and not of my behaving out of character, but I found it highly embarrassing, exposing a part of me that even I did not recognise – an exposure far worse than the hair loss.

In most other respects, the second cycle was a repeat of the first. At the start, I was unable to obtain a full night's sleep. I suffered from dyspepsia and severe burping and belching. For a short while, I became constipated but took measures in a timely manner to gain relief. At times, I felt weak and exhausted and in need of an afternoon nap. My mouth became sore and ulcerated, but there was no repeat of the sores on my buttocks and anus. The medicines prescribed and timetable for taking them were the same as for the first cycle, but with the addition of the lansoprazole gastro-resistant capsules to relieve the burping, and the nystatin suspension to safeguard against mouth infection.

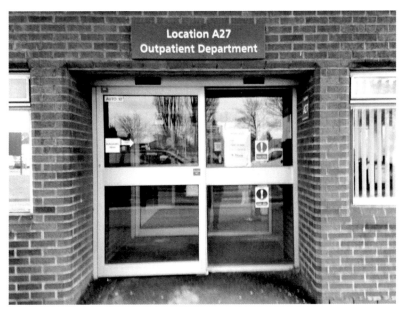

Newcross Outpatients' Department

Chapter 6

Urological interlude

Appointment with the consultant urologist

On learning of my failure to pass urine after my mastectomy, *Mr Venkatramanan* had referred me to the urology department. Nearly four months later, I was contacted by phone from the hospital and offered an appointment with a urologist. The date coincided with that of my second chemotherapy session and I had to decline. When I sought reassurance from the appointments clerk that my non-acceptance would not lead to further prolonged delay, she promised to rearrange within the next two weeks and, shortly afterwards, I received a text on my phone and a letter confirming an appointment a week later.

On Thursday 1st February, I went with Mel to the urology outpatients' department at the hospital to keep my 4.20 pm appointment with *Mr Hiyan Shome*, the consultant urological surgeon. As instructed, I took with me a specimen of urine which I gave to the attendant nurse. *Mr Shome* was well-spoken, good looking and cordial, and very much clued up on his specialism, making a habit of supporting his professional opinion by citing relevant urological research and paying close attention to my on-line medical history.

On his prompting, I told him of the reasons for my referral, starting with my mastectomy operation on the 22nd September 2017, the retention I experienced after waking up from the anaesthetic, my excessive consumption of fluid, my nocturnal frequency and eventual incontinence, the urinary infection and its duration, and the gradual return to normality.

He confirmed that an inability to pass urine was a recognised side-effect of anaesthetics, particularly among men, and that he strongly advised against the excessive intake of fluid to encourage micturition at such times. After an operation, one should drink normally. *Mr Shome* inquired about my current situation. Was I still experiencing frequency? Did I feel my bladder was empty after completing? Was the flow rapid, slow, or restricted? Did I finish cleanly or dribble afterwards?

I answered that I thought I was back to normal, able to empty, with a regular flow, and no leakage afterwards. Mel interjected, claiming that, in her opinion, I went too frequently especially at night, but admitted that it had always been my regular pattern. *Mr*

Shome said that medicines were available to regularise the flow and slow down the instances of urination.

He then conducted a digital rectal examination, inserting a gloved finger into my rectum, to assess the condition of my prostate gland. He judged it to be moderately enlarged (a 60 cc benign-feeling prostate)[1], but of an appropriate size for my age. I told him that a few years ago, a blood sample had been taken to perform a prostate-specific antigen (PSA) test. He found the result – a 2.1 reading in 2010 – in my computerised medical records (the 'Integrated Electronic Patient Record', or IEPR) on the screen in front of him.[2] On the basis of that information, he told us that the state of my prostate was in the range judged normal and that research showed very low rates of change in men of my age.

It was precisely at that moment that I began to appreciate the significance of my on-line medical record. Displayed on *Mr Shome's* screen were my medical history, my test results and all recent reports and documents relating to my health. The Integrated Electronic Patient Record was accessible at the touch of a key board to general practitioners and hospital consultants alike - an amazing professional silo-buster, focussing everyone's attention on me, the patient.

Already digitally versed in my oncological narrative, *Mr Shome* inquired in a sympathetic manner about the progress of my chemotherapy. He judged that I had a lot on my plate at the moment and that it was best to leave matters as they were until the end of my treatment. He would write to my GP with the name of the drug, tamsulosin, that might help with the frequency, if later I felt the need to have it prescribed.[3]

I was curious to ask *Mr Shome* about the origin and meaning of his name, which I suspected was Indian Bengali Hindu, as many years ago I had been friends with a Mr Mitra and a *Mr Shome* who organised an annual Bengali Durga Puja festival. However, I refrained from doing so, in the knowledge that Mel would disapprove of my infringement of protocol and unwanted presumption of familiarity at a first appointment.

As we left the room, I remember thinking how extraordinary it was that we had come through the interview without using any of the common colloquial terms for urination, such as 'peeing', 'weeing' or 'pissing'.

The nurse who had been present at my rectal examination led me to the lavatory to empty my bladder, before conducting a CT scan to see whether there had been any retention. A little urine indeed was still present but not enough to be of concern.

Breast cancer bias against men?

On Friday, 2nd February, I called in at the newsagent to buy *The Guardian* newspaper, but ended up purchasing the *Daily Mail* (a paper I rarely read) as well. The *Daily Mail*'s front page read: 'New figures show prostate is now a bigger killer than breast cancer which gets twice the funding. Is this a case of bias against men?' Ben Spencer, the paper's medical correspondent claimed that more than 11,800 men a year were killed by prostate cancer, compared with about 11,400 deaths from breast cancer among women, but that prostate cancer research received less than half the funding of breast cancer.[4]

Screening for breast cancer was routine – middle-aged women were invited for scans every three years – but prostate cancer had no national screening programme. Men with prostate cancer waited four times longer for diagnosis than women with breast cancer. From the early 1990s, campaigns such as *Pink Ribbon* and *Race for Life* had raised public awareness of breast cancer, but it was not until 2007 that the annual men's cancer campaign came to Britain.

It was no surprise that the story caught my eye, given that I was currently receiving chemotherapy for my breast cancer and had had my prostate checked out the day before. I knew from first hand that men could have breast cancer, and I had once read some esoteric article – I think, in a women's magazine I browsed in a dentist's waiting room – that women had a rudimentary prostate gland (was it called Skene's?) – that could become inflamed or encysted, and potentially cancerous, however rare or unusual that might be. I had always believed that men and women's bodies shared more features in common than those that differentiated them.

As a man with breast cancer, I found it difficult to give credence to the allegation of bias against men (that is of sex discrimination) arising from a greater expenditure on breast cancer research. Surely we were human beings first and shared mortality in common, whatever the form or location of our cancers? What was needed to address the disparity between the treatment of cancers of the breast and of the prostate, was to devote far more resources to prostate cancer awareness campaigns, better tests, systematic screening, and targeted research programmes. Blaming men for their reluctance to seek help, or failing to identify their symptoms early enough, was uncalled for and served only to excuse the NHS's neglect of the issues involved. The greater expenditure on breast cancer research was clearly a result of more effective campaigning and fund-raising by women's support groups.

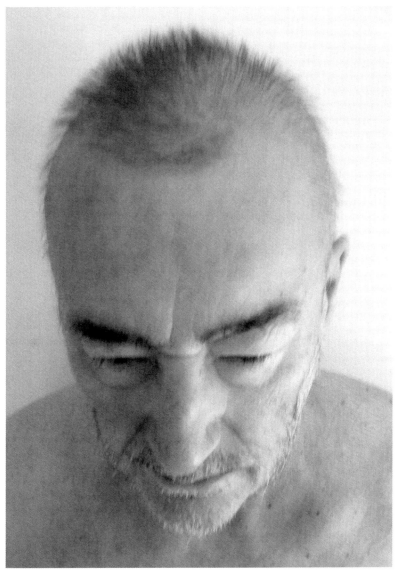

Hair loss by the third chemotherapy cycle

Chapter 7

Third chemotherapy cycle

Day 1 (Wednesday 14th February 2018)

St Valentine's Day, the 14th February 2018, was my daughter, Spartaca's birthday, but also the day on which I had to present myself at the Snowdrop Millennium Suite to be given my third round of FEC chemotherapy injections. The coincidence had its own compensations. Mel had sent me a Valentine card with the message "I'm so lucky that you're the one I get to share my life with," and our children had used the occasion to send birthday greetings to Spartaca and to wish me luck with my treatment.

As Mel and I walked into the Deanesly Suite, I recognised Derek Walsgrove, a friend and former colleague. He told me he was waiting with his partner for an oncology appointment, but the department was running three hours late. His partner was recovering from an operation to remove a large tumour from her abdomen – how large he indicated with a hand gesture. I reciprocated with information about my own cancer treatment. The sharing of personal or familial medical history is expected on these occasions as a means of conveying friendship and solidarity in times of distress.

Third session of chemotherapy at the Snowdrop Millennial Suite

Sister Jemima Holyoak, the same nurse who had treated me for the first cycle, came to collect us from the Snowdrop waiting area. I was asked to give my date of birth and address in order to make sure I was the very same Frank Reeves that they had treated before, and then invited to step onto the scales. She led us, as before, to a designated curtained unit on the u-shaped ward. Mel and I took our seats and I relaxed with my book, waiting for the procedure to begin.

Once more, *Sister Holyoak* put a hot compress against the back of my hand and gave me a 125 mg capsule of aprepitant. Once the veins became prominent, she searched for one that was suitable, announcing she had found "a fat juicy one" at the side of my wrist behind my right thumb. But when she inserted the needle, it caused me pain so intense that I told her I was about to retch. She immediately withdrew the needle, had a vomit bowl brought, and drew the curtains around my chair. I soon recovered and the feeling of nausea subsided, but *Jemima* would not continue until I voiced my consent.

Anxious to progress the procedure, I was pleased when she found another vein in the back of my hand and inserted the cannula without any further discomfort. My vein was then fed from a plastic bag of steroid fluid hung from the drip stand through a tube into the cannula, while I buried myself in my book.

A woman sitting next to a male patient, fitted like me to a plastic line, shouted out, leading me to glance across. The man's eyes had closed, his head had dropped, and he appeared to have lost consciousness. Her alarm led to nurses crowding around, the curtains being drawn, and two doctors quickly arriving. A bed was pushed in onto which the patient was placed and wheeled away towards the accident and emergency department.

That crisis, and a problem at the other end of the u-shaped ward, seemed to delay patient treatment across the suite. The machine on my drip stand began to beep and had to be silenced two or three times until *Sister Jemima Holyoak* returned at around 2.00 pm to administer my FEC injections. This time everything went to plan, helped along by an interesting and distractive conversation about recent television dramas, including *Trauma, McMafia, Hard Sun, Collateral,* and *Kiri* and the return of a new series of *Marcella,* which *Jemima* was looking forward to.

There was no repeat of the intense agitation I had experienced during the second chemotherapy session, and the cannula had been taken out and the dressings replaced before I had time to think about it.

As on the two previous occasions, we left the Snowdrop Millennium Suite with times and dates written in for the next blood count and the fourth round of chemotherapy, together with a package of medicines – a repeat of the second-cycle prescription – with the addition of extra steroids to be taken twice on the evening before the 4th set of injections. We came out of the hospital at 3.40 pm, much later than expected, and it was well after 4.00 pm by the time we reached home.

We rushed off almost immediately to collect our book proofs from the local printers, which had been finished more quickly than we had anticipated. By the time we got back, it was far too late for lunch, so we settled for a late afternoon pot of tea with shortbread and Viennese whirls, to keep us both going until supper. To ensure my stomach was settled, that I would have an appetite for my evening meal and spend a relatively restful night without hiccups, indigestion, belching or bloating, I took the ondansetron and lansoprazole anti-emetics. Mel cooked a tasty supper of potatoes, mince and broccoli, none of which required much mastication. She knew my gums were sore and hoped to avoid their deteriorating still further.

On day 1, I was tucked up in bed at 11.00 pm and had three hours sleep until 2.00 am, when I woke up with a febrile mind and could not doze off again. Bloated and burping, I went downstairs to make tea for us both, and returned to find Mel wide awake. By morning, she was truly exhausted. I had kept her awake all night, firstly, by snoring (which she admitted for me was atypical), secondly, with my restless tossing and turning and sitting up periodically to burp, and thirdly, by my non-stop exposition on artificial intelligence, the robot threat to jobs, and the cyborg[1] take-over of the planet. Mel attributed my alertness, articulation or, more properly, mania, to the steroids in my system, while I concluded that her reluctance to direct me to sleep in another bedroom revealed her truly to be my Saint Valentine.

Day 2 (Thursday 15th February)

I discovered more fallen hair when examining the shower sump after my shower. There was hair on my pillow, as well.

I referred to the third cycle schedule of drugs that I had drawn up to make sure I took my daily medicines on time – a sensible precaution given that I had been prescribed seven tablets/capsules to take on day 2 (see third-cycle timetable).

My notes for day 2's health report read: temperature am 37.2^0c, head buzzing with ideas and projects, irritatingly talkative, continuing hair loss, signs of constipation with only one sluggish bowel movement resembling rabbit balls, hot flushes to my face causing my cheeks to look red, continuous feeling of nausea, indigestion, bloating and belching, fatigue, light-headedness, giddiness, accompanied by agitation and the urge to scribble away, but not sufficiently exhausted yet to want to take a nap, temperature pm 36.7°c. It must be those soluble dexamethasone tablets again! Not the best of days!

Unsurprisingly, given the way I had disturbed her last night's sleep pattern, Mel retired to bed before me. I continued to write until 11.00 pm, when I turned off David Dimbleby's *Question Time*, and went up to join her. I slept soundly until 4.00 am when I woke up with a brain swirling with ideas, and found it impossible to doze off again. I went to make tea, which we both drank. Mel went back to sleep, but I got up and started to write where I had left off the night before, returning to bed at 7.00 am to lie down and listen to the *Today* radio programme.

Day 3 (Friday 16th February)

Before returning to bed at 7.00 am, I managed with difficulty to produce two small hard stools, defecating again a little more before I showered, but I was definitely becoming constipated.

After my shower, I examined my head and body in the mirror for hair loss. At that point, I had shed most of the hair on my head, apart from a mangy dark patch on the back of my crown. I still had my eyebrows, eyelashes, and beard, although all were much thinned. The hair on the back of my hands, on my arms, in my armpits, on my chest, my loins, and my legs, was still in place, but not, as before, in abundance. By now I had become used to my radically-altered appearance, and resolved not to hide Mr Hyde from myself any longer. I would leave off wearing my beanie indoors, henceforth exposing myself to myself, to Mel, and to visiting family and friends. During the day, the five scheduled doses of medicine - ondansetron, lansoprazole, dexamethasone, aprepitant and lansoprazole (again) – were taken at the right times and in the right order.

With the help of the anti-emetics, I ate well without feeling nauseous, but remained mildly indigested, with quite vigorous bouts of burping during and after lunch and supper.

The daily news broadcasts continued to highlight the story that, seven years previously in 2011, senior staff paid Haitian earthquake survivors for sex and hosted parties with prostitutes wearing Oxfam t-shirts, and that Oxfam had concealed the story, and had yet to take robust measures to clean up its act. As a consequence of the press exposures, Penny Mordaunt, the Secretary of State for International Development, announced that Oxfam would stop getting public funding until the government was satisfied it met the high standards expected of it.

I was infuriated by what I saw as an opportunistic attack on a charity that I had long supported and where my daughter had once worked as a diversity advisor. Knowing the right-wing objective of slashing the government target of spending 0.7 per cent of Gross National Income (GNI) on foreign aid, I immediately phoned up Oxfam and doubled our monthly donation to the surprise and delight of the call-centre recipient, who was expecting me to cancel my subscription like most other callers that day. Afterwards, I speculated as to whether my chemo-heightened emotions had contributed to my angry and abrupt response to the Oxfam crisis.

Shortly afterwards, the door bell rang. It was a parcel delivery man asking whether I would be willing to take in a parcel for our neighbours, Dev and Marie, at No 51, as they had not answered the door. Later, when I noticed their cars on the drive, I decided to take round their on-line delivery but first, out of habit, I put on my bright blue beanie. Dev came to the door, took the parcel and engaged me in neighbourly conversation. It may have been a figment of my imagination, but his eyes seemed to be fixated on my beanie. At that point, I chose to come clean and tell him on the doorstep about my cancer and chemo. As he worked as a consultant diabetologist at the hospital, himself, he asked me about the treatment I was receiving, the prognosis, and the consultants I was assigned to, reassuring me that I was in very good hands. He showed me genuine concern and sympathy. Afterwards, I began to question why I was still so reluctant to share the knowledge of my cancer with others – why had I been so keen to keep it a secret?

Mel cooked a tasty supper of garnished salmon, whole boiled potatoes and curly kale which I ate heartily, completing my meal by consuming a large navel orange, purposely aimed at my stiffening bowels.

As *Newsnight* finished around 11.00 pm, I went upstairs to bed, belching audibly on every tread. I continued to belch as I sat on the bed before falling asleep, only to wake up at 1.45 am to belch yet again. My belly felt and looked like an inflated plastic bag. From then on, I lay there, resting uncomfortably in an in-between state of semi-conscious, unable to distinguish between ideas that I dreamed and my waking thoughts, the time passing unbearably slowly and punctured occasionally by a hiccup or burp. At long last, at 6 00 am, I sat up to emit a series of belches and went down to make tea, thankful that the interminable dyspepsian night would soon be over, and the vertical posture of the day would offer relief.

Day 4 (Saturday 17th February)

I wanted to empty my bowels, but knew I was constipated, and sat in vain on the lavatory for a quarter of an hour before conceding defeat, and taking a shower. To settle my stomach, I took my first lansoprazole capsule around 8 am. I made sure I added four prunes to my oats porridge breakfast to speed up the chances of evacuation. I drank the dissolved dexamethasone tablet with my food.

After coffee, while engaged in a couple of Saturday DIY jobs about the house, I noticed that my head (now without the beanie and no longer insulated with a layer of hair) had grown cold, so I put on my beanie again – but merely on a temporary basis.

The DIY may have helped the downward shift of faecal matter for, shortly afterwards, I returned to the lavatory and, with much effort and straining, excreted a single 15 cm log of a stool, leaving me much relieved, yet recognising that, despite my increased consumption of prunes, I still had a looming constipation crunch.

The door bell rang. This time, it was a parcel delivery man with a parcel for David and Clare at No 55.

On checking my diary, I noted that Patrick Finucane, an old school friend of mine from 1963 who now lived in Faversham in Kent, was due to visit and stay for a couple of days next week. When I first told him of my cancer diagnosis, he had asked me whether I should like him to come to see me in Wolverhampton. I had jumped at the chance. Once more, it brought home to me the significance of family and friends – particularly such long-standing friends – when dealing with personal troubles and crisis. In eager anticipation of his visit, I phoned to check the time of his arrival at Wolverhampton station.

The day being mild and sunny, I followed Mel into the garden where she was digging potatoes for supper. She was pleased I had emerged to join her in the fresh air, and we paused to admire the snowdrops in flower under the magnolia tree. She pointed out an overgrown laurel bush that had to be pruned, whereupon I took up the challenge to gain much-needed exercise.

The cutting and shearing turned out to be more tiring than I had expected, but I was determined to finish the job, never imagining that I would so soon find myself with my heart thumping, giddy, light-headed, and out of breath. Mel ordered me indoors to lie down and rest. I made lunch for us both instead, before retiring to bed for a nap – a very short one – for it lasted for less than an hour. However, when I woke up, I was able to pass another firm stool, which I credited to my earlier bush-cutting exercise.

My indigestion persisted for most of the day, expressed in prolonged bouts of burping. Mel and I recalled that in the two previous cycles, she had resorted to making me mugs of real ginger tea, and, indeed, her herbal infusion helped a great deal. In addition, before supper, I took a further capsule of lansoprazole.

We went up to bed around 10.30 pm. I fell into a deep sleep almost immediately, only to wake up at 1am to belch and to visit the lavatory. I slept again soundly to 2 am, but thereafter, until 4 am, I only managed to rest. As on previous nights, my head swirled with wonderful ideas and magnificent schemes. I had made and drunk tea by 4.30 am, and fallen into a light sleep until the radio alarm came on at 7 am.

Day 5 (Sunday 18th February)

On waking, my principle concerns were the fear of a stubborn bout of constipation setting in, and the prospect of midday injection of filgrastim into my midriff. Mel made me cornmeal porridge before going out for her Sunday morning walk with Gem. I added at least four prunes and a date to my breakfast to fend off the constipation threat. The suggestive power of the prunes may have triggered the desired effect because, shortly afterwards, I achieved a colossal evacuation of firm, well-formed stools, and began to feel normal again.

I put on my coat and beanie to walk up to the shop for the Sunday papers. As I left the house, I saw cars on the drive at 55 and a little girl peeping out of the window, so I turned back to deliver our neighbours' parcel. Despite the cold weather, David and Clare kept their door open and engaged in a friendly chat. This time, I made use of the opportunity to tell them about my cancer and chemotherapy. Psychologists by profession, they took the news in their stride, pointing out how common the diagnosis was, with people living longer. They mentioning close relatives who were currently receiving similar treatment. As neighbours, they could not have been more sympathetic and supportive.

When Mel returned from her walk, we took coffee, and then retired to the bedroom for her to administer the dreaded filgrastim jab. After the initial impact of the needle, the injection could scarcely be felt, so how to explain my continuing phobia?

Before supper, I took another anti-emetic lansoprazole capsule, augmented by a steady flow of Mel's home-made ginger tea, the combined effect appearing to reduce the symptoms of indigestion considerably. I slept much better than on previous nights, but still woke up at roughly one-and-a-half-hour intervals before dozing off again.

Day 6 (Monday 19th February)

My temperature remained steady at around 37.2^0c, my hair continued to thin, my dyspepsia began to ease, and I felt distinctly constipated, although I managed eventually to pass a very firm stool. In addition, I experienced intermittent pain in the back of my right hand, which I attributed to bruising caused by the insertion of the cannula, but the chemo injections had occurred six days ago! Once more, I was fearful of the 300mg filgrastim injection, which Mel administered relatively painlessly to my midriff around 12.30 pm.

Patrick Finucane, my school friend for fifty-five years, was due to arrive at the station at 1.15 pm. I was cheered by the prospect of his visit, and arrived in good time on the platform to meet him and drive him home. Having resolved to 'come out' with my cancer, I had planned to greet him with a hug and a hairless head, but the weather was cold and so I kept on my beanie until I got home. When I took it off there, he looked at me curiously for a minute or two, and then, over a cup of tea, asked a series of sensible questions about chemo, the administration and duration of the treatment and its side effects, while simultaneously displaying his deep concern. I was so pleased that he had come all the way from Kent to stay for a couple of days. I realised immediately that the most effective form of therapy was the easy camaraderie, informal exchange, and natural rapport between two old friends who already understood each other's strengths and weaknesses in their entirety.

Notwithstanding Patrick's visit, I became very fatigued during the day and felt sick before supper. Mel urged me to take a lanzoprasole capsule before a grand supper of smoked haddock, mashed potato and broccoli, and afterwards made me a cup of her ginger-root tea. The three of us adjourned to the living room, to talk animatedly for a while before watching television. I fell asleep in the middle of a programme and was guided upstairs by Mel, where I went out like a light until 2.30 am. After that, I slept more fitfully, waking up every hour or so to belch or go to the lavatory. My sleep pattern seemed to be returning to normal, which I attributed to the diminishing effect of the dexamethasone steroid taken last on day 4.

Day 7 (Tuesday 20th February)

I woke up around 7.30 am, conscious that the back of my right hand still hurt, and there was pain in the crook of my right arm. My bowels remained sluggish, but I was able to evacuate sufficiently, before taking Patrick out for a drive around midday. After Mel administered the 300mg filgrastim injection around 11.45 am, I was greatly relieved that I had completed the third cycle's three subcutaneous injections.

Patrick wanted us to visit a local reclamation yard in search of a couple of inscribed house bricks to take back to Kent for incorporation into a patio he was building. We eventually located two suitable specimens in Tipton and then drove back via Bilston, so that I could show him Bilston High Street – the Bilston sculpture park, and the early 19th-century cast-iron tomb stones in St Leonard's churchyard. He showed a great deal of interest. We returned home for lunch, with me feeling extremely tired.

Soon afterwards, I fell asleep on the sofa, while Mel took Pat out into the garden to show him our vegetable patch. When they came back in, Mel persuaded me to go to bed for a nap. I flaked out immediately and didn't wake up until 5.00 pm, whereupon she made me a mug of root-ginger tea. Before supper, the three of us planned a holiday in Ireland in September 2018 to coincide with the end of my treatment. I retired to bed at 10.30 pm, still feeling tired, and fell asleep immediately. It turned out to be the best night's sleep of the third cycle, which I attributed to the effect of the steroid tablets wearing off.

Day 8 (Wednesday 21st February)

While drinking our morning mug of tea, Mel confided in me the substance of her conversation with Patrick the night before. He had expressed great concern for my health and questioned her closely about my prognosis. She had reassured him that the various x-rays and scans had shown no sign of metastases and that, with chemotherapy, radiotherapy, and tamoxifen, there were excellent odds on my living for many more years and making a full recovery. In the knowledge that Mel made periodic excursions to London to see our grandchildren, Patrick had offered to come to Wolverhampton to keep me company whenever he could be of help. Both Mel and I were much touched by this gesture of friendship, the mention of which almost reduced me to tears.

Over breakfast, we continued to scope the Ireland adventure, stressing to Patrick that we would prefer to leave the planning to him because of his superior historical and geographical knowledge and his insight into our characters and preferences. Then, sorry that his visit had to come to an end, I drove Patrick to the station to catch the 10.45 am London train. After purchasing items for the house and garden, I made my way home, feeling fatigued and nauseous – just as I thought I was well on the mend. Mel made me root ginger tea, which relieved the sickness and, just after midday, I retired to bed for a short nap.

When I woke up, I became conscious once more of a dull pain and soreness in the back of my right hand and crook of my arm. It seemed more oppressive and painful than on previous occasions, which I attributed to my anti-climactic mood following Patrick's departure. We had a late lunch of tomato and basil soup, bread, cheese and Krakowska sausage, after which we watched *East Enders* and *Holby City* on Catch-up. Patrick emailed from Faversham. He had arrived home safely and wanted to thank us for our hospitality. He would look further at planning the Irish trip and be in touch in due course, adding "I was most impressed by Frank's cheerful fortitude in the face of enormous challenge." It wasn't as if I had a choice!

My principal memories of day 8 were of nausea and physical exhaustion by midday and the dull aching of my right arm. I was fully expecting to be on the road to recovery. I refused to admit that the excitement of Patrick's visit might be partly responsible for the fatigue. That night, I slept relatively well at first, but woke at around 3.30 am feeling indigested and nauseous, and swallowed a lansoprazole capsule in the hope of relief. My arm became increasingly stiff and painful.

Day 9 (Thursday 22nd February)

All day my temperature hovered between 37.5^0 and 37.9^0 c. I had an excellent evacuation of my bowels prior to taking a shower. I noticed spots on my groin which I treated at first with antiseptic Sudocrem and then with Fucibet cream.

The back of my right hand and the crook of my elbow were still painful, so much so that I was unable to straighten my arm. On closer examination, I thought my forearm looked swollen and slighter redder than the surrounding areas of skin.

After breakfast of cornmeal porridge and prunes, I did a little DIY, but soon became tired, and retired to bed after lunch for an afternoon nap. That evening, I drank at least two mugs of Mel's root-ginger tea to deal with the continuing belches and indigestion. At this stage in the cycle, the home remedy seemed to work as effectively as the lansoprazole capsules and the domperidone. We were in bed by 10.45 pm, and I slept well, despite my high temperature.

Day 10 (Friday 23rd February)

Onset of thrombo-phlebitis

Day 10 turned out to be more eventful than expected. The pain I was experiencing in the back and crook of my right arm was slowly getting worse. On examining the area, Mel detected a line of redness extending almost from my shoulder to my wrist. It was so tender in places, it hurt when touched, and I was quite unable to straighten my right arm in comparison with the left. Furthermore, the thermometer showed a 7.00 am reading of 37.9^0c.

Mel felt the telltale signs were sufficiently ominous to report them immediately to the hospital in accordance with the advice booklet issued by the New Cross Directorate of Oncology[2]. When I phoned up to describe my symptoms, I was given an emergency appointment at the hospital, where I was to be diagnosed with thrombo-phlebitis, the serious consequences of which are described in the next chapter.

Days 11 to 21 (Saturday 24th – Tuesday 6th March)

Following the diagnosis of thrombo-phlebitis, I was put on a regimen of antibiotics, hydrocortisone ointment and anti-coagulant injections, which came to define my experience of the third chemotherapy cycle.

In regard to my general health, my temperature hovered around 37.4^0c – considerably higher than at the same stage in the second cycle. I went on feeling mildly indigested and belching at night, but believed I gained some relief from drinking mugs of Mel's root-ginger tea. My bowels returned to normal but, as a precaution every morning, I took a couple of prunes with my porridge. My energy levels and get-up-and-go were not as they used to be and, more often than not, I ended up taking a short nap in the afternoon.

I continued to shed hair from my head, but retained a much shorter and sparser coif, beard and moustache. By the end of the cycle, my hair had reduced to a fine soft down, no longer able to conceal the gleam of the pale white skin of my skull. When I looked in the mirror, I was reminded of a large joint of pork, skin and bristle attached, being prepared for the oven. I no longer sought to disguise my baldness, either in the house or in public, but had to put on my beanie when I went out because of the prolonged spell of extremely cold weather.

Apart from the thrombo-phlebitis, which I feared might delay subsequent chemo cycles, I experienced a number of minor side effects: sore buttocks which made it painful to sit on hard surfaces, sores in my groin (which responded to Fucibet cream) and a succession of mouth ulcers (which I treated with the prescribed nystatin solution). I might have weathered the third chemotherapy cycle just as I had the first and second, had it not been for the thrombo-phlebitis – the damage to the veins in my right arm – which threatened to disrupt the administration of any further drugs - if they had to be fed in through the back of my hand.

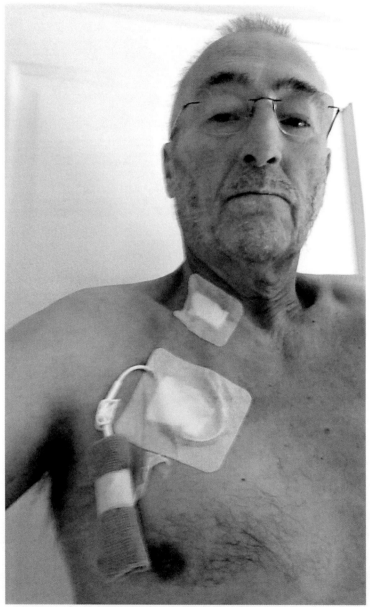

The Hickman line, 8th March 2018

Chapter 8

Thrombo-phlebitis and its consequences

On Friday 23rd February, day 10 of the third cycle, I woke with pains and skin rash running the length of my right arm, and with a raised temperature. I phoned at 8.30 am to make a same-day emergency appointment at the hospital's day-care Durnall Oncology Unit. We ate a hurried breakfast, de-iced the car windows, and drove to the hospital, arriving on the car park ten minutes before the appointment time at 10.00 am.

After a brief wait, I was weighed and measured and taken to a side ward, where a number of other elderly patients, most accompanied by a family member or friend, were already sitting patiently.

A nurse routinely prepared to take blood from my right arm, until Mel made clear to her that it was far too painful for that. Her attention then switched to the left arm which, following the lymph-node clearance, we had been told to avoid for that purpose. The nurse in charge, *Liza Warmington*, explained that blood samples would have to be taken and that, in this instance, she would be extracting fluid, not injecting it. She proceeded to draw from my left arm three samples for analysis to test, I believe, for FBC (full blood count), urea electrolytes and a platelet count. My blood pressure (132/82) and temperature (37.8^{0}c) were also taken and, shortly afterwards, because of my temperature, Mel and I were asked to wait by ourselves in a single treatment room.

At this point, *Nurse Warmington* told me to remove my beanie, as she thought it may have been responsible for raising my temperature taken from my ear. It had fallen slightly to 37.7^{0}c. I then asked the nurse to insert the thermometer into my right ear.

111

This time it showed up at 37.3^{0}c, a variation between ears of 0.4^{0}c. When taking my temperature at home, I had noticed for some time that my ear temperature on either side of my head could vary by as much as 1.1^{0}c.

At 11.30 am, we were visited by *Dr Yu Yan Qian*, a friendly and intelligent woman, who quickly contextualised the nature of my condition. On hearing that the worst pain was located in those places where the chemotherapy drugs had been injected, or the phlebotomist had taken blood, she suggested that the veins may have become inflamed as a consequence.

She ordered an ultrasound scan on my right arm and two further blood samples for culture in order to exclude or confirm infection but, at this stage, she did not think there was sepsis. Shortly afterwards, a haematology nurse took two further samples from my left arm, making a total of five in all. In the meantime, my blood pressure (132/60) and temperature (37.1^{0}c) declined towards normal.

The ultrasound scan was scheduled for 2.00 pm at the Imaging Department, towards which Mel and I duly made our way, stopping to buy sandwiches, crisps and Snicker bars to keep us going. After a 25-minute wait, I was led to a changing room to remove my upper garments, before being taken into a dimly-lit room to see the consultant sonographer, *Mr Anil Shergill*, a conscientious and courteous person, who took time to explain what he was doing and what he could see on the screen. The procedure lasted around 20 minutes. He reckoned my symptoms were consistent with a diagnosis of thrombo-phlebitis. By 3.30 pm, Mel and I were back in the same treatment room on Durnall, which we had been allocated that morning.

Half an hour later, we were surprised and delighted to see *Dr Tahir Raja* entering the room. He was the friendly oncology registrar, who had conducted my pre-assessment on the 12th February. He examined and marked out with a pen the painful and ruddy areas of my right arm, confirming that the phlebitis that was clearly visible on the surface of the skin was a side effect of the chemotherapy drugs.

He wrote a prescription for a course of flucloxacillin capsules, antibiotics to reduce the inflammation, and a tube of hydrocortisone cream to apply to the affected skin. He also made me an appointment for the following Tuesday (27th February) to review my progress.

We left Durnall at 3.45 pm and made our way to the hospital pharmacy to collect the prescription. We were told that the expected waiting time was 45 minutes (in reality, 50 minutes). We left the hospital at around 5.00 pm, and were about to drive off when my mobile phone rang. The screen showed 'no user ID', so I decided not to answer it, but it immediately rang again and, this time, I took the call. It was *Dr Tahir Raja*. Something had cropped up. Could I return to Durnall? We rushed back to meet him.

"Is it serious"?, I asked.

He took us to an interview room, and explained that *Dr Grigoryev* had been monitoring my record at a distance and had advised him to contact haematology. The outcome was that they wanted to put me on a course of anti-coagulant Inhixa enoxaparin sodium injections for at least two weeks. *Dr Raja* turned to Mel and asked her whether she would be able to give them to me subcutaneously on a daily basis in the same way as the earlier filgrastim injections.

A further appointment was made to review my condition after five days, when the prescribed medication would have had time to work. By 5.30 pm, we were back at the pharmacy.

The receptionist looked at the prescription and asked "What is the weight?"

Somewhat confused, I replied that the wait earlier that afternoon had been 50 minutes, and I hoped it would not be as long on this occasion.

Patiently, she explained that the doctor had not entered my weight on the prescription form, and that it was needed to calculate the appropriate dosage. Mel gave her the information immediately, as she had made a note of my weight on her phone when it was measured on the ward that morning.

This time, we waited for 18-minutes. When the prescription was at last prepared, the pharmacist explained that they had calculated from my weight that I needed 135 mg of the solution at each injection. Given the quantities of Inhixa enoxaparin available, this meant I would need each time to be given two injections, one of 100 mg and another of 40 mg. I winced at the prospect, but knew there was no alternative. We left the hospital at 6.00 pm and were home at 6.40 pm - an absence of nearly 9½ hours. I felt very tired.

We went to bed early, but not before I had taken two of the antibiotic capsules, my arm had been treated with hydrocortisone cream, and my belly jabbed with two syringes of enoxaparin solution.

Review of treatment for thrombo-phlebitis

On Tuesday 27th February (day 14), we woke to a very cold day and flurries of snow. I swept the snow off the car so that we could drive to the hospital. I was due to have a blood sample taken and checks at the Durnall Oncology Unit on the condition of the veins in my right arm. We arrived well before 10.00 am at the phlebotomy unit in the Outpatients Department (not the one in the Deanesly Suite, as before) and took the only available seats in the crowded waiting room, but not before a helpful woman nearby had advised us to take a numbered ticket from the dispensing machine.

As I waited there, it began to dawn on me that the hospital was extracting patients' blood on an industrial scale. Patients' numbers flashed up on an electronic board directing them to one of a number of booths, much like being directed to a cashier in a bank or supermarket. Despite the queue, my number came up in less than 5 minutes and I went to booth 3 where, after I told the phlebotomist about my thrombo-phlebitic condition, blood was drawn as before from my left arm. When I explained my appointment with the oncologist was for midday, she dispatched the sample immediately to the lab.

I asked her how many bloods she took on a shift: "150?"

"A lot more than that", she said, amiably.

I felt humbled to have met an individual whose working week consisted of drawing blood routinely and repetitively on a scarcely-imaginable scale, and yet who still took the trouble to respond so readily to me and my individual needs.

With two hours to wait until our next appointment, Mel and I walked to the coffee shop in the vicinity of the hospital's east entrance, hoping to while away the time in comfort over our cappuccinos. But it was a very cold day and we found ourselves sitting close to a window, chilled by the draught from the doors, every time people entered or left the hospital. We moved to a less draughty location nearer the centre of the site, but the heating of the hospital's public areas and corridors could barely cope with the cold weather outside.

At noon, we went to the Durnall Day Care Oncology Unit, and found the waiting room far warmer, but crowded. We stood until chairs became available, at which point a nurse called out my name and took me to be weighed and measured. We were led to a seating area on one of the side wards, where my temperature (36.7⁰c), blood pressure (132/89), and pulse were measured. The ward was busy with elderly patients like me, but many looking in need of far greater medical attention. Mel occupied herself with sudoku while I read the newspaper.

An hour and a half later at 2.00 pm, *Dr Maksym Maryniuk*, another oncology registrar, arrived, established my identity, and drew the privacy curtains around the seating area. He asked about the state of my arm and whether it was responding to the medication. I took off my shirt and he examined the swelling and discoloration of the arm. I told him that there had been an improvement: the veins were still sore but I could almost straighten my elbow. He advised me to continue the current treatment regime, and assured me that there were alternative ways of administering the fourth-cycle chemotherapy drugs if my arm did not recover in time.

We left the hospital by 2.30 pm and were home for 3.00 pm, when I felt in need of a nap. I continued the course of flucloxacillin antibiotic. Before I went to bed, Mel treated my arm with the hydrocortisone cream and injected me with the two syringes of enoxaparin sodium solution.

Review prior to the fourth cycle

On the morning of Monday 5th March (day 20 of the third cycle), we returned to the hospital in time for blood sample results to be ready for my scheduled appointment with *Dr Grigoryev* in the afternoon. An amiable phlebotomist at the Deanesly Centre, *Tina Rush*, saw me almost immediately, engaged me in effective distractive conversation, took my blood, and despatched the sample to the lab in time for my 2.00 pm appointment. The process took precisely 22 minutes from the time we arrived to the time we left the hospital.

Back at Deanesly in the afternoon, my name was called, and *Nurse Elspeth Hopkins* took us to a consultation room, where we met *Dr Hetu Charitha Gupta*, one of *Dr Grigoryev*'s registrars, whom we had first met in November. She inquired about my current state of health, particularly my phlebitic arm, and proceeded to inspect the phlebitis, the sores on my buttocks, and in my mouth. She listened carefully to everything I had to say, responding in a kindly and reassuring manner.

I asked how the fourth cycle drugs could be administered, given the phlebitic reaction during the third cycle. Painstakingly, she explained that there were other methods of introducing chemotherapy drugs, for example, through a PICC line (a peripherally-inserted central catheter) set in the arm, or a central or

Hickman line (a CVC, or central venous catheter) positioned to the right of my chest.

Before proceeding along this route, however, she thought it best to seek the opinion of the nursing team on the Snowdrop Suite, who injected the chemotherapy drugs on a daily basis. In the meantime, she wrote out a prescription for co-amoxiclav, another antibiotic, and enoxaparin, an anti-coagulant (administered in the form of an injection) to deal with the phlebitis, together with Difflam oral rinse and nystatin for my sore mouth. She recommended E45 body lotion to treat the rough cracked skin of my fingers.

Nurse Elspeth Hopkins, the nurse in attendance, then took me and Mel to the Snowdrop Suite, where we were asked to wait while she explained the issue of my phlebitic arm to staff at reception, before making her way back to *Dr Gupta*'s room. After a five-minute wait, a nurse holding a tourniquet strap came into the packed waiting room and called out my name. When I stood up, she walked over and, in a loud voice, asked me to explain my recent medical history, and to show her my arm.

Acutely conscious that other waiting patients were watching and that I had become the centre of attention, I took off my jacket and pullover and rolled up my sleeve to point out the red marks on my arm. I mentioned the pain that I was still having. She remarked that the arm could not be used, walked away, and then returned to ask the name of the doctor who had sent me, and for the form recording the date of my next appointment. I put back my clothes.

Mel responded angrily to the incident, seeing it as an infringement of a patient's right to privacy and to be treated with dignity, whereas I felt too anxious and too much of a victim to care. As we left the waiting room, Mel noticed an empty bay where we could have been taken aside, but pointed out to me that, even in a crowded waiting room, it was possible to huddle in a corner and talk quietly. When we returned to the consultation room, Mel made her annoyance clear to *Dr Gupta*, who promised to relay our concerns.

The upshot was that *Dr Gupta*, after consulting with *Dr Grigoryev*, decided to postpone my fourth cycle of chemo due on the 7th March, and book an appointment on the 8th for the insertion of a central line into my chest. This would allow the next three cycles of chemotherapy to be delivered more safely, although there was still a risk of infection and thrombosis.. Without more ado, and keen to keep the chemo on course, I immediately signed the consent form. Nevertheless, the delay caused by the additional procedure disrupted the regular end-on 21-day cycles, the fourth of which had now to be rescheduled. Initially, the only date on offer on Snowdrop was in a fortnight, unless we were prepared to travel to the NHS Trust's Cannock site, a proposal to which Mel strongly objected.

Dr Gupta and *Dr Grigoryev*, however, were keen to minimise the interval between cycles. The following morning, *Dr Grigoryev*'s secretary, phoned me at home, to give me the date of Wednesday 14th March at the Snowdrop Suite for my next chemotherapy, a gap of only one week.

Before leaving Deanesly, I was directed once more to the phlebotomist for a further blood sample to be taken in preparation for the line insertion on the 8th. The morning's dressing was pulled off, the blood sample taken and another plaster stuck on in the same place. Thereafter, we took the prescription to the pharmacy, where we waited around 45 minutes for my medicines to be dispensed. When I was called to collect the drugs, the pharmacist explained that the amount of the enoxaparin in one of the syringes was more than I should have, and some of the fluid would need to be squirted out prior to injection. Mel said that, for safety, she would prefer the syringes to contain the correct quantity for each occasion. The quantity was rectified and we received the drugs as prescribed.

Later that afternoon, when we got home, we received a call from *Mary McGrath*, manager of oncology, to ask whether we wished to lodge a formal complaint about the incident that had occurred in the waiting room at the Snowdrop Suite earlier that day. We told her that all we wanted was her best effort to ensure that an incident of that kind did not happen again on Snowdrop.

That evening, I started the new course of antibiotics, used the oral rinse, and resolved to continue the enoxaparin injections for the duration of my chemotherapy (that would be two syringes every evening for a further 65 days. Ugh!).

Insertion of a central line

Thursday 8th March was the day scheduled for the insertion of a central line (or central venous catheter) into the large vein in the right side of my chest to allow me to continue to receive chemotherapy drugs without further risk of phlebitis. We set the alarm for 5.30 am to reach New Cross Hospital Appleby Suite for day surgery by 7.00 am. By 8.00 am, Mel had said goodbye and I was seated in one of the bays set aside for male patients.

Staff Nurse Jean Wilson conducted the routine admission procedure, fixing an identity and tracking device onto my wrist and asking the standard set of questions (eg. Was I a diabetic? Did I suffer from epilepsy?), before checking that I knew the reasons for my admission. She was warm and friendly in manner and I opened my heart to her, whereupon she gave me a bear hug and told me that everything they were doing that day was only intended to make me better. She instructed me to get undressed, but retain my underwear, and put on a surgical gown and stockings, in preparation for the operation.

Around 9.30 am, I was visited by *Dr Guthrie Samuel*, a most friendly and sociable person, who was keen to learn the background to my case and to explain the surgical procedure she was about to undertake, which she referred to as placing a 'Hickman line'. (A Hickman line is a long plastic tube (of varying diameter), called a catheter, inserted under the chest wall into a large vein draining into the heart, and which could be left in place for the duration of my remaining chemotherapy cycles. It was named after Dr Robert Hickman, a paediatrician at Seattle Children's Hospital who, in 1979, modified the venous catheter for children, with the aim of reducing infection.)

Dr Samuel explained that she would numb a part of my chest with a local anaesthetic and then make a short incision (known as the entry site) through which she would insert one end of a plastic tube into my vein while, at the same time, threading the other end of the tube under my skin to another small incision at a lower point, known as the exit site. Both sites would then be sutured, but the tube or catheter would be left hanging from the exit site and bound to the chest with a dressing. I might feel a little discomfort at times but during the procedure, and afterwards, I was likely to find it relatively painless.

At around 10.00 am, a nurse asked me to walk across the corridor to an operating theatre where my identity was checked once more, before I was asked to lie on a padded couch, or operating table. *Dr Samuel* was assisted by five or six theatre staff dressed in theatre gowns, only distinguishable by their cheekbones and eyes She began to scan my chest, showing me the images on the screen of the ultra-sound scanner in front of her. A blue fabric was placed over my head, shielding me from any further sight of the procedure.

Dr Samuel and the theatre nurses engaged deliberately in distractive conversation about anything they thought might engage my attention – from my address in Tettenhall, to my previous occupations. It was at this point that I learned that *Dr Samuel* had once lived in Madras – Tamil Nadu, Southern India – but had originated on the southern seaboard of the sub-continent. I guessed that the needle pricks I felt were for the local anaesthetic that I had been told to expect, and the occasional jolting indicated the insertion of the line.

While the operation itself was relatively painless, I grew increasingly agitated as the procedure continued. I had no way of telling its duration. It must have lasted at least ten minutes, or perhaps even twenty-five minutes. I was shaking and my heart was pounding as it came to an end. When I was told that it was over and the cloth shield was removed from my head, I felt light-headed and giddy when dismounting from the couch, even with the help of a nurse. I was pleased that the Hickman line had been inserted and thanked *Dr Samuel* and the nursing team for their work. Aware of the common after-effects of surgical procedures, the nurse insisted I sit in a wheel chair, before pushing me back to the ward.

Here, I was cared for attentively by staff nurses, *Jean Wilson* and *Christine Bowker*, and student nurse, *Michelle Brock*, who offered me tea and biscuits and much friendly conversation. I was told to call my wife, Mel, and ask her to come and collect me at 11.15 am. Meanwhile, I was briefed on the care of my Hickman line and on what to do if it became displaced, damaged, cut, or dislodged, accidentally. It had to be cleaned on a weekly basis, with new dressings applied. When Mel arrived, *Nurse Christine Bowker* took us to a side room where she explained to us the use of an emergency kit (in case the tube became damaged) and the importance of keeping the Hickman line sterile and dry at all times, and 'flushed' on a regular basis.

Following my discharge, I remember feeling light-headed as we made our way to the car. Mel took me straight home where she inspected my newly-inserted Hickman line and the dressings around it. A bundle of tubing, sheathed in blue gauze, dangled from my chest like an array of military medals. After taking paracetamol for the dull pain in my neck, I went to bed and fell asleep. An hour later, Mel brought me a cup of ginger tea. Feeling hungry, I went downstairs for a light lunch of soup and bread. Then, taking another paracetamol, I went back to bed for most of the afternoon. I felt more uncomfortable, despondent and exhausted on this occasion, than I had since my chemotherapy began.

Aware of my despondency, Mel prepared a tasty meal especially to cheer me up. We relaxed watching television in the living room, retiring to bed after the ten o'clock news. Before we went to sleep, Mel anointed my phlebitic arm and sore buttocks, and injected my midriff with two syringes of enoxaparin anti-coagulant solution.

First line care on Durnall Day Care Unit

The next day, Friday 9th March, we returned to the Durnall Day Care Unit to have the Hickman line flushed and cleaned for the first time. I was apprehensive, as I did not know what to expect. On arrival, the waiting room was crowded with patients spilling into the corridor. The receptionist explained apologetically that there was a two-hour delay due to staff shortages, and suggested we went and had lunch and came back later.

We walked to Deanesly to rearrange some of my appointment times, now rendered obsolete by the rescheduled fourth cycle and, after whiling away an hour over lunch and tea, we returned to wait our turn at Durnall. Matters had improved dramatically and my name had already been called.

Soon after, we were led to a room, where *Staff Nurse Liza Warmington*, whom we had met before, took off the dressings surrounding my Hickman line and began to clean the blood off my chest with surgical wipes. Then, using the line, she drew off blood, which she disposed of, and then flushed the tube, first with saline and then with heparin.

"The Hickman line was the best thing you could have had done in the circumstances," she said, "From now on, you won't feel a thing". It was true. I had not realised that she had drawn off blood, nor experienced any sensation, as the saline and then the heparin were injected.

Whereas the use of the line was pain free, the spot where the line had been inserted continued to smart, especially when I coughed or stretched, and so, for the rest of the day, I went on taking paracetamol as a precaution. Nevertheless, *Nurse Warmington* afforded me much-needed relief when she expertly re-taped the line to my chest, dressing it in such a way that it no longer dangled or swayed. Before we left the hospital, she confirmed a further appointment at Durnall on Monday the 12th March, for line care and bloods in preparation for the fourth cycle of chemotherapy.

It was Friday afternoon but, fortuitously, the weekend afforded the perfect occasion for post-operative distractive therapy. Toussaint, our daughter, Luc, our son-in-law, together with baby Caio, and Robeson, our son, Tasha, our daughter-in-law, and grandchildren, Maxi and Genevieve, arrived that night to stay for the weekend and celebrate Mel's birthday, which happened to coincide with Mothers' Day. Both Mel and I were elated, as well as fully occupied, by their visit, which was further augmented by Spartaca, our daughter, and Patrick, our son-in-law's Sunday Facetime call from Kenya. It left me with no time to worry about the lingering phlebitis, the discomfort of the Hickman line, the nightly enoxaparin injections, or the sores on my buttocks. Only on Monday morning, as we prepared to leave for the hospital, did the mundane reality catch up with me.

Second line care on Durnall Day Care Unit

On the 12th March, Mel and I arrived at the hospital at 12.55 pm in good time for my 1.10 pm appointment at the Durnall Day Care Unit. Although the waiting room seemed crammed, we managed to find seats next to one another, but then had to wait until 2.15 pm – over an hour – before my name was called.

Nurse Rosie Puttock, whom we had not met before, led us to a side ward, where I was directed to a comfortable chair. Mel sat on the more upright seat next to me. I took off my cardigan, shirt and tie to expose the Hickman line on the right of my chest. Watched attentively by a student nurse, Nurse *Puttock* peeled off the surgical dressings from the entry and exit wounds and began cleaning around the line with what she referred to as "lollipops" – large swabs mounted on the end of plastic rods which the student nurse prepared for her by taking them from their sterile wrapping. Once the line and my chest had been wiped clean, *Rosie* drew off blood to be disposed of, blood samples for analysis, and flushed the line with syringes of saline and heparin. The line was then re-taped onto my chest in readiness for the fourth cycle of chemotherapy scheduled for Wednesday 14th March.

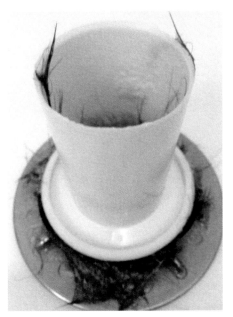

Inverted shower sump showing lost hairs
from Frank's head and body

Chapter 9

Fourth chemotherapy cycle with T

Preparation for the fourth cycle

On Monday night (12th March) before the Wednesday on which my fourth chemotherapy cycle was due to begin, I noticed redness and soreness on the joint of left big toe, and immediately diagnosed gout, which I had suffered from once before nearly ten years ago. To confirm, I waited till Tuesday morning before searching out the supply of 500mg colchicine pills and allopurinol tablets, which my doctor had prescribed in case of another attack of gout. This instance of gout, at least, could not be attributed to an excess of rich food or over-indulgence of alcohol for, in regard to the latter, I had now been teetotal for at least six months. As to my other complaints, the sores on my buttocks were still present and painful.

On Tuesday (13th March), I remembered to take four soluble 2mg dexamethosone tablets in the morning, and the same dose again in the afternoon, in preparation for the fourth cycle of chemotherapy, which would consist of docetaxel (Taxotere, the T drug).

Day 1 (Wednesday 14th March 2018)

The preparation continued with my taking four more 2mg dexamethasone tablets at 9.00 am on Wednesday (14th March), prior to my appointment at 2.00 pm at the Snowdrop Millennium Suite.

The death of Stephen Hawking

We had been woken with the announcement on BBC Radio 4 news that Stephen Hawking, the world-renowned physicist, had died early that morning at the age of 76. With my interest in cosmology, I had read his popular book, *The Brief History of Time*, in the late 1980s, and knew of his efforts to combine the general theory of relativity with quantum mechanics. I was also aware that, in the light of new evidence, he had revised his opinions that black holes sucked in and destroyed all information, and that the Higgs-boson would never be discovered. But what impressed me more than his ability as a scientist was his stubborn refusal at the age of 21 to accept that, following his diagnosis with motor neurone disease, he would be dead by the age of 23. Instead, he had persisted in living another 55 years, making use of new electronic gadgetry to engage in and contribute fully to theoretical physics. And here I was, at the age of 73, fretting about the administration and side effects of a fourth cycle of chemotherapy aimed at prolonging an already long life of normality!

Fourth session of chemotherapy at the Snowdrop Millennium Suite

Arriving at the hospital on time, we sat in the waiting room on Snowdrop for 25 minutes. *Senior Nurse Mary McGrath*, the manager of the oncology unit, greeted us in a friendly manner, before introducing us to *Sister Cassia Mainwaring*, who was to be in charge of my treatment that afternoon. After I had been weighed and measured, *Sister Mainwaring* took us to a curtained unit on the u-shaped ward, as before, and went through the usual checklist of questions. She was friendly, responsive, well-informed, and organised, with a business-like manner. We soon established that she carried considerable responsibility, being sister in charge of the chemotherapy unit of the Royal Wolverhampton Hospital Trust's hospital at Cannock, as well as working at the Snowdrop Suite.

Once I had unbuttoned my shirt, *Sister Mainwaring* removed the dressings on my chest surrounding the Hickman line and flushed the catheter by extracting blood and then injecting a small amount of saline and heparin. She then attached a tube from the drip-stand to feed in saline, steroid, and my first dose of docetaxel – the T drug, named after its trade name, Taxotere.

As this was the first time I had been given docetaxel, *Sister Mainwaring* also set up an electronic sphygmomanometer to monitor my blood pressure for any variation during the infusion, but it remained fairly constant over the hour at around 121/75. This time, I read and finished my book without interruption, which proved the effectiveness of the Hickman line and lightened my mood immensely.

Docetaxel has acquired a fearsome reputation for unpleasant side effects. During the administration of the drug itself, patients are told to report allergic responses, such as feelings of pyrexia, dizziness, breathlessness, itchiness, headaches, shivering, pains in the chest, and swelling of the face or lips. *Sister Mainwaring* warned me in advance of some of these symptoms and kept a watchful eye on me as the drug was fed in through the Hickman line.

In addition to the commonly-mentioned after-effects of chemotherapy drugs generally (nausea, vomiting, diarrhoea, constipation and fatigue), docetaxel is especially linked to the development of severe joint pains and to numbness and tingling of the fingers and toes – referred to as peripheral neuropathy – which may make it difficult for a time to tie laces, fasten buttons, or perform other delicate manual tasks[1]. More worryingly, Macmillan Cancer Support information on chemotherapy says that symptoms such as these 'usually improve slowly after treatment finishes, but in some people they may never go away'[1]. Broadcaster, Victoria Derbyshire, described how on day 5 of her fourth cycle after docetaxel: "I can barely move, am totally wiped out and find it difficult to get out of bed even to go to the loo because of agonising pains in my stomach and lower back"[2]. On day 7 she still felt poorly: "My throat is swollen, it hurts to swallow. I can't lie on either side in bed, because it's so painful"[3].

Around 4.00 pm, I took the prescribed four 2mg soluble dexamethasone tablets which, together with a bottle of water, Mel had thought to pack in her bag for the hospital.

A friendly nurse passing my chair remarked on the advantages of my Hickman line.

"All patients on the FEC-T course should have them," she said. "It prevents the veins getting damaged and makes it easier to take blood."

"If the benefits are so great," I asked her, "why isn't it routinely done?"

"All those minor ops would be judged too expensive," she replied. "Besides the phlebotomists aren't trained like us on oncology to deal with PICCs or CVCs".

"Do many of the patients on Snowdrop develop phlebitis?" I queried.

"The chemo drugs, especially the epirubicin, can easily damage the veins," she said. "It happens too often."

Mindful of my recent painful experience, I was thankful that I had submitted to the insertion of a Hickman line. Indeed, when the buzzer went off on the drip-stand monitor, I realised that I had experienced no pain, nor any allergic response to the drug and, for once, was feeling more normal than on the three previous occasions on Snowdrop.

After approximately half an hour, we were free to go, but not before *Sister Mainwaring* had reattached my Hickman line in a tidy fashion to my chest, explained and dispensed my medication for the fourth cycle, and given me appointment dates for the fifth and sixth sessions. Just after 5.00 pm, on the way back to the car, I felt frailer, weaker, and more out of breath than I had expected, and was glad for Mel to drive me home.

Mel and Toussaint, my daughter, cooked me an appetising meal of pork steak, broccoli and potatoes, which I was able to eat without nausea or indigestion, having prepared myself before hand with a 30mg lansoprazole gastro-resistant capsule.

At bedtime, Mel administered the two syringes (140mg in all) of the enoxaparin anti-coagulant to my midriff. At the same time, I took a 500mg paracetamol tablet to relieve the niggling soreness of my chest (the site of my Hickman line), my buttocks, and my midriff (where I had just been injected). I fell asleep almost immediately, but woke up at 3.00 am, tossed until 4.00 am, before getting up to make tea. I slept fitfully then until roused by the radio alarm. I blamed my early morning restlessness on the soluble steroids.

Day 2 (Thursday 15th March)

The course of dexamethasone steroid must also have energised me on day 2. I took four of the 2mg tablets in the morning and four in the afternoon. Although forced to reduce my normal routine to a snail's pace, and feeling light headed and faint, I pottered around the house, read the newspapers, and watched television, until retiring to bed at 11.00 pm. I continued to treat my sore buttocks with Fucibet cream, which, while relieving the discomfort, had so far had no discernible healing effect. In the evening, Mel injected the two syringes of enoxaparin solution. Thereafter, I slept soundly to 3.30 am, but got up to make tea for us both at 4.00 am. Throughout the day and for most of the night, I suffered from indigestion, having to sit up regularly to give vent to prolonged bouts of burping and belching. I imagined that the symptoms were worse than in previous cycles, because no aprepitant had been prescribed, but my diary proved otherwise.

Day 3 (Friday 16th March)

I woke up on day 3 feeling relatively pain free and optimistic, and relieved that, so far at least, I had experienced none of the possible unpleasant side effects of the docetaxel. That was not to say that I felt comfortable. My burping and belching continued and I had not slept well. Nevertheless, my temperature remained at between 37.1^0c and 37.2^0c, I emptied my bowels without difficulty, and ate breakfast, lunch and supper quite normally.

I spent the morning packaging and addressing books to send out to family and friends, and then drove to the post office at Tettenhall Green to post them. After successfully completing that task, I decided to drive to the shops in town. As I got out of the car and made my way into a store, I suddenly felt faint and weak. To stop myself keeling over, I was forced to sink to my knees and put my head on my lap. Other customers must have thought I was praying, for nobody seemed to notice. After a couple of minutes, I was able to rise to my feet and, slowly and warily, proceed with my shopping, much relieved when I returned to the car. I drove straight home and lay down for an hour.

Self-diagnosed gout

Around 5.00 pm, while drinking a cup of Mel's real ginger tea, I began to feel pain in my large toe joint, and took off my sock to examine the spot. It was indeed sore and red and, when I exerted pressure, the skin went white. I immediately suspected gout and took the precaution of swallowing a 500mg colchicine pill, followed thereafter, by a regular dose of allopurinol. At the same time, I googled 'Can chemotherapy cause gout?', the search leading me onto the Chemocare site. As I suspected, high uric acid levels (hyperuricemia) could indeed be brought about by chemotherapy agents causing abnormally high rates of cell death, and could, like gout, be treated with allopurinol.

Unlike in previous cycles, no capsules or tablets had been specifically prescribed for day 3, although I still had to look forward to the filgrastim 300mg injection to boost the white cell blood count, and the two syringes of enoxparin anti-coagulant. By bedtime, I felt very tired and slept well by current standards.

Day 4 (Saturday 17th March)

Woken by the radio alarm, I went to make tea, but felt stiff in my knee joints and faint and light-headed as I descended the stairs. Mel made an 8.00 am breakfast of cornmeal porridge, which I garnished with four prunes and a date in an effort to avoid constipation. Shortly afterwards, I realised that the recent excessive consumption of prunes, vegetables and fruit had eased my bowels to such an extent that my movements were now very loose.

The weather was windy and cold, with flurries of snow. We went up to shower, but ended up going back to bed and sleeping until 11.30 am, the first morning lie-in I had taken for many years – which I attributed to fatigue caused by the chemotherapy – although that did not explain Mel's extended slumber.

I took an allopurinol tablet as a precaution against gout and drank real ginger tea to deal with my dyspepsia. Mel injected me as before with filgrastim and enoxparin.

Cramp attack on evening of the fourth day

Just as I thought I had weathered the worst of the docetaxel side-effects, at 9.00 pm on the fourth day of the fourth cycle, I started to experience excruciating cramps in my calf muscles and abdomen, and spasms of pain across my chest and along my arms and legs. I tried to alleviate the aches by walking up and down, only to realise that the soles and heels of my feet were tender, too.

Mel gave me paracetamol and got me into bed, but the pain was persistent, and it took me some time to fall asleep. Every time I woke up, I could still feel the aches, and found myself trotting in pain to the lavatory. The clock seemed to dawdle and stop, and time to crawl backwards. I imagined the digital display to read 5.00 am but, on checking it said 3.00 am. When morning arrived, I lay there exhausted, still suffering from the cramps and the pangs.

Day 5 (Sunday 18ᵗʰ March)

It had snowed heavily during the night. Not surprisingly, I felt incapable of fetching the Sunday papers, and chose to spend the morning in bed, aided and abetted by Mel, who brought my porridge to me on a tray. To prevent any recurrence of the symptoms of gout, I went on taking the allopurinol. I remember the day for feeling unwell from exhaustion and cramps and, not least, from persistent heart burn, indigestion, and belching, which made me reluctant to eat.

Most of the afternoon and evening was spent spread out in front of the television in an attempt to escape from my bodily discomforts. When we went to bed, Mel gave me my three evening injections, and paracetamol for my various pains. It must have helped me to sleep, for I had a relatively good night's rest. The next morning, as I made my way to the lavatory, I recalled the pains that I had felt during the night in my legs and feet.

Day 6 (Monday 19th March)

I woke up around 7.30 am, still feeling fragile, but in less pain from cramps and dyspepsia. Mel brought me a glass of water and milk with which I swallowed the paracetamol and allopurinol tablets. She then made me breakfast of cornmeal porridge with dates, which I credited with helping to settle my stomach. I determined to wash and get dressed and return to some semblance of daily routine.

But while my mindset had undoubtedly improved for the better, my list of petty afflictions grew longer and longer. I still had the sores on my buttocks, feelings of nausea and indigestion, mouth ulcers, a hint of impending gout, a diminution of normal energy levels, and an irresistible fatigue.

Day 7 (Tuesday 20th March)

I woke on day 7 feeling rested and full of the best intentions. Philip came round in the morning and we began to work on preparing *Eastern Caribbean*, the fifth book in the Blue Bayou Series. His companionship and our purposeful activity cheered me up and diverted my attention away from my various bodily complaints.

When he left around lunch time, I felt a sharp pain in my belly and an urgent need to evacuate my bowels. That afternoon my motions became too loose and frequent for comfort, and I realised I had developed diarrhoea. As I sat on the lavatory bowl, I experienced a sharp debilitating muscular pain along my back, concentrated in my lumbar region. I felt nauseous and had difficulty in consuming a little meal of bread and soup. The combination of back and joint pain, stomach ache, dyspepsia and fatigue persuaded me to take to my bed, where I lay dormant and suffering until 4.30 pm.

The Trustee Board of Wolverhampton Citizen's Advice, which I had attended quite effortlessly during the second cycle, was scheduled to meet at 5.00 pm on the 20th March. I had already arranged for a fellow board member to drive me there. But I was quite unable to face the prospect and knew I was too ill to make a useful contribution. Reluctantly, I declined the lift and asked my friend to offer my apologies. I had not been expecting to cancel.

The extreme discomfort subsided and I spent the rest of the evening in the kitchen watching *East Enders*, or in the living room reading the newspapers. Mel and I discussed my recent complaints and concluded that they were the side-effects of the T, docetaxel, different from the previous cycles of FEC, and living up to its formidable reputation. The good news was that I had completed my five injections of filgrastim (for boosting my white blood count) and had only to contend with the two evening syringes of enoxaparin solution.

Day 8 (Wednesday 21st March)

Third line care at Durnall

My petty complaints persisted on day 8: sore buttocks, mouth ulcers, bleeding gums, indigestion, no sense of taste, unpredictable bouts of sneezing, the hint of an onset of gout, aches in my belly, and diarrhoea, of which diarrhoea came to the fore as the most pressing, as we had to attend a 9.50 am appointment at the hospital's Durnall Unit for line care and blood samples.

We drove through the ,morning traffic, anxious to arrive on time, arriving at 9.40 am on the hospital car park and at 9.50 am at Durnall. We then sat in the waiting room until 10.55 am, before my name was eventually called.

Encounter with *Dr Gill*

As Mel worked her way through her sudoku puzzles, somebody whispered her name, and she turned to recognise *Dr Chetpal Gill*, a GP at the Bradley Medical Centre, with whom we shared mutual friends. Accompanied by his wife, *Dr Gill* was also a patient on Durnall and had been suffering from cancer. The four of us fell into animated conversation, catching up on news from Bradley and sharing our recent medical histories. In common with me, *Chetpal* was experiencing chemotherapy-induced alopecia. We laughed at the hair strands still struggling to cling to our pates. More extraordinarily, *Chetpal* was a victim of breast cancer, too. Knowing that the incidence of male breast cancer was so rare, we marvelled at the odds of old friends meeting like this in the waiting room.– and that we were men who knew one another.

Eventually, I was taken to a chair space on a side ward, where Mel clarified with the nurse the routine purpose of our visit. It was to flush my Hickman line and take a blood sample. *Nurse Samantha Coburn*, who had worked in oncology for fifteen years, proceeded to remove the dressings from my chest. One of the plasters must have become attached to the line, for when she pulled at it, it tugged on the plastic tubing, causing me a moment of intense pain.

After flushing and sampling blood, she cleaned the spot with wipes and 'lollipops', and took out the sutures from either side of the entry wound, (but left in place the exit wound sutures for removal on a later occasion). She reattached the Hickman line to my chest and re-plastered the entry and exit wounds. In response to her questions about my health and the side effects of the chemotherapy, I listed a number of complaints, and she arranged for me to see one of the doctors before we left.

Meeting with *Dr Maksym Maryniuk*, registrar oncologist

Around 2.00 pm, *Dr Maksym Maryniuk* paid us a visit. I told him about the enduring nature of the sores on my buttocks, my severe indigestion and the signs of gout. He listened carefully, particularly to my confession of self-medicating my gout with colchicine and allopurinol. He suggested that, as the medicines had been prescribed originally by my GP, I should go back to the surgery to seek advice. In regard to my symptoms of indigestion, he wrote out a prescription for a week's supply of omeprazole 20mg gastro-resistant capsules (similar in effect to the gastro-resistant lansoprazole, but yellow in colour). On examining my buttocks, he remarked that the sores were relatively minor and contained.

He believed that I was coping well with the chemotherapy, compared with other patients undergoing the same treatment. He could try other remedies, but they might prove ineffective in the face of the two docetaxel cycles to follow. I was left with the impression that the chemotherapy singled out patients' historical weaknesses , tissue that had been previously damaged, and other predispositions to illness, and exacerbated them, and that, at 73 years of age, I was judged to be coping comparatively well.

We handed in the prescription for omeprasole at the pharmacy and sat for a further 45 minutes listening for my name to be called. Uppermost in my mind was the time we had spent at the hospital – around five hours – most of it waiting for hospital services beyond our control, but still to be paid for in car parking charges and in the tedium of wasted time.

That very same night I read in the local newspaper, *Express & Star*, that a new £3.5 million multi-storey car park was to be built at New Cross Hospital to provide for increasing visitor numbers, a project serving, no doubt to justify the exorbitant parking costs.

When we got home, I took the first of the omeprazole capsules and, feeling utterly exhausted, went to bed for an hour. That night, after the injections of enoxaparin, I slept soundly until woken at 3.00 am by severe stomach cramps and diarrhoea.

Day 9 (Thursday 22nd March)

The diarrhoea continued on day 9, with a liquid evacuation at 6.30 am and three more throughout the morning, but they failed to alleviate the stomach ache. In addition to most of the other complaints mentioned on day 8, I experienced a violent bout of sneezing when I woke up, followed by a persistent dripping nose, which I attributed to a loss of nasal hair. My eyelids felt sore, while eyelashes on my pillow convinced me that they, too, were falling out.

For lunch, I opened a can of Heinz's Cream of Tomato soup which I served with cheese biscuits and a slice of bread. I was expecting the soup to be mild and bland, but it tasted acidic and sour and so, after a couple of spoonfuls, I left it uneaten. I realised my taste buds were no longer working. Nothing tasted right.

I came to the conclusion that I was not very well and, after updating my diary, retired for an afternoon nap. Still feeling indigested and nauseous, I took an omeprazole capsule when I woke up, but at supper time, I was off my food and only ate a little of the chicken, potato and carrot meal that Mel had prepared for me. As usual, the meal looked appetising but, to me, it did not taste pleasant. Distinctly off-colour, with a dull ache in my gut, I sat slumped on the sofa in front of the television for the rest of the evening, before creeping upstairs at 10.45 pm in time for my enoxaparin injections. I took paracetamol for the stomach ache and any other odd pain, and soon fell asleep, only to be woken at 3.00 am by cramps in my abdomen, followed by a bout of explosive diarrhoea. Thereafter, I slept until 6.30 am, when I hurried to the lavatory once more for another malodorous discharge of faeces.

Day 10 (Friday 23rd March)

Day 10 was characterised by further stomach cramps, loose and gaseous faeces, continuing nausea and indigestion, and fatigue. Feeling confined and constrained by my condition, I defiantly ventured out around lunch time to go shopping, but, in recognition of my discomfort and unsteadiness, I soon returned home.

Feeling too sick to eat lunch, I went to lie down at around 2.00 pm and did not wake up until 5.30 pm, when I took a domperidone tablet to settle my stomach, but to little avail. At 6.30 pm, I had a further sudden bowel evacuation. Attempting to settle my stomach with a cup of Mel's real ginger tea, I managed to sip a small portion of home-made chicken soup for supper, but the little that I swallowed was tasteless. The stomach cramp, nausea and indigestion persisted.

At bedtime, I was injected again with the syringes of enoxaparin, took paracetamol, and then slept from 11.00 pm, waking up only occasionally to belch and urinate.

Days 11 to-21 (Saturday 24ᵗʰ March – Tuesday 3ʳᵈ April)

Waking on day 11, Saturday 24ᵗʰ March, I still felt physically weak, but far more optimistic, mentally alert, and intellectually active than on previous days. After a prolonged bout of audible peristalsis, I passed a reasonably glutinous stool, and the stomach cramp began to fade but, though much relieved, I was left with a premonition of constipation.

The feelings of nausea and indigestion began to subside and I was able to eat a bowl of cornmeal porridge (while foregoing the prunes). According to Mel, the sores on my buttocks were gradually healing, a result she attributed to her application of Sudocrem. To perk me up and for a change of scenery, Mel drove me in the morning to Dunhelm in Walsall to collect curtain cloth, to Lidl for groceries and, in the afternoon, to the Wyevale Garden Centre for plant supports. My life after the first cycle of docetaxel was improving, although I was still aware of my reduced energy level and tiredness. Nevertheless, we resumed our normal Saturday routines, retiring to bed around 11.00 pm, whereupon Mel gave me my injections, before we both fell asleep.

We slept soundly until woken on Sunday morning, the 25ᵗʰ March, by the radio alarm, the clocks having been brought forward an hour to British Summer Time. I had no problem eating a large bowl of cornmeal porridge, before venturing out on a bright spring morning for the Sunday newspapers – so different from the illness and heavy snow fall a week ago that had kept me indoors.

George Alagiah

Poor George Alagiah! *The Sunday Times* (25ᵗʰ March 2018) carried an article on the veteran television presenter's diagnosis with stage 4 bowel cancer in 2014 and his subsequent struggle with the disease ever since. He had undergone seventeen rounds of chemotherapy and five operations, but the cancer had now spread to his liver and lymph nodes. If he had lived in Scotland, he would have been screened for bowel cancer at the age of 50, rather than at 60, as in England. (The chance of surviving stage 1 bowel cancer for at least five years is nearly 100 per cent.) Understandably, he was supporting Bowel Cancer UK's campaign to make bowel cancer screening available at 50 to everyone in England.[4] As well as sympathising deeply with George Alagiah, I supported his argument that effective mass tests were needed for a wide range of cancers and that they should be deployed to detect cancer at its earliest stages.

Men were not routinely tested for breast cancer, either. The consequence was that diagnosis was later for males, with more than 40 per cent of men detected at Stage III or IV of the disease, a much later diagnosis, resulting in lower survival rates.[5]

I sat reading the Sunday papers in the conservatory, my grateful body soaking up the sunshine. The weather was improving, the daffodils were in flower, and the worst of the side effects – at least for the fourth cycle – seemed to have passed.

Review prior to the fifth cycle

On Monday 26th March (day 13 of the fourth cycle), Mel and I made our way to the New Cross Hospital's Deanesly Centre for *Dr Grigoryev's* regular review of my progress. Instead, we saw his registrar, the kindly *Dr Hetu Charitha Gupta*, who recognised me immediately, inquired how I had coped with the docetaxel, and showed her familiarity with the detail of my case, supported, as expected, by my Integrated Electronic Patient Record displayed on the screen in front of her.

I gave her a hurried account of my numerous complaints, the nausea and indigestion, fatigue, stiff joints, cramp attacks in calf muscles and abdomen, stomach ache, diarrhoea, loss of taste, loss of appetite, etc. and, last but not least, the symptoms of gout. She sympathised profoundly, but left me with the impression that most of what I had experienced were the side effects reported by most patients injected with docetaxel. The nausea and indigestion would respond to lansoprazole. The diarrhoea could be relieved with Imodium. Paracetamol and ibuprofen would control the pain. But this was the reality of chemotherapy, and I should expect and prepare for more of the same during the fifth and sixth cycles.[6]

I specifically asked her about my symptoms of gout and my self-medication with daily tablets of allopurinol. She referred to her screen, noting allopurinol's effect on liver and kidneys, and the dangers of using it in combination with other drugs. As I had not had gout as such, but only an intimation of it returning, she thought it best for the time being to rely on paracetamol or ibuprofen for pain relief. The situation could always be reviewed at a later date.[6]

As the sores on my buttocks had not grown worse and the antibiotics she had prescribed before had not cleared up the infection, she was inclined to rely on the body's natural defences, especially, if helped along – as advocated by Mel – with a regular application of Sudocrem.

After a full and careful consideration of my various complaints, *Dr Gupta* wrote out a prescription for further enoxaparin, and we hurried off before 6.00 pm (when the hospital pharmacy closed), to wait for it to be dispensed. The precise quantity needed of the drug proved difficult to calculate without further advice from the doctor, and so we agreed to collect the prescription on Wednesday, when I had to return to the hospital for line care.

Fourth line care at Durnall

On Wednesday 28th March, we arrived on the Durnall Unit well before my 10.00 am appointment for line care, but it had turned 11.00 am before *Nurse Shelley Seagrove* began to remove my dressings. Friendly and intelligent in conversation, *Shelley* inquired about my condition and why I had had a Hickman line inserted. When I told her of my rare breast cancer, she confided in us that her mother had also developed breast cancer, thus motivating her to pursue a nursing career in oncology.

Examining my chest, she decided it was time for the sutures on either side of my exit wound to be removed, which she accomplished quite painlessly with a blade and tweezers. A syringe of blood was taken, disposed of, and the line flushed with saline and heparin, before I was taped up again. As we left the unit, we made a further appointment at Durnall for line care and a blood sample on Friday 6th April. Then we walked to the pharmacy to pick up my consignment of enoxaparin injections.

Fourth cycle summary

My experience of chemotherapy in the fourth cycle, when I was injected with docetaxel (Taxotere), was different from those of the first three cycles of FEC (fluorouracil, epirubicin and cyclophosphamide). Many of the side effect turned out to be the same, such as the nausea, indigestion, weakness, fatigue and light-headedness, which persisted from day 1 to day 11. Additional side effects, in the form of cramps in my calf muscles, and abdomen and shooting pains across my chest and along my arms and legs (summarised in Macmillan Cancer Support notes, I assume, under the heading 'muscle and/or joint pain'[7]), occurred on the evening of day 4, and persisted, in the main, as severe stomach ache, until day 8. Unlike in previous cycles, when I had tended towards constipation, the stomach ache was accompanied by bouts of explosive diarrhoea.

It was on day 3 of the fourth cycle that I detected the first symptom of gout and became anxious at the prospect of a full-blown attack. Although this did not occur (whether or not as a result of my self-medication), it gave me further cause at the time to worry and fret.

The docetaxel also radically altered my sense of taste. My pallet was both dulled and distorted. Tomatoes and tomato juice, which I had always enjoyed, tasted bitter and sour, as did oranges, my favourite fruit. Parsnips and Swedes were pretty unpleasant, too, but potatoes, bread, and cheese biscuits tasted much the same as usual. For at least a couple of days I lost my appetite and ate only a modicum of food.

My regular complaints about belching, sore gums, buttock sores, and the nightly enoxaparin injections, persisted throughout.

The end of the fourth cycle coincided with the Easter break (from Friday 30th March to Monday 2nd April), with day 21 falling on Tuesday 3rd April, causing delay to the hospital's regimens and rhythm. My fifth line care session was postponed until Friday 6th April, and the fifth cycle of chemotherapy to the 9th, giving me a break of five days for recuperation.

My hair went on falling out, including the hair of my beard, my armpits, my eyelashes, and eyebrows. By the end of the fourth cycle, I was more bald and glabrous than ever, though still retaining the outline of my eyebrows, a scattering of hairs on my chest and legs, and a somewhat reduced fringe of pubic hair.

By day 11, I began to feel better, and much relieved that the worst of the side effects were over, and were unlikely to recur until the docetaxel of the fifth and sixth cycles was administered.

Easter was cold and wet, encouraging us to forego our customary early spring gardening endeavours and to stay indoors. The disruption caused by the bank holiday weekend led to a five-day postponement of my fifth cycle of treatment which, though delaying the date of completion, gave me more time to recuperate.

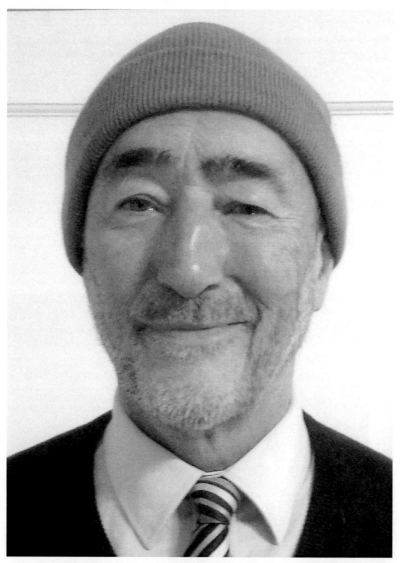

Frank wearing one of his beanies to disguise his hair loss

Chapter 10

Chemo-induced thinking on hair loss

Until chemotherapy in January 2018, and even at the age of 72, I had a full head of thick dark brown hair, bushy eyebrows, long eyelashes, a moustache and a beard, and was typically hirsute in a moderate but masculine way. Friends would express their surprise at how young I looked - like a man in his 40s - which they assessed chiefly in terms of the absence of greyness or hoariness in my head of hair. My hair grew vigorously, too. To keep myself tidy and presentable I had it trimmed at the hairdressers – grade 5 on top, grade 3 on the sides and grade 1 on the beard – at regular three-weekly intervals. The hairdressers joked about my youthful appearance, especially when giving me the customary pensioner discount.

Mel and I had been warned to expect the loss of hair on my head and face after chemotherapy. We had been talked through the side effects at length and in detail by *Sister Carys Jevons* and *Sister Donna Dobson* from the Breast Cancer Team, *Sister Natalie Edmunds,* the palliative care nurse, and by *Dr Grigoryev*, the gentle oncologist. The breast cancer nursing team also drew our attention to the extra services available at the Deanesly Centre, including a dedicated hairdressing and wig-fitting service, although it was never made clear, and I never asked, whether it catered for men.

After the first chemotherapy cycle, *Dr Grigoryev* had expressed interest in the fact that my hair had remained in situ, but warned me that it was almost certain to fall out during the second cycle. In fact, I grew progressively balder and balder throughout the second and third cycles, until my pate gleamed a ghostly white under moonlight in our conservatory. In addition to the verbal advice, we were given a copy of the hospital Oncology Directorate's *Patient Record Booklet and Advice for Cancer Patients having Chemotherapy Treatment*[1], the Breast Cancer Care charity's *Chemotherapy for Breast Cancer Treatments and Side Effects* [2], and the Macmillan Cancer Support guide book on *Coping with Hair Loss*[3]. Systematically laid out and very well written in non-technical language, these books dealt comprehensively with what was most likely to happen to me in the hair department. Significantly, the cover illustrations of both Breast Cancer Care and Macmillan publications showed women with head scarves stylishly wrapped, suggesting their tresses had already been shed.

The emotional impact of hair loss

Neither Mel nor I needed to be told by word-of-mouth, or by means of the printed word, that one consequence of chemotherapy was the loss of hair and temporary baldness. Of the adverse side effects of chemotherapy for cancer, particularly for breast cancer, chemically-induced alopecia has passed into popular culture as the defining and universally-recognised image of the terrifying 'c' disease[4], which I had heard on a number of occasions referred to as the 'curse' or 'mark of chemo', in deference, no doubt, to the biblical 'mark of Cain'. The Genesis story (Ch 4, v 11-16) tells how God put a physical mark on Cain for killing his brother, Abel, at the same time making him an outcast, but affording him divine protection.

The Macmillan Cancer Support guide, *Coping with Hair Loss*[3], is written for both women and men and contains informative sections on the way cancer treatments affect hair loss and growth, the impact of hair loss on the emotions, and practical tips for preparing oneself to cope with it, including wearing a wig, a wrap, or a hat.

The section on feelings and emotions explains that, for many people, their hair is an important part of their appearance, and a means of expressing their identity. Thus, they are likely to find the loss of their hair upsetting, as it radically changes the way they look and raises doubt about how they will be received and treated by family, friends or in public. For some, losing their hair is the very worst aspect of their cancer treatment, making them anxious, depressed, shy, vulnerable, and fearful of others. If eyebrows, eyelashes or pubic hair are lost, the impact may be even more traumatic. As a visible indicator of cancer, the sight of hair loss may cause close friends and kin to become distraught and unable to hide their feelings, thus confirming and reinforcing the patients' fears about the way they look.

To help chemotherapy patients gain greater control of their lives when their hair falls out, the guide recommends that they talk to family and friends to gain their support, cut their hair short prior to its falling out in longer clumps, and cover up their alopecia with a wig, hat, scarf, or other headwear. The guide is made up of around hundred pages, of which fifty, or half, are given over to ways of concealing the hair loss caused by chemotherapy.

Hair loss and covering the head

I studied the guide book closely, but was unable to establish to my own satisfaction the reason, or reasons, it offered for covering the head. Was it to help patients come to terms with their sudden shocking change in appearance? Was it to deal with their anxiety over how others might see and treat them? Was it about their right to keep private their illness and medical treatment? Was it their need to keep their heads warm and protected, or some complex combination of all of those issues?

Chemotherapy patients may offer their own alternative personal reasons, too. In her book, *Dear Cancer, Love Victoria* (2017), television broadcaster and journalist, Victoria Derbyshire, tells her readers " I definitely don't want ...people turning on the TV to watch our programme and being distracted from the story we're covering by my loss of hair or me wearing a scarf round my head. And the only way round that is to get a wig"[5].

With a background in social science, I, too, could provide a set of general hypotheses, but I had no means at hand of establishing which, if any of them, were true. What was it that the disguises and camouflages (in the form of wigs and hats) were meant to conceal and from whom? Could it be the disease, the damage, or the stigma of cancer? Or the fact that the individual was undergoing chemotherapy? Was it to prevent the upset, grief, shock or rejection of significant others, such as family members, friends or, more generally, members of the public? Was it simply an attempt to restore one's former recognisable appearance, in order to pass oneself off as normal –'normalisation', in social scientific jargon? (Victoria Derbyshire's explanation falls into that category.) Was it done mainly for personal contentment and peace of mind – to help patients themselves come to terms with their sudden and shocking change in appearance?

Instead of encouraging the wearing of wigs and hats, it is, of course, possible to conceive of alternative approaches: for example, to display a hairless or shaven head to promote pride, self-esteem, or defiance in facing up to the disease, or, in political terms, to 'normalise' cancer, by encouraging the millions[6] it affects to 'come out', in order to raise awareness of the scale of the current cancer crisis, and put pressure on government to resource more lavishly cancer research, diagnostic testing, and treatment.

How I, as a man, responded to hair loss

As for myself, why did I stubbornly cling to my beanie, deriving great comfort from it, and wearing it even when I was by myself at home? I concluded that, in my case, it was primarily to help me come to terms personally with my sudden and shocking change of appearance, but I was conscious, too, that I liked to dress smartly and present myself at my best to family, friends and in public. I was now very relaxed about letting people know about my cancer and chemotherapy, and quite overwhelmed by their compassionate and supportive response.

In reading the medically-approved guidance on breast cancer and chemotherapy, I came to the conclusion that, though written for both sexes, many of the suggestions had been made with only women in mind, most probably for the very sound reason that women formed the bulk of those receiving chemotherapy for breast cancer. However, some of the leaflets on display at the Deanesly Centre were less inclusive in their approach. *Pampering Therapy*, with a shocking pink cover, described the benefits of a 'look good feel better programme', helping to support women with cancer by offering them free skin care and make-up workshops: 'After the shock of being diagnosed with cancer, many women can dramatically change their appearance and body image – loss of hair, eyebrows and eyelashes can be particularly difficult to cope with.'[7] Were men more able to cope?

I was aware of the widespread belief that women were far more distressed by their hair loss than men. Women, it was reasoned, lost their hair when they were ill, became run down or stressed, underwent chemotherapy, or were approaching extreme old age. Men, on the other hand, went bald or experienced a receding hairline quite naturally as they advanced in years. For women, their hair, in common with the shape of their figure and breasts, was regarded as a sign of their beauty and sexual attractiveness. For men, hairiness, or the lack of it in the form of baldness, seemed unrelated to perceptions of their masculinity or virility. Indeed, well-known film stars with bald or shaven pates, such as Telly Savalas (who played Kojak), or Yul Brynner (who played the king in *The King and I*) were regarded in their days as sex idols. These generally-accepted assumptions seemed to form the basis of many of the popular articles appearing in women's magazines, written from a woman's perspective, and aimed at a female readership.

Many took their arguments further by asserting that women and men experienced cancer, chemotherapy, and chemically-induced alopecia, in radically different ways. For women, breast cancer, mastectomies, and hair loss during chemotherapy constituted an assault on the essence of what it was to be a woman, with drastic consequences for their mental health and wellbeing and sense of worth. For men it was different: the outward signs of surgery, including mastectomy, could be proudly displayed as manly battle scars, and the hair loss attributed to the ageing process.

While, at a cursory glance, I was able to locate several qualitative social scientific studies of the impact of breast cancer and hair loss on women, I never found any comparative study of a varying impact on men. An anthropological study in Denmark confirmed that women equated hair loss with the loss of womanhood, sickness and death, and that they took to wearing wigs and make-up to minimise those effects[8]. This finding seemed already to be taken for granted, judging from the content of the Macmillan Cancer Support guide, *Coping with Hair Loss*[3].

In considering this issue, I was conscious that the risk of developing breast cancer increased with age simply because age increased the likelihood of abnormal changes occurring to the cells. Very few women under 40 were diagnosed with breast cancer, (5 per cent of those diagnosed), the highest rate occurring in women over 70, a profile almost identical to that of men. Given the modal age of people with breast cancer, of which I was a fine example, I doubted whether most older women who lost their hair would be any more concerned than I about their physical appearance, beauty, or sexual attractiveness, but in the absence, or ignorance, of further social research, my assumption could well be wrong.

Another puzzling aspect of the literature on breast cancer and chemotherapy was its deficiency in dealing with the damaging effect of the chemo drugs on both women's and men's fertility, in contrast with the emphasis placed on what I regarded as the less-serious matter of chemically-induced alopecia. I suspected this, too, related to the post-menopausal age at which most breast cancer patients were diagnosed.

I chose to focus instead on my own experience of mastectomy and hair loss. Once over the initial shock of the cancer diagnosis, I saw the mastectomy scar and, similarly, the lymph node clearance incision, as a reassuring sign that the tumour had gone. The replacement of my nipple with a neat 12 cm scar did not trouble me and, in any case, all was concealed by my clothing. But what of the hair loss?

Initially, I bought into the Telly Savalas and Yul Brynner line – bald man were not unattractive. My brother-in-law had considerably less hair than I, and he didn't seem to worry! If the truth were told, I was far less relaxed about the prospect of my eyebrows, eyelashes and beard falling out. My pubic hairs were of little consequence to me or my sex life. I was also consoled by the realisation that I no longer had to shave under my chin or visit the hairdresser at two-weekly intervals. The other side effects of chemotherapy were of far more concern: nausea, vomiting, diarrhoea and constipation and a dangerous rise in temperature. If the alopecia was not painful, why all the fuss about hair loss?

Buying beanies

Notwithstanding these observations, I followed ritualistically the advice in the Macmillan guide[3], buying an unnecessarily large number of beanies in assorted colours, and a hair trimmer and cutter, in preparation for the time when my hair would fall out. In the first cycle of chemo, nothing happened, and I began to believe I was one of the very few whose hair was unaffected by the drugs. *Dr Grigoryev* knew better. Between day 1 and day 10 of the second cycle, my hair thinned and fell out, at first very gradually, then building up to a sump-choking cascade on day 6 until, like Autumn leaves in December, few remained to drift down.

Much to my surprise, I soon discovered that I was far more perturbed by my changing appearance than I could ever have predicted. My hair line receded at a frightening speed, leaving my forehead and the sides of my head, looking bald, and my ears exposed and alone, like deforested peaks in Snowdonia. While my beard remained discernible, it grew noticeably thinner and the whiskers on either side of my lower lip fell out.

The sight of a stranger

I could scarcely recognise myself when I looked in the mirror. The face that I had lived with for 50 years or more had been replaced by a stranger, a chemically-induced Mr Hyde, and that total transformation had occurred in just over a week. Fortuitously, I could avoid the mirror, and turn to my beanies for an effective disguise. No one was any the wiser when I met family or friends, went shopping, or attended a meeting at Citizens Advice, although people must have wondered as to why I went on wearing my beanie pulled down to my ears in centrally-heated rooms. However, the beanie disguise would have been far less effective if my eyebrows, eyelashes and beard had been lost. That was to come later.

I did not like my alopecic appearance and found it difficult to come to terms with it, yearning for my hair to grow back to what I was used to. What was more, I tried by any means possible to keep my Mr Hyde hidden, private and secret. I even surprised myself by my response to exposure and my reluctance to reveal myself. With the benefit of hindsight, the intensity of my feelings may have been heightened by another side-effect of the drugs: the dreadful sense of emotional vulnerability, helplessness, fragility, and loss of control.

Extreme sensitivity

The following incident serves as an example of my extreme sensitivity. When the family were eating supper at the dining table, Mel noticed that my beanie had slipped over my eyebrows, and sought to pull it back up. Not knowing the reason for her intervention, I reacted angrily by pushing her away and pulling my hat down hard. I had wrongly assumed that she had been about to expose my recent loss of hair to my children and grandchildren. I was surprised by the vehemence of my response. Was it really of consequence if my son and daughter-in-law saw the extent of my alopecia? I deliberately removed my beanie to show them.

After that incident, I realised that among family, friends and members of the public, my chemically-induced alopecia elicited mostly sympathy, kindness and respect for what I was going through. Indeed, it bestowed on me the biblical 'mark of Cain' – a shield of protection from my feelings of emotional vulnerability. I also had the consolation of knowing that the loss of my hair was merely a temporary phase - temporary perhaps, but currently deteriorating, personally disturbing, and constantly protracted.

By the 10th day of the sixth and final chemo cycle, with only a few remaining centimetre-long strands on my head and a smattering of irregular bristles on my chin, I decided at last to make use of my recently-acquired Philips Styleshaver and take everything off. As I peered in the circular shaving mirror, I was horrified by the wrinkled and haggard old man staring ashamedly in my direction. Was that really the same debonair 72-year-old man who once sported a full head of brown hair, a smart well-trimmed beard and a styled moustache? It was not my appearance in public, or in front of my friends, that dismayed me, but the loss of my familiar, pleasing, pleasant and presentable face. The real me had gone missing, abandoning me in an ugly unrecognisable alien body.

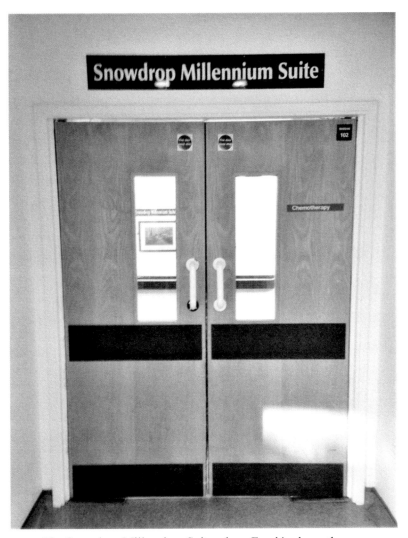

The Snowdrop Millennium Suite where Frank's chemotherapy
was administered

Chapter 11

Fifth chemotherapy cycle

Speeding up cancer diagnosis

On Tuesday 3rd April, we woke up to the news that NHS England, Cancer Research UK, and Macmillan Cancer Support were opening 'one-stop shops' to speed up the diagnosis of cancer and catch the disease at an early stage. GPs would be able to refer people with indeterminate symptoms, such as unexplained weight loss, reduced appetite, abdominal pains, fatigue, or night sweats, to a single centre, where they would undergo a battery of diagnostic tests, instead of their being dispatched separately and in turn to specialist units – thus leading to unnecessary delay. The approach had been developed in Denmark, and was now being trialled in ten areas of the country – none, so far, in Wolverhampton, or the West Midlands. Nevertheless, we were pleased that the issue of prompt diagnosis was being addressed, thus contributing to an improvement in cancer survival rates.

Coffee morning with Geoff

On Wednesday 4th April, I met Geoff Hurd for morning coffee at the Wolverhampton Art Gallery cafeteria. On learning of my cancer, Geoff, a long-standing friend and a former deputy vice chancellor at the University of Wolverhampton where Mel once worked, telephoned and asked whether he could help out in any way – suggesting that we talk over coffee. He also volunteered to drive me to hospital appointments, should I require him to. We spent a most amicable morning catching up on news of our recent histories, holidays, children and grandchildren, discussing current political issues and, in the course of our conversation, exploring my experience of the mastectomy operation and chemotherapy. Always gentle, modest and considerate, Geoff did his utmost to draw me out of myself. His company did me a power of good and we agreed to meet again soon towards the end of the next chemotherapy cycle.

Reminded of Darwinian principles

Mel and I noticed a pair of Mallard ducks settled on the little bog pond at the end of our garden, a male with an iridescent green head and grey on its wings and chest, the female with brown-speckled plumage, and wondered what had attracted them there. They stayed in our garden for a couple of days, refusing to move even when we approached. Every hour or so, they waddled up and down the lawn as if taking possession of a territory. Believing them to dabble and to dine mainly on water weed, at first we were pleased to see that they were making our garden their home. On closer examination, we realised that they had gobbled up all the newly-hatched tadpoles, and deprived us of the next generation of garden frogs. It was a timely reminder of the Darwinian principles of natural selection which operated without reference to moral or aesthetic considerations - similar indeed to the spread of my breast cancer. My mastectomy and subsequent chemotherapy demonstrated my commitment to waging an all-out personal war against natural selection.

Fifth line care on Durnall, Friday 6th April

On Friday 6th April, Mel and I returned to the Durnall Oncology Day Unit to have my line checked and flushed, and for blood samples to be taken, prior to Monday's fifth cycle of chemotherapy. On the advice of the receptionist, on ward A24, we had made the appointment early at 8.30 am, in the hope of a shorter waiting time, and sure enough, my name was called by 8.45 am.

We recognised *Sister Natalie Edmunds*, the lead palliative care nurse, who greeted us warmly and engaged us in lively and informative conversation. I opened the front of my shirt and she skilfully removed the dressing around my Hickman line. The tube was flushed and blood samples taken in a jiffy, almost without my noticing. Aware of my interest in books on the patients' experience of cancer and cancer treatment, *Natalie* recommended John Diamond's book, *C. Because Cowards Get Cancer* (1999). An English journalist and author, John had been married to Nigella Lawson, the food writer, until he died from head and neck cancer in 2001. We left Durnall by 9.30 am, just over an hour's stay. We would still have incurred a parking charge of £3.40, if it were not for the oncology £1.50 concession.

That evening Mel, my loving wife and nurse. gave me my regular nightly injections of enoxaparin, and then proceed to inspect the sores on my buttocks. She inquired as to whether it still hurt at that spot, as I had not complained of discomfort in recent days. When I said it did not, she confirmed that the sores had healed up and there was nothing to see. More good news!

Upset at hearing of others' death

On Saturday 7th April, Ed, the child of Trevor, my recently-deceased cousin, phoned me from Bristol to say that Margaret, his mother (my cousin-in-law), had passed away in hospital that morning, following a massive stroke. She was in her eighties and had been devastated by her husband's death, so Ed's news was not wholly unexpected. Worse was to follow. Later, I received an email from Wynne Moran to tell me her husband, Mick Moran, had suffered a massive heart attack on Easter Sunday and had died soon afterwards. Mick was a friend from my school and Lancaster University days, and would have reached his 72nd birthday later in the month. He was more than a year younger than I, and as far as I knew in good health, and so the news shocked and upset me. As young men, in the 1960s, we had campaigned together against the racism of Peter Griffiths who was elected as the Conservative MP for Smethwick. Allegedly aided by the slogan, 'If you want a nigger for your neighbour vote Labour', he was famously denounced by prime minister Harold Wilson as a 'parliamentary leper'. Mick's death reminded me once more of our mortality, and that people could be struck down, often suddenly and without warning, by diseases other than cancer. This news forced me to think of myself as one of the lucky ones.

On Sunday 8th April, in preparation for the fifth cycle of chemotherapy on the 9th, I had been prescribed four soluble 2mg tablets of dexamethasone – a corticosteroid used, in my case, to prevent nausea and vomiting following chemotherapy, but also given when breast cancer has spread to other parts of the body. Having taken Glensoludex dexamethasone at the start of the four previous chemo-cycles, I had already experienced some of the recognised side effects: particularly the over-active brain or mania, problems in going to sleep, irregular sleeping patterns, hot flushes, and red rosy cheeks. My erratic behaviour kept Mel awake and made her very tired.

Day 1 (Monday 9th April 2018)

I took another four tablets of dexamethasone with my cereals on Monday morning, the 9th April, in preparation for my 1.30 pm appointment on Snowdrop for the injection of docetaxel at the start of the fifth chemo-cycle. Just as I finished breakfast at 9.00 am, I received a telephone call summoning me to the hospital for an urgent repeat neutrophil blood test. We reached the Snowdrop Millennium Centre for 10.05 am and were seen immediately. It was explained that the neutrophil count for the blood taken on Friday was worrying low and it would have to be checked again before they could proceed with the fifth drug cycle. The amiable *Sister Jemima Holyoaks* drew off, through my Hickman line, a further blood sample to test for neutrophils, which came back about ten minutes later with the result (at 6.9). The count had risen to an acceptable level over the weekend and we would now be able to proceed with the fifth cycle previously booked for 1.30 pm that afternoon. In the meantime, we went home for coffee and a light lunch.

Fifth session of chemotherapy at the Snowdrop Millennial Suite

Returning to Snowdrop to start the fifth cycle, we waited until 2.00 pm to be taken to a narrow cubicle at the u-turn of the u-shaped ward. We were met by the friendly and efficient staff nurse, *Michelle McLean*, who inquired about my experiences during the fourth cycle, and then prepared me for the second docetaxel infusion by connecting my Hickman line to a bag of saline solution hung on the drip stand to my right. When the saline went through, it was replaced by a bag of steroid solution which, I assumed, was more of the dexamethasone. This was followed by a much larger bag of the real McCoy – the docetaxel – yet another clear transparent fluid, but sheathed in a black plastic hood, to distinguish it and protect it, from deterioration under the light. *Nurse McLean* also connected me to a sphygmomanometer, as before, to monitor my blood pressure and pulse, and to alert the staff to any possible allergic reactions during the infusion. I reassured her – or was it myself – that I had taken the docetaxel on a previous occasion without any problem.

Bubbles in my drip tube

As the docetaxel drained out and was coming to and end, I noticed little bubbles entering the drip tube and, having read about venous air embolisms, I became anxious. Mel summoned the nurse, but not before some of the bubbles had entered the line in my chest. *Nurse McLean* reassured me that small bubbles of air – and these were very small – often got into the body through intravenous fluid lines, but were stopped at the lungs and were unlikely to cause me harm. She uncoupled me from the drip stand, flushed my line with heparin to prevent the possibility of clotting, and re-taped the tubes onto my chest. Mel had brought my 4.00 pm dose of soluble dexamethasone, which she dissolved in a plastic cup of water for me to drink while I munched at a couple of ginger biscuits.

Buying Difflam

From Snowdrop, we walked to the hospital pharmacy, where we had been told we could buy a replacement bottle of Difflam oral rinse (benzydamine hydrochloride), which I had previously been prescribed for the sore mouth caused by the chemotherapy. The pharmacy assistant was very helpful, confirming that they did supply Difflam, but that I could only obtain it from the hospital pharmacy on a hospital doctor's prescription, as it was part of the hospital's stock. The Boots Pharmacy consisted of two sections, each with its own stock. She could sell Boots stock over the counter to me there and then, but the hospital stock – of which the Difflam was part – could only be obtained on a hospital prescription. She asked me if I would be prepared to walk over to the Boots Pharmacy at the Bentley Bridge Retail Park, where I could buy Difflam without prescription over the counter. She phoned up to check on its availability and had a bottle put aside for me to pick up. Sure enough, when we arrived at the store, I was able to collect and pay for the Difflam.

Mel went into the Bentley Bridge Aldi to buy some food for the evening meal, but we did not arrive home until after 6.00 pm, with both of us feeling tired after the stressful events of the day. I suggested that I went out to buy us both fish, chips and mushy peas, which we eventually consumed hungrily, but late in the evening, while watching *East Enders*.

Indigestion from eating late

The choice of meal eaten so late after the day's chemotherapy was a grave mistake. Mel had noticed on previous occasions that I seemed to digest food more easily when it was eaten at an earlier hour. I started burping before bedtime and the enoxaparin injections. It would be an understatement to say that I did not sleep well. No doubt aided by the dexamethasone steroids, I woke at three-quarter-hour intervals and sat up for twenty-minute bouts of violent hiccups, before settling down uncomfortably to wait for the next onslaught. The hiccups and belching lasted till 6.30 am when I went downstairs to take a gastro-resistant lansoprazole capsule, and paracetamol to control a developing headache, before making our early morning tea.

Day 2 (Tuesday 10ᵗʰ April)

The lansoprazole seemed to have been effective, for I was able to eat my oats porridge without further belching and indigestion, while using the intake of food to sip the now-dissolved dexamethasone tablets. The dexamethasone kept me busy and active all day, but I became light-headed and giddy at times. Philip called round to assist me on the computer in laying out the Blue Bayou Series, *Eastern Caribbean*.

In the afternoon I drove to the IKEA store in Darlaston in search of a rug, but saw nothing to my liking or of an appropriate size. On return, I dissolved the four remaining dexamethasone tablets and drank the resultant brown-tinted liquid.. It dawned on me that the dexamethasone was meant to deal with the side effects of the docetaxel on the digestive tract, just as the Emend aprepitant had been used in the earlier FEC cycles. As in previous cycles, I noticed my eyes had become dry and sore and, as before, resorted to self-medication with Xailin carmellose sodium eye drops, which eased the dry-eye sensation.

For supper, we ate smoked haddock, home-grown pink fir apple potatoes, mushrooms and broccoli – a favourite meal of mine which Mel prepared especially to please me, but it didn't taste as appetising as usual, which I blamed on the chemotherapy. This time we ate earlier in the hope of a better night's sleep, then watched BBC1's *East Enders*, *Holby City*, the last of the series of *Come Home*, and the *News at Ten*, one programme after the other. This was an attempt to blot out the prospect of my three evening injections, the first of filgrastim to stimulate the growth of white blood cells, and then the two enoxaparin anti-coagulant jabs. Once Mel had administered them, I relaxed and fell asleep easily, waking only at 4.00 am to make tea, before dozing off again.

Day 3 (Wednesday 11th April)

Morning came with mild indigestion, which I attempted to offset with a lansoprazole capsule, following which I breakfasted on a bowl of cereals: shredded wheat, harvest crunch and cornflakes, accompanied by a date and a couple of prunes, to prevent constipation. To be frank, while I had varied my diet, I was unable to distinguish the cereals from the porridge I had eaten on Tuesday. Apart from the texture, they tasted the same. Some of the harder cereal granules lodged themselves between my dentures and gums, resulting in my mouth becoming sore. At this time in the cycle, I should have stuck with the porridge.

What's in a name?

The *Express & Star* (11.4.2018) carried the headline, 'Compton Hospice changes its name'. The local hospice had decided to rebrand itself after a consultation exercise with patients, families, staff, volunteers, and referral agencies revealed a widespread fear of referral for end-of-life care, seeing it as a place where people were sent to die. Henceforth, it would be known, not as 'Compton Hospice' with the strap line 'caring together', but as 'Compton Care', with the strap line 'making everyday extraordinary'.

Given Compton Hospice's role and function, made apparent by its charity shops and fundraising activities, I wondered whether the change of name would make any difference. Would it merely make a familiar local brand more obscure, in the same way that the 'Consignia' rebrand had damaged the Royal Mail, one of the most well-known institutions in the commercial world? There was no doubt, however, that the public had an appetite for euphemisms. At the hospital, I attended the Snowdrop Millennium Suite for my chemotherapy. The name gave no clue whatsoever as to what went on there. I suppose it could have been called the 'Chrysanthemum Chemotherapy Centre', or even the 'Orchid Oncology Garden', but what was the point of drawing attention to the awful carcinogenic reality? Come to think of it, should the name of New Cross

Hospital itself be changed in order to improve the chemo experience and make it 'extraordinary', along the same lines as the hospice, to "New Cross Care and Well-being'?

As the weather was cold, wet and dismal, I spent most of the day updating my breast cancer diary. In the evening, I took 500g of paracetamol 40 minutes before the filgrastim and enoxaparin injections and, though still apprehensive, imagined the jabs were less sharp.

Day 4 (Thursday 12th April)

In the morning, I noticed that my temperature had risen to 37.4^0c from the average of 36.6^0c over the first three days. Day 4 began well but deteriorated sharply as the afternoon progressed, initially with stomach cramps and aches, followed by three violent evacuations in the form of loose explosive stools and noisily-emitted flatus. Feeling tired and fatigued, I retired to my bed for a rest, but aching joints, and continuing stomach cramps made it difficult to sleep.

Mel did her best to liven my mood by cooking me sausage, bacon, sweet potatoes and broccoli for supper, but I suffered from a loss of taste, as if my mouth had been scalded. Most morsels were uniformly bland, although the broccoli was slimy and unpleasantly sour. As before, paracetamol before bedtime relieved the pain of the injections, but I slept very badly, and woke up tired.

Day 5 (Friday 13th April)

With my early-morning appointment for line care, I set the alarm for 6.40 am, and tried to spring out of bed. I had felt distinctly uncomfortable for most of the night, with aches and pains in my muscles and joints, and severe stomach cramps, which soon translated into a bout of loose stools and later to diarrhoea. To avoid Mel having to wait needlessly at the hospital, I had planned to drive myself to my 8.30 am line care appointment on Durnall, and then to walk over to Deanesly for 10.30 am to attend a visualisation and relaxation group organised for cancer patients by the Cancer Psychology and Counselling Service. As I staggered in pain around the bedroom, I realised that I was not well enough to drive myself, let alone to spend most of the morning in a meeting at the hospital. Mel readily agreed to resume her normal routine and drive me to my line care appointment and then take me home immediately afterwards. Weak and vulnerable, I would not have coped that day without Mel as a minder and advocate.

Sixth line care on Durnall, Friday 13th April

We arrived at Durnall at 8.25 am. My name was called out, along with two others, at 8.55 am. *Sister Natalie Edmunds*, a favourite of ours, led the three patients and their companions to the treatment bay, where curtains were drawn, and the procedures administered in turn. I was able to engage in an informative conversation with *Natalie* and Mel, as my line was flushed. Soon afterwards, still aching and weak, I made my way back to the car, and Mel drove us both home for 10.00 am. I took paracetamol and went back to bed, where I stayed until 2.00 pm.

As I lay there wretchedly, I began to list my numerous complaints, chief among which were the muscle and joint pains, the stomach cramps, the sore heels and soles of my feet, and sensitive finger tips and toes, as if I had stubbed each of them, individually. As the day progressed, my stomach ache got worse and by late afternoon regular bouts of explosive diarrhoea had set in.

And this was by no means all that the docetaxel had inflicted on me. I still had indigestion and wind. Despite regular use of the Difflam, the gums under my dentures were sore, making hard food difficult to masticate. I continued to shed hair and my head looked balder and shinier than ever. I found fine hairs sprinkled on my porridge – so fine I couldn't avoid eating them. Were they whiskers, eye brows, eye lashes, nasal hairs or straight from my head? I had long given up trying to identify them and no longer had the energy to care. The three evening injections into my midriff followed as inevitably as night follows day.

Day 6 (Saturday 14th April)

Feeling weary, I woke to the worrying news that the United States, the UK and France had launched multiple air strikes on Syria in order, they claimed, to deter the production, spread, and use of chemical weapons. Out of sorts to begin with, I was annoyed that the UK government had engaged in military action without the approval of parliament, that it assumed the right to dish out punishment to other sovereign states, that diplomatic channels had not been exhausted, that by arming the rebels in the first place it had fuelled the Syrian civil war, and that it showed no concern for killing more Syrians, risking a third world war, or causing yet more 'collateral damage'.

In the context of my cancer, my government was prepared to allocate £3.16 million to bunker-busting Storm Shadow cruise missiles to kill and destroy Syrians, in comparison with the £10,000 (excluding the cost of the day-patient care) it was prepared to spend on chemo-medicines for prolonging my life. I was only counting the RAF's fire power. According to the news, at least 110 cruise missiles had been used to attack Syria during the night, most of them Tomahawks, at a total estimated cost of nearly £800 million – and that sum included only the missiles.

At 37.5^{0}c, my temperature remained worryingly high, and the cramps in my calf muscles and sore heels and soles reduced my mobility to a slow lumbering stroll. After breakfast of cornmeal porridge, prepared by Mel, I imagined improvement and chose to accompany Mel to the B & Q Garden Centre (with its offer of a 20 per cent reduction on spring garden plants) in search of Avalanche clemates, a favourite of ours. With mission accomplished, we went and did further shopping, which used up all my remaining energy. In the hope of recovery, we bought a quarter-pounder meal at McDonalds and sat down to eat. For all that my taste buds were able to tell me, I could have been eating a cherry bakewell tart.

I sauntered sluggishly out of the shop and Mel drove me home, where I retired to bed for the afternoon. My sense of taste at supper was as poor as at lunch. That evening, Mel gave the last of the five filgrastim jabs for the fifth cycle, henceforth reducing the nightly injections to two syringes. The sharps box was now full and on Monday would be exchanged for an empty one. I did not sleep well and at 4.00 am went to make tea..

Day 7 (Sunday 15th April)

The good news was that my morning temperature had fallen to 37.0^{0}c. After a lansoprazole capsule followed by cornmeal porridge, I walked to Tettenhall Green, to purchase my Sunday papers. I found myself lumbering slowly along and soon out of breath. Far from coasting through the fifth cycle of chemo, I was more tired, debilitated, and unfit than ever before. By pacing myself and regularly stopping for breath, I eventually made it to the shop and back again – a distance of about two miles. Nevertheless,

I was thoroughly alarmed by the deterioration in my physical condition, and in the expectation that the sixth cycle would only make it worse.

By the time Mel returned from her walk, I had read the headlines on Western missile strikes on Syria, undertaken a few DIY jobs, and had coffee. Yet I felt so fatigued that I was forced to go back to bed, where I slept to 2.00 pm. When I woke, I had soup and a roll, and pottered around the house still feeling tired. I began to feel a severe back pain in my lumbar region, so debilitating that I had to take paracetamol. The pain eventually subsided, whether as a result of the passing of time or the effect of the paracetamol. For supper, we feasted on oxtail, rice and peas and sprouts, a meal which Gem, our friend, had cooked and sent round, in a conspiracy with Mel to cheer me up. My enjoyment of the treat was constrained by my impaired sense of taste, mild indigestion, and back ache. I retired to bed after my usual nightly enoxaparin injections.

Day 8 (Monday 16th April)

After lansoprazole and porridge, I worked on a glossary of medical terms for much of the morning. My health report read: 'feeling weak, easily fatigued, sores on my buttocks, loose bowel, mouth ulcers, loss of taste, further hair loss, but marginally improved and more optimistic than at the weekend'. We had an early lunch before driving to the hospital for a 3.00 pm appointment with *Dr Grigoryev*, but meetings rarely run to time, and we were not called in to see *Dr Gupta*, his registrar, until 4.10 pm. While in the waiting room, we met Frank Lewis, our friend Essie's son, and Tina, his wife, who were waiting like us for an oncology assessment –once more, a camaraderie of cancer.

Dr Gupta was her normal warm and welcoming self, inquiring after my health during the fifth cycle, expressing her sympathy when I listed my side effects, and agreeing apologetically that I was most likely to encounter the same problems again in the final 6th cycle. In preparation for the final lap, she began to compile a prescription of the medicines I would need: more enoxaparin injections, to last until the 23rd May, more lansoprazole to settle the stomach, a further bottle of Difflam oral rinse, and an initial supply of tamoxifen tablets to start taking on the 30th May, around ten days after the completion of the 6th cycle of chemotherapy.

In response to my queries, *Dr Gupta* spent much of the time explaining the arrangements for the forthcoming radiotherapy and the planned removal of my Hickman line. I also sought advice about overseas travel and a return to swimming. When the five-year course of tamoxifen was mentioned, I inquired about the impact of the medication on my long-term survival rate. Expertly, *Dr Gupta* turned to her computer screen, typed in the type, size and stage of my breast cancer and showed me a bar chart showing the combined effect of chemotherapy, radiotherapy and tamoxifen hormone therapy on overall breast cancer survival rates. The overall survival rates were 87 per cent after 5 years and 69 per cent after 10, reassuring, no doubt, provided that any one individual was not part of the 13 per cent or 31 per cent who died. We thanked *Dr Gupta* for her help and advice and made our way to the pharmacy, eventually leaving the hospital at 5.30 pm.

Walking to the car park, I became breathless and giddy and was glad that Mel was able to drive. We ate supper, but with my sore gums and a marked diminution of taste, I did not enjoy it as much as I would normally have done. Later, Mel gave me my enoxaparin jabs.

Day 9 (Tuesday 17th April)

I slept well but woke at 5 am with a head full of ideas that I had to write down. I made tea for us both, then put on my glasses and scribbled away until 7 am, when the radio alarm came on. After a breakfast of cornmeal porridge, I went out into the garden to mow the lawn, drank coffee, and then worked with Philip on the computer for the rest of the morning. After this treble whammy of early morning writing, lawn mowing, and time at the computer, I began to fall asleep and, when Philip left, I went for a nap. Apart from tiring easily, continued indigestion, sore mouth and distortion of my sense of taste, I realised my mood had begun to improve and that I had surmounted the worst of the 5th cycle.

Day 10 (Wednesday 18th April)

Day 10 was beautifully bright – the warmest and sunniest of the year to date and so, after breakfast, I went into the garden to catch up on some of the jobs. It was hot, and the sun caught my face, despite having a hat on my head. Mel reminded me that I had been warned to keep out of the sun because, with the ongoing chemo, my skin was likely to burn easily, and so I retired indoors. Feeling very tired, I took a short nap in preparation for that evening's first mindfulness course in Tettenhall (described in Chapter 12). When I returned from the class, Mel had prepared a light supper of a baked potato and beans. I told her what I had learned of mindful meditation and listening. That evening, while administering my enoxaparin injections, she asked me if the mindfulness course had helped, and whether I would still need paracetamol.

Days 11 to 21 (Thursday 19th – Sunday 29th April)

The general state of my health and of my petty side effects remained very much the same for the rest of the cycle. Periodically, I got indigestion, sometimes my mouth was sore, and I regularly became fatigued after only minor activity and exercise. I gained minor relief from the fact that the sores on my buttocks had now healed.

A glance in the mirror after my morning wash, showed me to be just, if not more, bald-headed, then before. The change that this cycle had brought was that my eyebrows had begun to fall out, giving me an owl-like mottled appearance. With the weather turning warm, it became uncomfortable to wear a beanie outdoors, although I still needed to shield my head from the sun. Instead, I would select a cap, broad-brimmed fedora, trilby, or panama for the forthcoming summer months.

Seventh line care on Durnall, Friday 20th April

On Friday 20th April, I made my way to the Durnall Day Centre for an 8.30 am appointment for line care. *Nurse Liza Warmington* eventually flushed my line around 9.35 am. I asked her politely, why the hour-long wait? Why not give me a 9.30 am appointment instead? She told me how busy they all were on Durnall. They were nearly always short-staffed and appointment slots from Monday to Friday were filled to overflowing. We agreed that demand for the service was outstripping supply and would continue to do so with the increasing number of elderly cancer patients. I remained unclear as to whether the shortage of nurses arose from understaffing, a failure to fill vacancies, or staff phoning in sick.

I was reminded of my conversation with *Liza* about three weeks later, when I read an article in *The Observer* (13.05.18), reporting on a national dossier compiled by the Royal College of Nursing on nurses' concerns at the risk to cancer sufferers of staff shortages on hospital wards. One nurse wrote that 'A lack of trained chemotherapy nurses means we are treating patients every day in an unsafe manner, mistakes are being made, and managers have no answer to the staffing crisis'. Another stated 'Our (cancer) patients may have to have less psychological support, as we do not have the time to sit with them and reassure them...Today's shift, where we were fully staffed with the majority of our own staff, was a very rare event'. These views were echoed by an earlier Macmillan report which found that there were widespread shortages of specialist cancer nurses. Hospitals in England had vacancies for more than 400 vacancies for specialist cancer nurses, chemotherapy nurses, palliative care nurses, and cancer support workers.[1]

Out of darkness cometh light

With the Wolverhampton Wanderers clinching the Championship title on Saturday 21st April by beating Bolton Wanderers, the spirit of the people of Wolverhampton grew noticeably lighter. The city expressed its gratitude to club manager, Nuno Espirito Santo, and celebrated in style a return to the Premier League (despite the announcement shortly afterwards of a rise in the price of a season ticket). Our son Robeson, Mel, and I were delighted. Wolves' victory and their supporters' joyful exuberance were infectious, giving me an unexpected, yet welcome, psychological boost on the 13th day of my fifth cycle.

On Monday 23rd April, Mel and I returned to the hospital for a CT scan of my chest and for me to be marked and tattooed in readiness for the course in radiotherapy, planned for when I had completed and recovered from the sixth cycle of chemo. Chapter 14 provides more detail

Baby Caio therapy

When we returned home, we prepared for the next visit of our daughter, Toussaint, and our grandson, baby Caio. Their presence was guaranteed to lighten the long-lasting burden of the chemotherapy cycles, and the next few days provide a delightful distraction. I participated nightly in the bathing-of-baby routine, and gained a great deal of fun from Caio's joyful and vigorous kicking and splashing. He grinned and giggled and wriggled and dabbled and paddled, making Toussaint and me damp but delighted with his naked display of vitality. As soon as Caio was physically soaped, sponged and rinsed off in that bath, I let out the bath water. The mental contamination of my cancer disappeared mysteriously down the plug hole!

Meeting friends

On Tuesday 24th, I met Geoff Hurd, again at the Art Gallery, for morning coffee. He had gone to the trouble of reading a draft of the early chapters of *Breast Cancer Man,* and gave me some helpful feedback and suggestions. On the evening of the 25th, I attended my second mindfulness class, and on the 26th, Anna, my friend and former colleague, visited, as arranged, to take me for a further therapeutic session of industrial history (for both occasions, see Chapter 12).

Eighth line care on Durnall

On Friday 27th April, I returned to Durnall for the eighth spell of line care and, on this occasion, to have blood samples taken in preparation for the sixth chemo cycle. As before, I arrived in good time for my 8.30 am appointment, but was not shown to the ward until 9.15 am, where I waited once more until 9.50 am for the procedure to begin.

Staff Nurse Liza Warmington introduced me to *Nurse Janice Trainer*, who had been sent from the Deanesly Ward that morning to help out on Durnall. While being willing, *Janice* soon made it clear that she had not undertaken the procedure before, and *Nurse Warmington* agreed to stay with us and oversee the line care.

Janice removed the dressing, drew off some blood and disposed of it, filled two syringes with my blood samples, injected saline and heparin and then re-taped the line to my chest. I buttoned up my shirt, put on my tie, jacket and coat, and went to reception to make further appointments for line care. I left the ward at 10.15 am to walk over to Deanesly, just in time for my visualisation and relaxation group (see Chapter 12).

Chemo-induced displacement of activity, ambition and aspiration

My memory of cycle 5 is chiefly one of nostalgia - nostalgia for a past life of political activism in race relations and the realisation that, because of my chemo-induced feebleness, I no longer had the strength to participate in the events of the moment. In the 1960s and early 70s, I had campaigned against Enoch Powell's poisonous anti-immigrant rhetoric but was now quite unable to find the energy to participate in the debate triggered by the 50th anniversary of his 'river of blood' speech. While Mel had assumed British citizenship soon after our marriage, she and I knew many Jamaicans in Wolverhampton of the so-called Windrush generation, and were horrified at the bureaucratic cruelty unleashed in the government's pursuit of its policy of creating 'a hostile climate' for so-called illegal immigrants, many of whom had lived for most of their lives in the UK. Pre-occupied with the demands of my chemotherapy, we never got round to publicly expressing our anger. The same went for the 25th anniversary of Stephen Lawrence's murder.

We had always been active in campaigning against racial injustice and corruption in the police force, but our current preoccupation with cancer, restrained our participation. This displacement of activity, ambition and aspiration is an important feature of cancer treatment – a significant side effect - which rarely receives the attention it deserves. The involuntary withdrawal from political life (for example, in my case, from political campaigning and from attending the trustee board of Citizens Advice) revealed the true extent of my loss of personal autonomy and control.

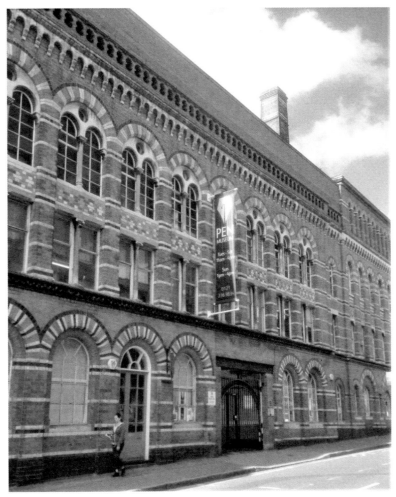

Industrial history therapy with Anna, the Birmingham Pen Museum,
Jewellery Quarter, Birmingham

Chapter 12

Chemo-induced thinking on therapy

For most patients, chemotherapy is an ordeal, voluntarily undertaken, in my case to reduce the risk of cancer returning by targeting any remaining cancer cells - so-called 'adjuvant chemotherapy'. Chemotherapy is invariably perceived and experienced as an ordeal because of its numerous unpalatable side effects and the prolonged duration of treatment. For me, the course was originally scheduled to last for over four months but, because of set-backs and delays, extended from January to May 2018 - a significant test of endurance. I could cope with the chemo for much of the time, responding to fatigue and weakness by taking a nap, but the belching and nausea were more debilitating, reducing my normal activity levels and making me bored, frustrated and bad-tempered. Though of comparatively short duration, other side effects were far more unpleasant and painful, preoccupying my thoughts and preventing me engaging in any purposeful exercise. I found the thrombo-phlebitis of the third cycle, and the side-effects of the docetaxel of the fourth, fifth and sixth, particularly unpleasant and distressing.

At such times, chemotherapy patients look for ways of coping with their daily experiences, and of alleviating the tedium of their mostly uncomfortable and unpredictable existence. The strategies that they adopt, often spontaneously, are commonly referred to as therapies, from the Greek word, *therapeiã*, meaning 'treatment'. As my six cycles of chemotherapy progressed, I, too, discovered activities that distracted me from routine aches and pains and provided me with a modicum of relief and comfort. I went on to develop ideas of my own on the therapies that would best suit me.

Recognising the importance of family

In the third week of the first chemotherapy cycle, when I thought I might be less tired, I allowed my sister, Annie, to pay us a visit. From the time she learned of my illness, she had pressed to drive over, but I had procrastinated until I felt in recovery mode. I was touched by the trouble she had taken to see me, and by her heartfelt concern for my welfare. The day she spent with me gave me a palpable psychological boost, and I realised once more the importance at such times of family support – confirming the maxim that 'a trouble shared is a trouble halved'.

Reflecting later on the impact of Annie's companionship, I became conscious of the numerous messages of solidarity and support I had received from family and friends, and how these had helped me, resulting at times in an overwhelming and painful sense of gratitude. Such expressions of companionship and empathy appeared to be a spontaneous and collective response to individuals' illness, infirmity, pain or misfortune, giving them an actual emotional, and possibly physical, stimulus or fillip. The lesson for me was to draw on the power of that goodwill over my remaining cycles of chemo- and radio- therapy.

On Friday 26th January, day 4 of my second cycle, Robeson, Tasha and grand children arrived from London. After my grandchildren, Maxi and Vieve, had been put to bed, they inquired after my health and I told them about the routine of the chemotherapy. They showed a genuine interest in my condition, but I held back on the detail in case it disturbed them. Robeson and Tasha had been very supportive of me and had sent me kind messages. It was wonderful to see them and to catch up on their lives.

I found the weekend visit of my son, daughter-in-law and grandchildren a tender and joyful occasion, in which they paid close attention to my welfare. When the grandchildren played in the back garden, I noticed that the snowdrops had started to flower. The garden and grandchildren were growing and blooming and, at that instance, the chemo transformed itself, like a newly-opened purple crocus, into the prelude for a cancer-free future.

On Saturday 10th February, day 18 of the second cycle, we received a Facetime call from Spartaca, our daughter in Kenya, and Patrick, our son-in-law. They gave us the best news of the year so far, namely that Spartaca had recently gone for a scan and was in the early stages of pregnancy. Mel and I rejoiced with them at the prospect of welcoming another grandchild into the family. I found the news particularly poignant in the context of my current cancer diagnosis and treatment, and was brought close to tears. It provided Mel and me, as an aging couple, with vitality and hope in the face of our inevitable long-term decline and eventual death.

Being open about cancer

I have mentioned already my initial inclination to confine the news of my cancer to close family members, and then to have changed my approach in the light of the overwhelming sympathy and support I was offered by friends, neighbours, and people who barely knew me. I came very quickly to appreciate the strength of the family and community in lightening the burdens of cancer and chemotherapy. The values of openness and honesty far outweighed the covert confidentiality of the stereotypical nuclear family unit. I told people - even the window cleaner - that I had cancer and was undergoing chemotherapy and continued to be amazed by the generosity of their response. I no longer felt the need to wear my beanie among friends, or even in public, removing it in the hospital without hesitation. I was thoroughly convinced of the beneficial effects of exposing my cancer to anyone who happened to notice it.

Nevertheless, I did not foresee the inevitable consequence of my openness, or my intuitive responses when faced with it. The extended circle of friends, neighbours and acquaintances constantly inquired after my health, either by asking me directly how I was feeling, or by taking Mel to one side for a professional carer's briefing. They assured me that I looked well considering everything I was going through, they urged me to stay positive, and they told me I was being brave, all these at times when I did not feel well, had no good reason to adopt a positive outlook, and knew that I wasn't being brave in a matter over which I had no control.

Responding to well-wishers

As anyone who has undertaken chemotherapy will know, the severity of one's debilities and complaints varies considerably from day to day. While willing to tell it as it was, I was reluctant to talk in detail, or for long, for example, about the sores on my buttocks and groin, my mouth ulcers, my feelings of anxiety or exhaustion, my constipation, stomach ache, or gout, the details of which, I guessed, nobody really wanted to hear about. Instead, in accordance with the time-honoured cultural norms among men of my generation, I resorted to euphemism, litotes, and understatement. Conscious of the quintessential features of such discourse, I began to record the expressions I used, of which the following provide a representative list. When asked about my health, I replied:

As well as can be expected under the circumstances.

At times, it hasn't been easy.

I am doing ok.

I am fine but my gym subscription is still on hold.

I am not about to drop, you know.

I am not at my best.

I am still up and running, as you can see.

I can't say that I always feel up to it.

I've been a bit up and down recently (but currently up, now that I've seen you!).

I won't be running the (Wolverhampton) marathon just yet.

It can be a little uncomfortable.

It could have been better.

It's not the greatest of fun.

It's not without complications.

It won't be a gold in the Winter Olympics.

I've been a bit under the weather.

I've felt better.

They are taking good care of me.

They're fixing me slowly.

You have to look on the bright side. It'll soon be over.

The profusion of my obfuscatory responses came as a surprise even to me. They probably reflected my varying moods, but said little, if anything, about my health, although they seemed to satisfy, or even please my inquirers. It occurred to me that the effectiveness of the social therapeutic process depended not only on a resounding expression of good will and support from friends, neighbours and acquaintances, but on reassurance from patients that they were facing up courageously to their treatment and coping with it to the best of their ability. Anything less would have unbalanced the fulcrum of reciprocity on which all social therapy was based. Patients had to be seen to be optimistic, and to play a full and brave part in their own recovery. It was considered bad form to moan or complain unduly. On reflection, I concluded that this was a general cultural trait and not merely a 'man thing'.

The downside of positive thinking

It dawned on me that it went further than this. Personally and privately, I wanted to think objectively and base the evaluation of my bodily condition on facts. My moods and emotions would follow accordingly. I was never a fantasist. The unrelenting insistence on positive thinking, optimism under any circumstance, and the power of the will in determining outcomes, undermined patients' ability to project their true moods and feelings, to assess dispassionately their condition in the light of the medical evidence, and to reflect on the reality of their lack of control over the course of their cancer.

Worse, it was clear that some of my well-wishers - I hope a minority - really believed that positive thinking had a contribution to make in curing the cancer, or at least arresting its progress. I found the implications of their belief deeply troubling. By attributing agency to positive thinking or to the strength of my resolve to combat the cancer, any blame for the deterioration of my condition could be shifted away from the damaging effects of abnormal cell growth and onto my shoulders. I suppose it wasn't very different from blaming disease or death on a sinful life, or on my failure to believe in God and the power of prayer. But there was no scientific evidence to support the view that positive thinking (or for that matter, prayer) had any impact whatsoever on the outcome of a cancer diagnosis. That was why I was subjecting myself instead to a course of chemotherapy, for which evidence of efficacy did exist.

Industrial roots therapy

On Tuesday 13th February, the final day of the third cycle, I planned a break and a change of scenery to buoy me up. I arranged to meet my friend and former colleague, Anna, in the Jewellery Quarter in Birmingham. While on holiday in Myanmar, she had bought a ruby, and was having it set in a ring by Becka, a jewellery designer with a traditional workshop at 31 Hilton Street.

After collecting the fine-looking ruby ring, we paid a visit to the Birmingham Pen Museum at 60 Frederick Street. The collection of steel nibs, pens, and the various tools that were used to make them, were arranged to demonstrate the role that Birmingham factories played in the 19th century in supplying 75 per cent of the world's steel pens, the writing implements responsible for penning three quarters of all that was written at that time. In the late 19th century, there were a hundred pen factories in the Birmingham Jewellery Quarter, employing 8,000 people, 70 per cent of them women. The museum commemorated the names of the famous

Birmingham pen factory magnates, who pioneered the manufacture of steel pens: John Mitchell, Joseph Gillott and Josiah Mason, the last, a noteworthy philanthropist who built an orphanage and a technical college for the city.

One of the museum's current curators, who had donated his personal collection of nibs to the museum, explained the manufacturing process, bringing alive the harsh conditions of the lowly-paid women workers, with his detailed knowledge and enthusiasm. Anna and I learned a great deal from our visit. We speculated as to why the entrepreneurs of the 19th century had failed to invent or adapt to 20th century innovations, such as the typewriter, or Lásló Bíró's ball point pen. It related, we thought, to the division between share holders, who were prepared to settle on a steady return on their capital, and the factory managers left to oversee that return, but without the power or incentive to innovate and invest in new machinery. Bíró, we knew, had ended up, not in Birmingham, but in Buenos Aires, Argentina. We continued our conversation on political economy, in which we shared a common interest, over a lunch of fish and chips in the House of Fraser restaurant. Anna listened patiently and therapeutically as usual, as I did most of the talking.

My visit to Birmingham, the city of my birth and upbringing, did me a power of good. I continued to identify strongly with its industrial townscape, the railway, blue-brick-lined tunnels and cuttings, the canals with their hump-back bridges, the workshops of the Jewellery Quarter, the cast-iron Chamberlain Clock Tower, the Council House, the Museum and Art Gallery, the Art School, the Town Hall, St Philip's Cathedral, and Colmore Row and Corporation Street. My family was rooted there - three generations of Reeves on my father's side from 1892, and six generations of Fortey on my mother's from 1841.

With its intimation of mortality, my cancer diagnosis resulted in a greater awareness of my place in an historically and geographically-anchored family network, a stronger affection for the familiar local landscape, and a renewed appreciation of the security and tenacity that they continued collectively to afford me. The time I had spent exploring the Jewellery Quarter and my industrial roots had lightened my mood, made me more optimistic, and proved unexpectedly therapeutic.

Conscious of the therapeutic benefits of our earlier excursion, I met with Anna again on the 26th April, for a trip to the Black Country Living Museum in Dudley - 26 acres of former industrial land, studded with historical buildings, street furniture and other memorabilia, reassembled on that site from all over the Black Country. The museum's collection included houses, outbuildings, shops, workshops, a school, a chapel, wharves, canal bridges, narrow boats and trams. Having visited the museum on a number of occasions, I knew it was likely to give me a significant therapeutic boost.

Despite the bitterly-cold wind, Anna and I wandered the site, exploring the Newcomen Engine, the Providence Chapel, the Bottle and Glass Inn, the Anchor Forge, and the Rolling Mill, among others, to end up in the warmth of the Cradley Heath Workers' Institute, described in the guide as 'a monument to the struggle of the women chain makers of Cradley Heath' who, in 1910, had come out on strike for a living wage. They were led by the Scottish suffragist, Mary Macarthur (1880-1921), a committed trade unionist, who devoted her life to the struggle to improve conditions for women workers and to win them a living wage (in the case of the women chain makers, of $2\frac{1}{2}$d (1p) an hour for a 55 hour week). The appalling conditions and hardship brought a lump to my throat, while the fact that Mary Macarthur had died from cancer at the age of 40 upset me still further. (Her death was due not to breast cancer, as I first feared, but to cancer of the stomach.)

The visualisation and relaxation group for cancer patients

While waiting for line care on the Durnall Day Unit, I noticed a leaflet publicising the existence of a 'visualisation and relaxation group for cancer patients', arranged every fortnight by the hospital's Cancer Psychology and Counselling Service, to help patients feel more relaxed and less anxious, relieve their tensions and stress, and deal with any unhelpful thoughts they might have. Believing that I might benefit from being more relaxed, I planned to find out more by joining the group on the 13th April, day 5 of my fifth chemotherapy cycle, but at that stage felt so tired and ill that after visiting the hospital for line care, I went home instead to lie down. Two weeks later on the 27th April, I was feeling much better and turned up at the right place and time along with three other cancer patients. The Friday-morning meeting, held in a first-floor room next to the Deanesly Ward, was scheduled to last for $1\frac{1}{2}$ hours but continued for an extra 20 minutes, as patients appreciated the session and were reluctant to leave.

The group was facilitated by the vivacious *Columbine Cornwallis*, a member of the hospital counselling team, a friendly, warm, and compassionate woman, thoroughly expert at putting her patients at ease and drawing the best out of them. To prepare the room, she removed a scarf from her neck and spread it on the table in front of us. The brightly-coloured cloth was decorated with a peacock motif. She produced an amethyst crystal candle holder, lit a candle, and placed it at the centre of her improvised table cloth, the overall effect enhanced by the amethyst pendant that dangled from her neck. *Columbine* began by engaging her four patients in a 'relaxation exercise'.

We were told to sit casually with eyes closed, loose shoulders, loose hands, loose feet, and to listen to the sounds inside and outside the room. *Columbine*'s voice was calming and soothing, but all other noise was drowned out by the whirring of an extractor fan. Nevertheless, I found myself very rested, at ease, and barely awake.

Each of us was then given a picture of outline human figures in a tree, climbing or perched in varying postures, and asked to select and identify with one of them. Was I climbing, falling, holding, hanging on, or helping others? No. Bizarrely, I saw myself with a chain saw, cutting away at the trunk (an image derived I believe from the recent visit of a tree surgeon to lop the beech in our garden). Needless to say, other group members envisaged their arboreal existence differently.

Columbine asked us next to introduce ourselves and explain our reasons for attending the session, which triggered a spontaneous outpouring of personal information about our respective cancers, our treatments, prognoses and circumstances. Simultaneously, we identified our own reactions, hopes and fears in the responses of our fellow patients, and derived solace and comfort from the dialogue. Recognising the burst of empathic emotion, and the benefit of the ongoing bonding, *Columbine* intervened subtly to draw out the traits and the themes that her four cancer patients shared in common, and allowed the discussion to occupy much of the session.

In conclusion, she moved on to a 'visualisation exercise', described in the leaflet as 'a form of relaxation' using 'the power of imagination'. We were encouraged to sit at ease with our eyes closed, while *Columbine*'s gentle voice guided us on an imaginary pastoral journey through an ideal landscape. We emerged from woodland into a bright meadow of wild flowers. We wandered, ever onwards, through dunes to a sandy shoreline lapped by the deep blue ocean. We peered into rock pools and explored caves concealing hidden treasure. We picnicked on the beach and walked back in rapture the way we had come. *Columbine* brought us back gradually from our shared Shangri-La to the reality of the Deanesly Cancer Centre and our current bodily afflictions. We speculated as to what part of the country her visualisation had been based. She admitted that she had derived much of her imagery from the Cornish landscape. I recognised immediately that visualisation afforded endless opportunity for escapist fantasies, well beyond *Poldark* and Ross and Demelza's Cornish adventures. I hastily averted my gaze from the amethyst pendant. Visualisation was merely a scholarly approach to Walter Mitty's 'fantastic daydreams of personal triumphs'.

The lesson to be learned was that the deliberate recollection of an event or location associated with freedom and happiness could serve as an effective distraction from the pain, distress and worry of cancer. I realised as I left the hospital that I had gained comfort from the visualisation and relaxation group, but not so much from the actual visualisation and relaxation exercises (which, nevertheless, I had found useful and instructive), as from the frank, honest and heart-to-heart conversations I had had with my fellow cancer patients - what turned out to be a successful group therapy session, so ably facilitated by *Columbine*, a hospital counsellor.

Two weeks later on the 11th May, day 12 of my sixth cycle, I attended a further session of the visualisation and relaxation group led by *Charles Ridley*, a clinical psychologist working with the New Cross Cancer Psychology Service. On that occasion, four cancer patients turned up, three of us - Rod, Veronica[1], and me - from the previous group. The session followed much the same pattern as before, with relaxation and visualisation exercises and time for a group discussion, but with the addition of a 'body-map exercise'. Body mapping involved marking where we experienced psychosomatic sensations, for example, neck pains, shoulder tension, nervous breathlessness, and sinking feelings in the pit of the stomach, on a picture of the body, , It was obvious to me that what we all enjoyed most was the discussion and sharing of our cancer experiences and treatment, in other words, the chance of a group therapy session.

The nature of therapy

What, indeed, is therapy and what is it meant to do? I was aware that the ancient Greeks saw it as treating persons to restore them to mental or physical health, in a civilisation that accepted the principle of the unity of mind and body. The problem with deriving the meaning of therapy solely from Greek is that, since the late-19th century, the word has become inextricably associated with psychotherapy and its less intimidating offspring, counselling. As such, it carries with it the baggage of well over a century of professional and institutional practice and malpractice, including well-documented instances of socially-sanctioned abuse.

Psychotherapists and counsellors have, for example, been variously accused of:

creating a multi-million-dollar business profiting from other people's misery,

misusing the power and authority of their role and profession to impose their values on clients, deny the authenticity of their accounts, and distort their reality.

accepting implicitly the status quo, and displaying a singular lack of interest in social justice.

rarely ever treating clients' problems as a natural consequence of their broader economic or social environment, but as arising from personality defects or the pathology of an individual's choices, experiences, or intimate family relations.

claiming professional skills, expertise and beneficial outcomes that have never been subject to rigorous scientific testing and evaluation, thus revealing psychotherapeutic practices to be no better than quackery.[2]

Therapy and power

Some critics go so far as to claim that the therapeutic relationship always entails an imbalance of power, and that even when therapy is undertaken voluntarily, it results in some form of emotional and mental coercion.[1] In the case of contemporary established therapies on offer from outside agencies, therapeutic transactions raise questions of why and how people undertake the treatment of others, and why and how people end up being treated, and which party to the therapy benefits, or loses, more from the outcome. The key is understanding the power dynamic: who is in charge, who has the authority, is the therapy being used to manipulate, control, or determine the outcome, to what purpose, and in whose interests? (For instance, I signed up voluntarily to 'mindfulness' but, throughout the course, felt that a spurious philosophy of dualism (a complete separation of mind and body) and an insistence on the superior benefits of 'living in the moment' were being imposed on me, without allowing me an opportunity to question those assumptions.)

However, a complementary, psychological, or self-help therapy may be developed and practised by an individual without the help of others (as in the case of my industrial history, or Baby Caio therapies). More commonly, in the context of cancer treatment, a therapy may be offered to patients by approved practitioners (as with the visualisation and relaxation group), in which case the question of the practitioner's power and ideology can always be raised. What are they up to and why? The mindfulness course was marketed and run for the general public by *Mindspan*, a private agency, but I had a good idea of what to expect.

A therapy for me was any activity that made me, as a chemotherapy patient, feel better by stimulating my interests and occupying my thoughts with prospects other than the side effects and anxiety caused by my illness and treatment. Having spontaneously stumbled on the power of industrial history as a therapy for myself, it occurred to me that current popular or fashionable lists of therapies and psychotherapies were incomplete, focussed unduly on middle-class leisure pursuits, and had been largely devised and marketed for women, whom I assumed, were also their main participants.

Complementary therapies

At the hospital, the oncology and clinical haematology department advertised a series of complementary therapies, available on the NHS. They included aromatherapy, reiki (an ancient Japanese energy-based treatment undertaken by the laying on of hands), reflexology, and Indian head massage. Classed as 'complementary' because they were offered in addition, but not as an alternative, to medical treatment, they were aimed at improving the quality of sleep, reducing nausea, pain, anxiety, stress and depression, and getting patients to feel better and more relaxed.[3] For most people, I guessed, they succeeded because they shared in common the social relational and purposeful activity of other psychotherapies, yet to me they sounded to be mumbo-jumbo.

As a man, I was not instantly drawn to many or most of the recognised physio- or psycho-therapies I saw advertised, such as aroma, art, colonic, crystal, dance, detox, dietary, drama, herbal, hydro, inner relationship, manicure, massage, mindfulness, mud, music, pedicure, person-centred, play, poetry or spa (although I had experienced for myself the seduction of retail therapy, characterised as a female weakness, but indulged in by both men and women).

Therapies for men?

Some therapies, such as behavioural, contemplative, family, group, or relationship therapies, were more general or abstract in scope and might appeal equally to men and women, depending on their content. But what mentally stimulating, pleasurable, entertaining, mood improving, or distractive therapies might prove more appealing and effective for men with cancer, like me?

By focussing on my own interests and those of my male friends, it took me less than ten minutes to compile a list of thirty alternative therapies: angling and fishing, antiques, astronomy and science-related, car and car-driving, card-playing, collector, conservation project and ecologically-related, cross-word puzzle, cycling and spin, digital and computer apps., gadget, gaming, gardening and horticultural, gym, hobby, horse racing and book-maker, industrial history and archaeology, machine-repairs and engineering, martial arts and boxing, painting and decorating, political interest and involvement, sports and sport-spectator, stocks and shares (shadowing), swimming, sudoku and number, television programme appreciation, films, vegetable growing, walking and rambling, weight-lifting, whisky-appreciation. (Many of these - for example, cycling, gardening, or walking - would also appeal to women but, as far as I could ascertain, few if any were being marketed as therapies for either sex.) The number of popular and enjoyable pastimes that could be pursued as therapies, or in a therapeutic fashion, was simply immense. Indeed, most hobbies could easily be re-construed or reconceived as therapies.

Nevertheless, many of the activities listed above might have to be avoided or restricted after an operation, or to reduce the risk of infection following chemotherapy. In my case, I was advised to suspend my gym membership and to stop swimming during the course of my treatment. In reality, of course, my feelings of weakness and physical fatigue de-motivated me, and transformed the prospect of the more physically-demanding therapies into phobias. When experiencing the very worst side effects, I really did not want to do, nor was capable of doing, anything.

Holiday therapy

When Patrick Finucane, a friend from my schooldays, travelled from Kent to visit us for three days in the third cycle, the three of us embarked on a plan, aimed largely, I believe, at raising my spirits and aiding my recovery. We talked of taking a holiday in Ireland in September 2018, twelve months after my cancer diagnosis, when I had completed the chemo and radiotherapy, and once I had had time to recover from their side effects. Ireland was chosen because of Patrick's Irish heritage and his vast knowledge of and interest in Irish history, and because it was geographically close, which would allow us to return home easily if anything went amiss.

Patrick and Mel decided on provisional dates and travel arrangements. Patrick traced out a possible route on a large Ireland touring map. I was delighted at their initiative and at the prospect of spending a holiday in Ireland under the guidance of my well-informed and historically-erudite friend. This, again, constituted another form of therapy, devised deliberately for my benefit and recuperation.

My kind of therapy

The satisfaction I derived from Patrick's visit, together with my previous excursion with Anna, made me reflect once more on the essence of therapy or, more precisely, the most suitable psychotherapy for me to pursue during the course of my treatment. I knew it was the chemotherapy that made me feel tired and unwell and so was not expecting to discover a therapy that worked along medical lines to relieve the unpleasant side effects and make my body feel better. Rather, I had come to see therapy in humanistic terms, as establishing a stimulating social environment in which I could engage in worthwhile activities by myself, or with others, thus providing me with projects, purpose, and hope.

It was obvious to me that my kind of therapy had two essential features: (1) an intellectually-invigorating activity that (2) was undertaken in the company and with the support and encouragement of like-minded others – preferably family members, or enduring friends, such as Patrick and Anna.

George Monbiot and the the beneficial effects of community

On the same day that I wrote this, I read an article by George Monbiot in *The Guardian* (21st February 2018) reporting on research on the Somerset town of Frome (published in *Resurgence & Ecologist*).[4] It found that when isolated people with health problems were supported by community groups and volunteers, emergency admissions to hospital fell dramatically. Illness reduced people's opportunity to mix socially, which led in turn to isolation and loneliness, which made their condition worse. Other research showed that people without social connections were more prone to inflammation, while those who were thoroughly imbedded in the local community had a much better chance of survival. Monbiot concluded that, on the basis of this evidence, 'social contact should be on prescription'. I was left thinking that if the therapies available on the NHS had been developed on the basis of a social or community model, rather than on a psychology-derived one-to-one or small group basis, they might have been more effective and would have appealed to a greater number of patients.

Excluded by pink ribbon?

But many of the smaller group therapies –especially those aimed at breast cancer patients – had not been devised with people like me in mind, which I found entirely understandable and justifiable given the rarity of my complaint. Nevertheless, the predictable consequence was that advertisements for their services were not directed at me and, indeed, could well be interpreted as excluding me.

For example, at the Deanesly Centre, a pink leaflet, carrying the pink ribbon logo of breast cancer awareness, advertised the services of the Wolverhampton and District Breast Cancer Action Group, which aimed to provide its members with the opportunity to share experiences, learn from each other, and give and receive help. Inviting breast cancer patients to join, the charity claimed to be 'a friendly group of women, who also enjoy some social outings together'. To improve breast cancer services, the group had campaigned for counselling and complementary therapies 'to help women through their cancer journey'.[5] Recognising the value of their fund-raising work, as well as the name of one of the leading lights in the organisation, I knew that, were I to phone the contact number, I would be offered a sympathetic ear, but was reluctant to do so. A breast cancer group centred exclusively on women had its own intrinsic intimacies , merits and strengths.

George Monbiot's prostate cancer

Three weeks later on the 13th March, another article by George Monbiot appeared in *The Guardian*, entitled 'I have prostate cancer. But I am happy.'[6] From writing detachedly about the role of the community in the treatment of cancer, the author now gave a graphic account of his recent diagnosis with prostate cancer and the dangerous radical surgery he was about to undergo. His claim to be happy, he said, was supported by his adoption of three principles:

- Imagine how much worse it could be, rather than how much better (or in the words of the proverb, "cheer up, it could be worse").
- Change what can be changed, but accept what cannot (for sometimes an obstacle is insuperable and has to be accepted as such).
- Never let fear rule your life (for "fear hems us in, stops us from thinking clearly and prevents us from either challenging oppression or engaging calmly with the impersonal fates").

Monbiot made no apology for describing the grisly details of his condition because the more familiar they became, the less horrifying. He wanted to 'socialise' his condition, in the knowledge that, last month, he 'discussed the remarkable evidence that a caring community enhances recovery and reduces mortality': "In talking about my cancer with family and friends, I feel the love that I know will get me through this. The old strategy of suffering in silence could not have been more misguided".[4] I had reached exactly the same conclusion from my own personal experience.

Monbiot went on to point out that prostate cancer had overtaken breast cancer to rank as the UK's third highest 'cancer killer'. Because the standard PSA blood test for cancer was now considered to be of limited use, he urged support for Prostate Cancer UK's campaign to develop a better test. He believed "breast cancer has attracted twice as much money and research as prostate cancer, not because (as the *Daily Mail* suggested) men are the victims of injustice, but because women's advocacy has been so effective".[6]

I considered that his personal stance towards his cancer mirrored my own stoicism, but he had expressed it so much more succinctly than I - the mark of a very committed and capable journalist! I, too, shared his preference for collective social action as a means of tackling ill-health and as an alternative to psychologically-based individual self-help programmes. Monbiot, I was sure, was familiar with the association between mental health and poverty, highlighted, for example, in recent research sponsored by the Joseph Rowntree Foundation.[7] There was convincing evidence to show that mental ill-health, in the form of anxiety, depression, and suicidal thoughts, was shaped by the social, economic and political environment which impacted unequally on various categories of people, such as those on low incomes, adults who had experienced domestic violence or abuse, the homeless, or isolated older people.[6]

For me, this meant that for most ordinary people, their states of mind, especially their moods - their levels of fear, anxiety, stress, depression, optimism, energy and motivation - were intimately and predictably related to the reality of their immediate personal circumstances. If they were exposed to an incident that was painful or frightening, they would quite properly experience pain or fright.

Seeking relief through therapy: a personal quest

Nevertheless, the psychological self-help hypothesis continued to fascinate me. Was it possible to train myself to adopt a personal strategy of mind, or psychological technique to reduce, or avoid, my customary responses to some of the distressing circumstances I found myself in? The thought of the misery brought about by my third-cycle thrombo-phlebitis and fourth-cycle docetaxel side-effects spurred me to find an answer. In search of information, I went online, first to the macmillan.org.uk and then to cancerresearch.uk.org websites.

Macmillan made a distinction between two kinds of therapy: complementary, on the one hand, and psychological and self-help, on the other. Already sceptical of the former, I turned to the latter, to be told that 'many people use psychological and self-help therapies as a source of support during and after their treatment'. Macmillan was particularly keen on the efficacy of sharing thoughts and feelings by means of cancer support groups and self-help groups. But it also named two other therapies, both starting with the enigmatic term 'mindfulness'.[8]

'Mindfulness meditation', Macmillan explained, was a therapy "that aims to help you change negative thoughts to more positive ones". Mindfulness therapists used various techniques to change patients' thought patterns in order to reduce stress and anxiety. They brought about that change by using meditation and breathing techniques to focus patients' attention on 'the present moment'.[8]

In addition, there were mindfulness specialities with more refined psychologically-sounding names, such as mindfulness-based cognitive therapy (MBCT), and mindfulness-based stress reduction (MBSR). They aimed to change thought patterns through meditation, yoga and breathing, by focusing on 'here and now' difficulties to change the individual's current state of mind, so thoughts became more positive.[8]

Meditation

The Cancer Research UK website focused on meditation as a means of improving the health, wellbeing, and feelings of people with cancer.[9] Meditation could assist in calming and relaxing the mind and body. It could reduce anxiety and stress and help control problems such as pain, sleeplessness, tiredness, feelings of nausea, and high blood pressure. According to Cancer Research, there were many different types of meditation, most of them involving being still and quiet, but some, such as tai chi, chi gong, and walking meditation, that entailed movement. Seven forms were listed in the following order: mindfulness meditation, mindfulness-based stress reduction (MBSR), focused meditation, visualisation and guided imagery, transcendental meditation, prayerful meditation, and meditation and movement.[9] That mysterious word, 'mindfulness', kept reappearing. Could it be what I was looking for?

Mindfulness

Curious to discover more, I googled 'mindfulness'. Wikipedia told me it was 'the psychological process of bringing one's attention to experiences occurring in the present moment'. Derived originally from Buddhist teaching and meditation techniques, its modern manifestations had been developed in the West by John Kabat-Zinn, an American academic and founder of the Stress Reduction Clinic and Centre for Mindfulness at the University of Massachusetts.[10]

Kabat-Zinn's best-selling books included: *Wherever You Go, There You Are: Mindfulness Meditation in Everyday Life; Mindfulness for Beginners: Reclaiming the Present Moment and Your Life;* and *Guided Mindfulness Meditation: A Complete Guided Mindfulness Meditation Programme.* It was widely believed that his purposely-developed techniques, involving meditation and mind exercises, were effective in reducing the anxiety and stress that were thought to exacerbate and cause much mental distress and illness. Kabat-

Zinn's stress reduction programme was referred to as 'mindfulness-based stress reduction' or 'MBSR'.[11]

Further reading informed me that mindfulness involved mental exercises to help me live in the moment, rather than to spend time thinking about what had already happened in the past, or what was about to happen in future. It was about fully experiencing today's sensations in the present, and not ignoring them in favour of yesterday's memories, or tomorrow's anticipations. It required me to concentrate on my breathing and bodily senses of seeing, hearing, feeling, smelling and tasting. It meant enhancing my ability to pay attention to what was happening to me in the current moment and stopping my mind from wandering. I needed to master my mind – being 'mindful' – to avoid letting it fritter itself away in 'mindless' meandering. I had to be non-judgmental and less critical of the circumstances and conditions I faced – noticing and becoming more aware of my experiences, rather than evaluating or proscribing them.

My life span was limited and ebbing away by the moment. Yet I spent most of my time thinking regretfully or nostalgically about past events, or speculating, planning or worrying about what was going to happen to me in the future. It would be far better to concentrate my efforts instead on living a fuller and richer life in the experiential stream of my current consciousness, in the heightened awareness of the present moment. In so doing, so the theory went, the practice of mindfulness had the capacity to diminish the impact of stressful thoughts and feelings and promote balance and tranquillity.

My initial assessment of mindfulness in relation to chemotherapy

Did the practice of mindfulness have the potential to reduce or avoid the pain or distress of the chemotherapy I was currently undergoing? In as far as I had grasped its principles (at this stage, I accepted my reading and understanding could only be superficial), I remained highly sceptical, especially of any application that I could conceive for the alleviation of the pain and distress caused by the chemotherapy's side effects. For example, it struck me that the common practice of distractive therapy, employed by phlebotomists, nurses and other medical personnel, was aimed especially at mitigating the pain of the moment, by forcing patients to think of holidays they had taken or were about to take, or of family events – grandchildren or ruby weddings, perhaps. Were not the visualisation techniques practised by the hospital's counselling team based on the same principle - deliberately fixing the mind on vivid images from the past? Similarly, on each occasion that the nurse injected the chemotherapy drugs, I had deliberately chosen to engross myself in a book and to do my best to avoid thinking about the immediate sensations in my arm and veins. Indeed, the most effective technique that I had discovered for coping with chemo was to tick off the cycles and think of the time when the course would be completed. Why, when I was currently going through such an unpleasant patch would I wish to dwell on it, rather than choose to contemplate a far more pleasurable past or future?

If this critique of mindfulness's preoccupation with the daunting present in preference to a more comforting past or reassuring future was so obvious to me, had I totally misunderstood the theory and practice on which it was based? I came to the conclusion that the only way to find out more and to put mindfulness's psycho-therapeutic claims to the test was to enrol myself on a mindfulness course.

Enrolment on a mindfulness course

I found an eight-week beginner course – "Mindful – increase focus, reduce stress'- located a mile or so from our house at the Newman Centre in Tettenhall, paid the fee and duly enrolled, with the first session scheduled in April. I would learn mindfulness meditation in eight one-hour sessions, entitled: mindful listening, mindful body, mindful breathing, mindful mind, mindful movements, mindful eating, mindful sleep, and mindful heart.[12]

On Wednesday evening, the 18th April (day 10 of the fifth chemo cycle, I attended my mindfulness class, entitled 'mindful listening', the first in the eight-week beginner course, held at the Newman Centre in Tettenhall. (Should mindfulness have a beginner course implying, as it must, the focus of the mind on a further course in the future, with attendant anxieties about progression?) While I arrived early, the car park was already full, and there was a queue of people at the door, waiting to enrol. As I had already registered and paid in advance, my name was ticked on the list and I entered the hall along with other students and sat on one of the flimsy plastic chairs, already set out in rows. At the scheduled 7.30 pm starting time, 55 students had assembled, joined afterwards by a further 3 late-comers, making a total of 58, of whom four fifths were women. Most people, I judged, were aged between 40 and 60, and I may have been one of the oldest.

The tutor - or class leader - was *Aaron Dharma*, the founder of *Mindspan* who, according to the course flyer, had once been a Buddhist monk. He had practised and taught mindfulness meditation for over 25 years and, judging from the number and locations of classes advertised, the size of our group, and the fee being charged (a £9 fee on the night), his mindfulness teaching was earning him a very good income. For most of the hour, he addressed the group as a whole.

Aaron told us he had been teaching mindfulness since 1996 but had written the particular course we were taking in 2016. He had a face with a smile and a soothing relaxing voice, and spent time reassuring his audience that his course was for everyone, and would not involve having to stand up and say, "My name is Alan and I am stressed out". The class would not take the form of a group therapy session. One of the advantages of the group's size was that people could choose to conceal themselves in the crowd.

The aim of the class, he explained, was to reduce personal stress and anxiety, by learning to live in the moment - the present. Being mindful was a non-judgmental awareness of the present, because most stress and anxiety arose from worrying about what might happen in the future. Our problems could be sorted out simply by bringing our attention into the present moment. We needed to train our minds and take responsibility for our own mental health. We could prevent our minds wandering, and bring them back into the room along with our bodies. At least, that is what I thought he said. I found his stream of assumptions difficult to accept unchallenged, but my philosophical insistence on reason, and rejection of his preposterous dualism, had no place in the context of the mindfulness class, where many held on to his every word.

Towards the end of his lengthy monologue, two occasions were provided for student participation. We were expected to improve our listening skills by pairing with a person sitting next to us and talking for two minutes about ourselves, while our partner listened. We then had to swap roles and to listen to our partner. I paired with a lively good-natured woman called *Tessa*, aged 41, who worked for a housing association in Walsall. I found our conversation the most enjoyable and stimulating part of the class. The idea, I assumed, was that the very act of listening carefully forced the listener to focus exclusively on the moment.

Another exercise involved the whole class sitting in silence and listening to background noises, which certainly had a relaxing and settling effect on me, for I almost fell asleep - or was that the fatigue of the chemo?

Over supper, Mel asked me how I'd got on. I told her that I had found the listening exercise instructive and would be listening to her more attentively in future. I recalled using exactly the same listening exercise with my own class of students some fifty years previously.

Mindful body

One week later on the 25th April, I returned for the second class entitled 'mindful body: learning to live in the moment'. This time 54 people turned up. Sitting in front of us on the platform, *Aaron* declared that the human mind was "naturally distracted", and urged us to listen to the sounds inside and outside our bodies, and bring our minds back into the room again. We must sit in comfortable posture, allowing our hands to loosen, closing our eyes if we chose and, by listening to the sounds around us, bring our attention into the room. All I could think about was the discomfort of the plastic chair, digging into my thighs and back. *Aaron* asked that we connect moment by moment with the sounds of the present, not allowing our thoughts to rush forward or stay stuck in the past.

Outside, I could hear the sounds of the traffic and bird song, and inside, coughing, audible peristalsis and worse.

Aaron congratulated us on completing the exercise, telling us that "keeping a happy mind is the kindest thing we can do for ourselves". We should realise that we had everything we needed learn to appreciate it. This week, we were going to use our bodies to live in the moment, for "if we can have a mindful relationship with our body, we can be happy".

He used the rest of the session to instruct us in mindfulness practices, the chief of which he labelled "mindful standing" (when we were shown how to relax in a standing position), "mindful hands" (resting our hands in our lap and concentrating on their rising and falling as we breathed in and out), and "mindful body scan" (when we focussed on the sensations in the parts of our body, working down from the head to the feet). Irrespective of their dimension of mindfulness, I found some of these meditative and yogic-like exercises very relaxing and might have dropped off to sleep, if not for the discomfort of the plastic chair. Our homework was to practise these mindful techniques and to persuade our family and friends of their beneficial effects.

Mindful breathing

My third mindfulness class on mindful breathing was held on the 2nd May, day 3 of my sixth chemotherapy cycle. I was tired, but relaxed and by no means incapacitated, as I entered the Newman Centre to join the class, now 46 strong in number. We were introduced to "the world of breath", as *Aaron Dharma*, our tutor put it, and "you'll be on cloud 9 by the time you're through". The third class, in the main, consisted of his usual light-hearted monologue and three meditation exercises, each lasting about 7 to 15 minutes:

starting with a 'mindful body scan' (as practised last week) and progressing to 'the natural breath' and 'mindful breath counting'. The stimulus of the steroids was wearing off on me and, perhaps because of that, I found the breathing exercises remarkably relaxing.

Aaron repeated the wise words of the Buddha on breathing as he sat in the shade under a bodhi tree in northern India: "If your breath is long, focus on it; if your breath is short, focus on it", which was explained as meaning "if you are breathing deeply, continue to breathe deeply; if you are breathing shallowly, continue to breathe shallowly". The "natural breath" was all-important, in contrast to instructions to "stop and breathe deeply". We had to become "at one with the flow" of our breathing. Breathing was important, hence the expression, "take a breather", when we exerted ourselves. As befitting a former Buddhist monk, *Aaron* had a great deal of respect for the Buddha, Siddhattha Gotama - 'the one who has achieved his aim'. I was aware that the Buddha had founded a religion that was primarily concerned with releasing the individual from discontentment and suffering but, under my current circumstances, was yet to be convinced that he could do more for my pain relief and breast cancer than paracetamol, or the NHS,

Aaron recounted how Thich Nhat Hanh, a Vietnamese Zen-Buddhist monk, had visited Birmingham in the 1990s, telling his listeners about 'the mindful bell', or gong, which was rung across the Vietnamese countryside to remind the monks and the people not to be distracted by thoughts of bodily need, and to bring their thoughts back to the moment. *Aaron* suggested that in modern-day Britain, the ringing of one's smart phone could be used to the same effect: "turn your phone into a mindful bell". Before responding to the phone or firing off an email, "take a few breaths - get emotionally ready through breathing".

All well and good, but for me the mindfulness add-ons were beginning to jar. Why if your mind wanders, should you insist on dragging it back "into the present moment", or "into the room"? At that point, I realised that *Aaron Dharma* was the dog walker and I was the dog, straining at the leash in pursuit of my own freedom of thought. He also kept telling us that the average human attention span was three minutes. In my case, I knew I couldn't be average. By the end of his class, I had been listening with critical attention to him for more than an hour.

Mindful mind

The fourth class on the 9th May took much the same form as the previous three, this time including a 'smiling Buddha' breathing exercise, a 'just sitting' meditation, and various 'thought watching' and 'simplification of daily life' practices. As before, I felt relaxed and would have fallen asleep, if some of *Aaron's* monologue had not simulated my critical capacity. What sense was I to make of *Aaron's* instructions to 'sit and do nothing' and to 'watch thoughts'? According to him, the former might be challenging, if I were used (as I was) to doing things and ticking them off on a mental list as soon as I completed them. Instead, I should spend time "being", that is, "being in the moment", "abiding in the present moment", just sitting, watching and welcoming my thoughts as they came and went. As a person who gains fulfilment and a sense of achievement from completing the tasks that I set for myself, I judged *Aaron's* exercise in doing nothing or, from my perspective, of letting my tasks accumulate and overwhelm me, not as a means of relaxation, but as way of encouraging idleness, which would result in the frustration, agitation and stress I sought to avoid.

The important point to make here is that I plan my work load beforehand and make sure that my list of jobs is manageable, the very opposite of tackling my tasks by dealing with them only in the moment. Anticipation and planning ahead are key human facilities essential to survival and civilisation, necessary for chess players, architects, generals, breast-cancer surgeons, oncologists, and radiotherapists, alike. In my book, stress and anxiety are caused by inadequate preparation. Only monks, nuns, tramps, prisoners, patients stranded in hospital waiting rooms, and the terminally ill can afford to live in the moment. Mindfulness therapists (or philosophers) can sit and interpret the world to their heart's content, but my satisfaction and well-being derive from engaging, controlling and determining my situation, which would include active participation in any cancer recovery plan.

Having dwelt on the subject for nigh on 3,000 words and becoming increasingly dissatisfied, I will spare the reader any further account of my mindfulness course, which continued along much the same lines for another four classes (mindful movement, eating, sleep, and heart). While I felt I had benefited from some of its constituent parts, such as the yoga, meditation, relaxation and visualisation, I was convinced that mindfulness by itself was unlikely to improve by one iota my current personal circumstances or state of mind. That is not to say that others, less critical than I, might not find it of benefit to them. Indeed, on a number of occasions, I overheard fellow students telling each other how much they were helped by the classes and had been using the techniques they had been taught in their everyday lives. Not for me. While I could see the relaxation exercises had value, the mindfulness gobbledegook about living in the moment was of no use whatsoever in alleviating the pain, distress and anxiety brought about by the chemotherapy.

Music and earfulness

On reading a draft of this chapter, our friend, Geoff Hurd, told me I had spent far too many words on the topic of mindfulness, and recommended an alternative therapy that worked for him. When he was stressed, he turned to the music of Johann Sebastian Bach. He brought round a CD and played me some of Bach's mathematically-constructed but soothing compositions. I found that baroque music therapy of the early 18th century both agreeable and relaxing, but was aware that I was more of a Miles Davis man and that I, personally, would prefer listening to *Kind of Blue*.

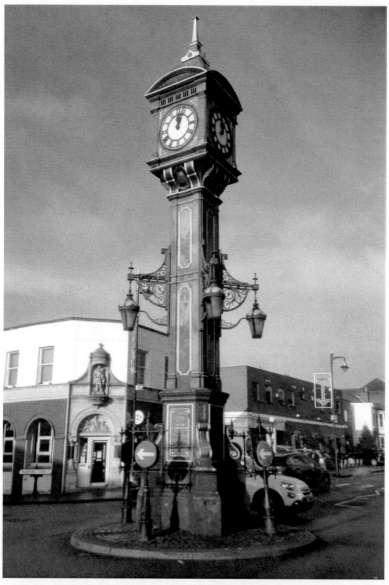

Industrial history therapy, Chamberlain Clock (1903),
Jewellery Quarter, Birmingham

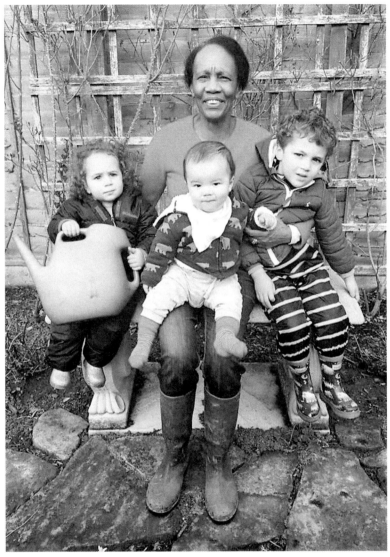

Grandchildren therapy, Mel with Genevieve, Caio and Maximus

Chapter 13

Sixth chemotherapy cycle

Following the blood samples taken on the morning of the 27th April, I was telephoned in the afternoon by *Sister Jemima Holyoak* at the Snowdrop Chemotherapy Suite to tell me the result of my blood count. The neutrophil reading had come back unexpectedly low, with a figure of 2.8, under the minimum of 3.0 considered safe for a further session of chemotherapy. I was asked to turn up at Snowdrop at 8.30 am on Monday 30th April to repeat the blood test, prior to my scheduled docetaxel infusion that day at 10 am. I found it difficult to live with the prospect of further delay and was desperate for the sixth cycle to proceed on time. Mel and my daughter, Toussaint, reminded me of a similar occasion before my fifth cycle, and the rapid recovery of my neutrophil level in just three days.

On Sunday the 29th April, I prepared for my final session of chemotherapy by taking the prescribed dexamethasone steroids – four soluble tablets in the morning, and four in the afternoon, knowing the preparation would be wasted if the chemotherapy was delayed.

Day 1 (Monday 30th April 2018)

On Monday, Mel and I woke early for my 8.30 am appointment on the Snowdrop Suite. I took a further four dexamethasone tablets with my breakfast. Mel drove me to the hospital. We kept thinking about what the neutrophil test would reveal. Soon after we arrived at Snowdrop, we were taken by *Nurse Michelle McLean* to a chair on the u-shaped ward where my blood sample was taken from the Hickman line and sent for analysis. About 15 minutes later, the result came back showing, to our immense relief, that my neutrophil count had risen to an acceptable level, allowing my sixth and final chemotherapy session to go full-steam ahead..

Sixth session of chemotherapy at the Snowdrop Millennium Suite

At about 9.15 am, *Nurse Michelle McLean*, connected my Hickman line to a bag of saline on the drip stand, replacing it, when it had gone through, with an infusion of anti-emetic. When the alarm bell went on the drip stand, another nurse, who had not treated us before, came over to see that all was well. *Nurse McLean* soon returned and prepared to give me the black-bagged docetaxel infusion, but not before attaching my arm, as before, to the sphygmomanometer to warn her in case I showed signs of an allergic reaction during the treatment.

As the docetaxil infusion was due to last for around an hour, I turned to my latest read, *The King's Revenge* (about the manhunt and violent retribution Charles II exacted from the men who had signed his father's death warrant), while Mel took up her sudoku challenge. I scarcely noticed the time as the docetaxil emptied through my Hickman line and into my vein and heart. Mel kept a watchful eye on the liquid visible at the bottom of the bag. Once the bag had emptied, further saline and heparin were given before *Nurse McLean* taped my Hickman line carefully back onto my chest.

As this was the last and sixth session of my chemotherapy treatment, I felt in a celebratory mood and congratulated *Michelle* on helping me all the way to completion. I had brought a box of chocolates to share with everyone on the team and gave it to *Michelle* to smuggle to the reception desk. I asked her to make sure she saved a few for herself, but she told me she did not eat chocolates. Neither, unfortunately, did *Sister Jemima Holyoak*, another of the chemotherapy nurses who had treated me.

As we had arrived and started early on Snowdrop, we left the hospital around 12.00 noon and went shopping – perhaps in my case, 'retail therapy' to celebrate my final chemo session – starting at Bentley Bridge and gravitating later to Wolverhampton. By the time we arrived home, four more dexamethasone tablets were due, which I drank down with water and ginger biscuits. Still firing on steroids, I went into the garden to edge and tidy the lawn. After supper, we watched *The Woman in White* by Wilkie Collins, and the news. Before we went to bed, Mel gave me my enoxaparin injections.

I slept relatively well until 1.30 am when I was woken by severe indigestion and heartburn and a prolonged bout of hiccups. Thereafter, I was woken every half hour by fits of belching and hiccups. In discomfort and unable to sleep, I went downstairs and sipped at a cup of hot water and read at the kitchen table in the hope that the upright position would afford relief.

On returning to bed, I tried out a mindfulness exercise – mindful listening – to help me to relax and sleep. While listening to the sounds inside and outside of me, I became alarmed by the din of the dawn chorus, which started at 4.50 am, and became louder and louder, overwhelming the faint noise from the bed of Mel's gentle breathing. By then I was tired and even the occasional burp and belch could not prevent me from sleeping, until the radio alarm woke us with John Humphry's voice on the *Today* programme.

Day 2 (Tuesday 1ˢᵗ May)

May Day! I woke with a relatively low temperature of 36.5c, a slight headache, a feeling of the onset of constipation, and a continuing but lessening indigestion. Mel made cornmeal porridge which I consumed with two prunes and a date, a paracetamol capsule, a lansoprazole 30mg gastro-resistant capsule, and the scheduled four 2mg soluble tablets of dexamethasone, in the hope that, in combination, they might relieve some, or all, of my miserable symptoms.

Mel left to attend Norman Davis's funeral service at St Leonard's in Bilston, held there and then, appropriately, as he had represented a Bilston ward as a Labour Councillor and the funeral had been arranged for the 1ˢᵗ May – International Labour Day. Pat MacFadden, the MP for Wolverhampton South East, gave the oration. Mel explained the reason for my non-attendance to Mary, his widow, and Councillors Roger Lawrence and Pete Bilson, friends of ours in the Labour Party. I vividly recalled the last time I had seen Norman alive, when he called out my name from his hospital trolley.

A male friend asked me today in a roundabout way about the impact that my cancer and chemo had had on my sex life. I felt flattered at first, until I recalled that Silvio Berlusconi, former Italian premier of bunga bunga party fame, was nine years my senior! As this was my private domestic business and not merely a medical matter, I was not prepared to answer his question directly, or commit to print. Suffice it to say that a man of 73 is not driven so intensely in that quarter as a 32-year-old, but that the breast cancer itself and the subsequent mastectomy had no effect whatsoever on my normal drives. The same could not be said of the chemotherapy which at times, during a cycle, left me in such discomfort that I would defy any man to rise to the occasion. Time soon passes and before the next bout of chemo approaches, a bounce returns to the step, a twinkle to the eye, hope to the mind, and possibilities beckon like the bulging buds of May. I can't yet speak for the radiotherapy, or the tamoxifen.

In the afternoon, I took my final four tablets of dexamethasone. Later, before supper, I took a further capsule of lansoprazole in the hope it would prevent a repeat of Monday night's severe indigestion. I made sure I ate early and moderately. Mel prepared a baked potato, baked beans and cheese. At bed time, she administered three syringes to my midriff, two of the anti-coagulant enoxaparin, and one of filgrastim to help with my white blood cell count. I was unable to decide whether it was the dexamethasone steroid, or the indigestion caused by the chemotherapy, that kept me awake for most of the night. I rose to make tea at 4.00 am, but slept for an hour or so afterwards.

Day 3 (Wednesday 2nd May)

My temperature remained constant, averaging 36.6^{0}c for the day, but I felt very weak, unwell and unsteady. I noticed the tips of my fingers and thumbs were cracked and sore, and rubbed them with the E45 emollient cream. Mel insisted that I should check them and apply the cream on a daily basis.

After breakfast, I loaded the car with baskets of garden waste to take to the tip but, before driving off, found my heart pounding, lungs panting in search of breath, and head faint and giddy, and was forced to sit on the stairs for at least five minutes to recover my composure.

On reaching the civic recycling centre, I unloaded and emptied the baskets into the skip at a steady and leisurely pace, quite shaken and shocked by my sudden loss of strength. The experience was insufficient to deter me from further activity – my various errands and normal Wednesday shopping at B & Q. By the time I returned home, I was utterly exhausted and went for a nap in the afternoon, before reviving myself with real ginger tea and ginger biscuits, prior to setting out for my mindfulness evening class.

When I got back, Mel told me of a telephone call she had received from my second cousin, Helen Curtis (née Lewis), informing us of the death of Joy Ettridge (née Wiggins), her mother (my late father's cousin). Joy had died, aged 96, near Grimsby. I returned Helen's call to express my condolences and learn more of her mother's death. I told her about my current treatment for breast cancer but promised to attend the funeral if, on the day, I felt well enough. Helen and I both agreed that Joy had had 'a good innings' – a good deal longer, I thought, than I was likely to bat! Mel and I ate supper late, a prelude, I feared, to another night of burping and belching (which turned out as predicted).

That evening, we learned from the news that a computer failure at Public Health England had resulted in 450,000 women aged between 68 and 71 missing out on routine breast cancer screening, which may have led to the avoidable deaths of between 135 to 270 people. Jeremy Hunt, the Secretary of State for Health and Social Care, told the House of Commons that an independent review had been launched into the blunder, but the extent of the damage caused by the delay in diagnosis was not yet clear.

The story brought home the importance of breast cancer screening programmes for catching the disease early. There is no screening for male breast cancer because of its rarity, which meant that men were diagnosed later, with poorer prognosis rates. For the unfortunate women, 'the computer algorithm failure' had resulted in lethal consequences, with 'lives cut short'. I suspected, however, that the issues involved were more complicated. The mass breast screening programme for women did not extend beyond their 71st birthday anyway, and there had been no trials on its effectiveness beyond that age, while there was little evidence that screening prolonged the life of older women. The screening programme might prevent premature death from breast cancer, but it also resulted in three times as many women being treated unnecessarily for a harmless cancer that would not have affected their life expectation.

And so to the bedroom for my enoxaparin and filgrastim injections. Once again, I slept poorly, waking up regularly to belch.

Day 4 (Thursday 3rd May)

The morning light came with a list of jobs in my head and the best of intentions. Not willing to wait for porridge, I had shredded wheat, pecan and maple crisp, and cornflakes for breakfast, but found chewing hard work, and soon developed very sore gums, which affected my eating for the rest of the day.

I went into the garden to plant ornamental bushes, a job I completed after an hour, but it left me totally exhausted. I was annoyed at my weakness and inability to tick off my jobs. Slowing my pace, I managed to edge the lawn, before going indoors to collapse in an armchair. After coffee, I staggered upstairs and fell sound asleep on the bed.

After a nap, I pressed on with my tasks, removing the tarpaulin from the fountain and adding a new coat of concrete sealant. I felt unnaturally tired and had to sit down again. By the end of the day, my fatigue and frustration were downright and dire. I knew that I should have spent the day taking it easy, or staying in bed. Drowsy and drained, I was damaging my health in my determination to defy the chemotherapy's debilitating side effects. I should have learned by now that the side effects of the docetaxel were at their worst on day 4 and day 5.

The night of the 3rd May was atrocious. I lay on the bed aching all over with cramps in my joints. When I made my way to the lavatory, I felt bruising on the heels and soles of my feet. As I groaned with pain, Mel urged me to take a paracetamol capsule, which afforded relief to both me and her, and helped me sleep until the alarm went off.

Day 5 (Friday 4th May)

Fragile and weak and still with joints aching, I crept to the bathroom, knowing I had to reach New Cross's Durnall Ward, for my line care appointment at 8.30am. Mel drove me to the hospital, but then I had the job of crossing the car park and making my way to Durnall. Mel offered to take me to the nearest hospital entrance to Durnall but I refused, saying that I had to walk. I walked very slowly, stopping occasionally for breath, and felt a sense of relief when I got to the lift. Here, on our way up to the ward, we met *Nurse Shelley Seagrove*, who recognised us and greeted us warmly, as we did her.

Ninth line care on Durnall

Despite waiting times and routine procedures, I found Durnall a warm and welcoming place due, in the main, to the friendliness of the receptionists, nurses and supporting staff. I especially recall *Amber Hepworth*, the ever-helpful, amiable ward clerk, and *Dean Eden*, the smiling young ward assistant, who was always on hand to make us tea. Amie, who had the most remarkable searching blue eyes, would do her best to fix my appointments at times that suited me.

On this occasion, we did not wait long. By 8.40 am, *Staff Nurse Liza Warmington* called my name and we were led to a side room. My line was quickly cleaned, flushed and dressed – no need for blood samples on this occasion.

Visit of Robeson, Tasha, Maxi and Vieve

On our return from the hospital, Mel went to join her 'Costa Club' friends for coffee and I went into the garden to fix up the fountain ready for the bank holiday weekend, when Robeson, our son, Tasha, our daughter-in-law, and Maxi and Vieve, our grandchildren, were due to arrive from London to stay. By now, Mel and I were well aware of the happiness and therapeutic benefits their visit was likely to bring.

Once the fountain was flowing, I came indoors and made coffee, conscious that even the slightest exertion contributed to the sensitivity of my heels and soles, the aches in my joints, and my enduring fatigue. I drank coffee, read the newspaper, and lay on the bed for a while, suddenly aware that my gums were sensitive and that sores had returned to my buttocks.

Robeson, Tasha, and our grandchildren arrived at around 9.45 pm. The young ones, looking drowsy, were put straight to bed We sat round the table discussing family matters and the side effects of my current round of chemotherapy, for which Robeson and Tasha expressed their concern. Everyone was pleased that I had now completed the course. By now feeling utterly exhausted, I excused myself and went up to bed. Mel followed shortly afterwards to administer my enoxaparin and filgrastim injections. I slept well, but felt excruciating aches in my leg joints when I got up in the night.

Day 6 (Saturday 5ᵗʰ May)

May bank holiday weekend weather was gloriously sunny and warm, the sky forget-me-not blue, without a cloud in sight. Robeson, Tasha, and the children sat or played games in the garden and then went out with Mel for an afternoon stroll around Tettenhall, while Maxi and Vieve scooted alongside. I wanted to join in the fun, but was stricken by the restrictive effects of my chemo-cycle.

From the time I woke up, I experienced stiffness and pain in my joints, a loss of energy and drive, and extreme fatigue, which annoyed and frustrated me greatly, as I measure my health and fitness by the number of tasks I achieve. I filled my time by sitting, reading the newspaper, and word processing but, by lunch time, I was defeated, and crept upstairs for an afternoon nap. Other discomforts included stomach cramps and frequent bowel movements, sore gums and sore finger tips – as if I had stubbed my fingers and thumbs on a brick.

I woke at around 5.30 pm, and went out into the garden to edge the lawn. I found it hard-going and was about to give up, when

Robeson spotted me and insisted that I stop while he finished the job, assisted by Maxi, his little helper.. I went indoors, said goodnight to the children, ate supper with the family and then curled up in front of the television. Tasha made me a real ginger tea. At bedtime, Mel gave me the enoxaparin and filgrastim injections. Once more, I slept well and woke believing that I was now over the worst of the side effects.

Day 7 (Sunday 6th May)

Sunlight illuminated the bedroom curtains as we welcomed another warm and sparkling day. I was optimistic that the worst of the nausea, fatigue, joint aches, and stomach cramps were now over, and sprang up to engage in my normal Sunday routines. I walked to Tettenhall Upper Green and back for the Sunday papers, returning for oats porridge breakfast and a relaxing read. Robeson and Tasha were busy in the kitchen, preparing Maxi and Vieve's breakfast.

Robeson, Tasha, Mel and the grandchildren drove out to Essington farm to walk in the bluebell woods, which had been opened for three days to raise money for a local breast cancer support group. It occurred to me that bluebell woods might feature quite prominently in breast cancer patients' visualisation exercises. As soon as the bluebell walkers left, I went into the garden to mow the lawns, back and front, knowing full well that, had family members been present, I would have been forbidden to exert myself at all, but especially in the glare of the mid-morning sun. I managed the task before the walkers returned.

They came back with news of the Wolverhampton and District Breast Cancer Action Group, whose members had been out in force at the venue, raising money for their charity. Was it merely a coincidence that early spring flowers, such as snowdrops and bluebells, featured so prominently on the Wolverhampton breast cancer scene? I was told that the group no longer consisted exclusively of women – one man now attended the meetings, and there would be two, were I to accept the invitation from group members to join, relayed enthusiastically to me by Robeson and Tasha

As a measure of changing times, the Breast Cancer Action group had produced a new leaflet deleting its former reference to women. The sentence, 'We are a friendly group of women...', had been reworded to 'We are a friendly group who also enjoy some social outings together'. The picture of women in pink skirts, black tights and pink socks participating in the 'Race for Life' had been replaced with one of New Cross breast cancer surgical consultants, *Mr Tajim Shastri* and *Mr Suri Venkatramanan*. The aim was now 'to help men and women throughout their breast cancer journey'.[1]

"Will you join?" Mel asked me. I agreed to consider the request.

After lunch, my earlier vigour was spent, and I went to bed for the afternoon. Robeson and Mel cooked us all an excellent supper of roast chicken, rice and peas, green beans and carrots, as well as sticky toffee pudding. It smelled delicious, but for me alone, it had almost no taste or texture, apart from sweet fermenting pap..The sticky toffee pudding and custard were clearly discernible and enjoyable After our meal, we watched the television news of the heat wave, before nightly routines followed their inevitable course (apart from the filgrastim injections that finished last night).

Day 8 (Monday 7th May)

229

Because Robeson, Tasha and our two grandchildren had come to stay in fine weather on a bonny bank holiday weekend, I became convinced that the worst of the sixth cycle of chemotherapy was over. I should have referred to my record for the fifth cycle to remind me of what day 8 might be like.

Two side effects were particularly acute. I had only just stumbled out of bed, but I felt very tired, weak and floppy, like Genevieve's blue Peter Rabbit. When I spooned up my porridge, my dentures rubbed on my gums, like chewing on gravel, the sweetness of the honey and date being the only noticeable taste in my mouth. Add on to that the sores on my buttocks, pains in my stomach, and cramp in my calves.

Robeson, Tasha, Mel and the grandchildren wanted me to go for a walk but I hadn't the energy. Instead I collapsed in a chair on the veranda and dozed off to sleep until they returned after they had had lunch at a café in Tettenhall. I woke up and paid them attention, until they had packed and departed for their drive back to London. I was frustrated and sad that I had not been well enough to accompany them on their bank holiday weekend adventures, and must have left them with the impression that I was a frail and grumpy old man.

Thereafter, I sipped at some soup, experienced soreness once more as I chewed on a slice of soft bread, and then retired back to bed, not rising again until 5.30 pm. Exhaustion is painless but, for a man like me, used to assessing his life on activity and outcome, it is one of the most depressing and vexatious side effects of the chemotherapy.

Mel attempted to revive me by making a tasty Jamaican soup (stew) from the remains of the chicken carcass. My gums remained super-sore, but I could taste the heat of the pepper   We watched *East Enders*, *Woman in White,* and the *BBC News,* before bedtime, after what had turned out for me to be a totally inactive, futile, and ineffectual day.

Day 9 (Tuesday 8th May)

Day 9 was another fine day, but forecast to be the last of the heat wave, with cool westerlies and rain sweeping in during the afternoon. Robeson and Tasha's visit and the recent weather, I believed, had improved my mood, if not noticeably reducing my continuing tiredness, indigestion, soreness of mouth and distortion of taste. I made a mental list of jobs to be done, and ticked them off as the day progressed. I went shopping for slippers and clothes, worked on the computer with Philip, wrote my diary and, in the afternoon, visited a garden centre to buy climbing plants. I did not take a nap, but sat proof-reading at the computer.

My nemesis came at supper. Mel had prepared a tasty paella, mainly of rice and bacon, which I would normally relish. Each mouthful I attempted to chew caused my dentures to rub on my gums. I managed three or four forkfuls before being overwhelmed by the pain. What I succeeded in consuming tasted sour, rank and rotten. Still feeling hungry, I sucked at a slice of soft bread, and spoonfuls of salmon and mushy peas.   I cleaned my teeth immediately afterwards and washed my mouth out with Difflam and nystatin.

Th 8th May was the day that President Trump announced that the US was withdrawing from the 2015 Iran nuclear agreement, against the advice of the UK, France and Germany, and the continuing support for the deal from Russia and China, the other signatories. In my view, this would make the Middle East, indeed, the world as a whole, a more dangerous place. For the rest of the evening, I speculated on the relationship of scale, importance, significance, etc., for me of my breast cancer diagnosis, and the potential for war, conflagration and death in the Middle East. For me, personally, the breast cancer was of greater concern. How selfish was that?

Day 10 (Wednesday 9th May)

I should point out that, since the insertion of my Hickman line, I had been using a flannel on my face, head and chest and a shower head to wash my lower body. Following my ablutions this morning, I looked at myself in the mirror, and decided to use my Philips 'Styleshaver' to remove, with Mel's help, the few remaining centimetre-long strands on my head and the irregular bristles on my chin. At this stage in the sixth cycle, the few hairs I had left were unevenly scattered and patchy. The haircut had little effect. I still looked like an elderly ET – an extra-terrestrial, but not nearly as lovable.

Wednesday took its habitual course. We drove to B&Q and spent time in the garden centre buying compost and plants, with the Diamond Card ten per cent discount, and then went to Lidl for groceries. Feeling exhausted in the afternoon, I went to bed for a nap, hoping to refresh myself for the evening mindfulness class. I continued to suffer from indigestion, sore gums and a distorted sense of taste. Worse, I started to sneeze and my nose ran, leading me to suspect the hay fever season had started early, for which I took an anti-histamine cetirizine but, by evening, the tablet had had no effect.

Day 11 to 21 (Thursday 10th May – Sunday 20th May)

On the 10th May, the sneezing and runny nose continued without let-up, and by evening my temperature had risen to 37.6^0c. I concluded that I must have caught a cold and considered the option of staying in bed, but had an appointment booked at 11.00 am with a radiotherapy practitioner/lymphoedema therapist at the Deanesly Centre. An account of that meeting can be found in Chapter 15.

My nose went on running and I sneezed intermittently for the rest of the day. My gums remained sore, making it painful to eat. I felt very fatigued and again went to bed for an afternoon nap.

On Friday 11th May, my temperature remained at 37.6^0c but I imagined that, as it was day 12 of the cycle, my health was improving and I should proceed as if business were normal.

Tenth line care on Durnall

I made my way to the hospital for my tenth session of line care, on this occasion without Mel, as I also had a group session afterwards. I arrived on Durnall at 8.25 am and, shortly afterwards, at 8.35 am, my name was called and I was led to a chair, where my chest was cleaned with a 'lollipop', blood was drawn off, heparin injected, and my line was reattached with a dressing patch. It was 8.50 am when I left Durnall, the earliest that my line care had been completed.

Visualisation and relaxation group

Having an hour and half to spare before the visualisation and relaxation group was due to begin on Deanesly, I made my way to the hospital coffee bar, bought a coffee, and settled down to write my diary. Glancing at my watch some time later, I realised that time had flown, and rushed down to join the visualisation and relaxation group (see Chapter 12). Unfortunately, I disrupted the session twice, first by coming in late, and second, by sneezing and coughing right in the middle of a visualisation exercise.

A cold goes from bad to worse

As the day progressed, my coughing became louder, more prolonged and bronchial. I felt tired and ill. After the group, I drove straight home and took paracetamol. I realised I had a very bad cold and hoped that it would not deteriorate into the pneumonia I had caught on holiday in 2017.

By mid afternoon, I flaked out on the bed and slept soundly for a couple of hours, by which time my temperature had risen to 37.7^0c, my bouts of coughing had become more frequent, my nose was dripping like a leaking tap, my eyes were streaming as if I was peeling onions, and my voice was as gravelly and gruff as a pneumatic drill.

I came down for a while to eat supper and then returned to bed, only raising myself to blow my nose and receive my enoxaparin injections.

By Saturday, the 12th May, I felt much the same, but I dosed myself initially with paracetamol and, later, with Max Strength Cold and Flu capsules, and accompanied Mel to the optician for her eye test. We had coffee in town, before returning home for lunch, after which I went back to bed feeling utterly depressed and exhausted.

I woke later and sat in the conservatory, but was surprised by how what started as a minor sniffle had progressed to a serious cold, with prolonged bouts of chesty coughing, fits of sneezing, a sore throat, a handkerchief heavy with mucus and catarrh, and fluctuations in temperature of between 36.6°c and 37.7°c (I guessed the lows might be related to the paracetamol I was taking). With Durnall and Deanesly day centres and the Castlecoft Surgery closed, there was little I could do at the weekend except self-medicate. We watched television for a while after supper, but I did not have the energy to concentrate, and made my way up to bed, where Mel gave me two more Max Strength flu capsules and my enoxaparin injections.

I woke on day 14, Sunday, to a beautiful sunny day but, despite the good weather, the bad cold kept its gloomy grip on me. I swallowed a further dose of the Max Strength, and arose at the usual hour for my breakfast of cornmeal porridge, before setting out for Tettenhall Green to purchase the newspapers. I paced myself, managing the two-mile return journey, with only minor fatigue.

After reading the papers for half an hour and making myself a cappuccino, I went into the garden to cut the lawn. I took the mowing slowly but, by the time I had finished, I knew I had to take off my Wellies and go back to bed for a nap. I slept for three hours, waking up with a croaking voice and a feeling of intense gloom and despondency. Philip and Gem called round to say hello, but I barely had the energy to communicate.

Realising how seriously the bad cold was affecting me, Mel urged me to make a GP appointment at the Castlecroft Medical Practice as soon as the surgery opened after the weekend. What happened to me after I phoned the surgery on Monday 14th May (the 15th day of the cycle) is described in Chapter 14. In brief, the symptoms of a bad cold or influenza are similar to those of impending neutropenic sepsis and demand urgent medical investigation and precautionary intervention. I found my subsequent admission to the New Cross Emergency Department and Acute Medical Unit a terrifying episode, during which I felt utterly powerless and at the mercy of the medical profession. I explore the events of day 15 (Monday 14th May) and day 16 (Tuesday 15th May) in greater detail in the next chapter, and take up the story of the sixth cycle again on day 17 (Wednesday 16th May), when hospital tests had eliminated the possibility that I was succumbing to neutropenic sepsis.

On Wednesday morning, the 16th May, I still felt unnaturally tired and weak, but was determined to accompany Mel on our regular outing to B&Q, where we used our Diamond Club discount to buy yet more plants for the garden, and then went on to Lidl for groceries, before Mel drove us home for lunch. Mel went to work in the garden, while I retired to bed for a nap.

Hickman hallucination

Early on Thursday morning around 4 00 am, I went downstairs to make tea, but imagined I felt a pain in my right shoulder as I prized the lid from the kettle. The parallel with the detection of my breast lump was unmistakable. Was I dreaming? Had I merely recalled the Monday night drip pump and the 2000 ml Hartmann's infusion, and fantasised about the unnecessary abuse of my Hickman line and the risk of it becoming infected? (See chapter 14.) I looked in the bathroom mirror and fixated on the vein in my neck, realising that it was accentuated by the presence of a plastic tube. I then woke Mel and convinced her, too, that my neck was swollen and that I was in pain. With both of us worried, we resolved to make our way at the earliest opportunity to Durnall to have the Hickman line cleaned, flushed and examined for infection. But we managed to go back to sleep.

Eleventh line care on Durnall

Mel and I arrived on Durnall on Thursday 17th May at 8.30 am and explained to *Amber*, the ward clerk, the reason we had turned up without first making a telephone call. By 8.45 am, the motherly nurse, *Liza Warmington*, led us to the triage suite. Mel then had to leave for an appointment elsewhere. *Liza* soon returned to strip off the make-shift dressing applied on the Acute Medical Unit, clean my chest meticulously with a 'lollipop', draw blood, inject saline and then heparin, and re-dress the site. She could see no sign of infection, but thought that, to be on the safe side, I should stay and be seen by a doctor.

Dean Eden, the amiable ward assistant, made me at least two cups of tea and, not long afterwards, the lively and animated *Dr Haripriya Narayani* arrived to examine my neck, shoulder and chest. She could see no sign of swelling but agreed that the Hickman line always carried the risk of infection. Since I had completed the final cycle of chemotherapy, she inquired as to when it was planned to remove it. She offered to take it out herself later, on Durnall, if my consultant agreed. Why had it been inserted in the first place? I told her of my phlebitis. I suspect she went away to study my patient record.

Dr Narayani returned to ask whether I was still receiving enoxaparin and, on learning that it was being injected on a nightly basis, told me that the course would have to cease for at least a day prior to any operation to remove my Hickman line. We agreed that I should contact *Dr Grigoryev's* secretary to arrange a convenient date for the Hickman line to come out. (I contacted her on the following Monday, and she phoned me back shortly afterwards to tell me *Dr Grigoryev* had given the go-ahead.) I also mentioned to *Dr Narayani* that I was feeling abnormally tired and asked her whether my haemoglobin level was low. She assured me that my haemoglobin and other blood count readings from the morning's sample were within the normal range. I left Durnall in a more optimistic state of mind than when I arrived.

I met Mel downstairs in the hospital. She had been to her appointment and returned to drive me home. When I got back, I took my midday co-amoxiclav antibiotic tablet. This was the third day of taking the oral antibiotics but my congestion, blocked nose, and coughing up of mucus showed no signs as yet of improvement. Mel thought to supplement our medication by searching out the Clenil Modulite inhalers we had been prescribed to treat breathing difficulties and coughing when we both caught pneumonia the previous year, but both cartridges were almost exhausted. Believing the inhalers might help alleviate our coughing, particularly at night, Mel visited the Castlecroft Medical Practice for further prescriptions, which she collected the very same day. I still felt abnormally tired and went for an afternoon nap.

On Friday the 18th May, Mel went with Gem to their 'Costa Club', while Philip came round to work with me on the computer. After lunch, I worked in the garden for half an hour but, with the coughing and physical exercise, soon became very tired again and went for a nap around 4.00 pm, waking up in time for the news at 6.00 pm. Even by the weekend, my cold had not shifted - I was still blowing my nose and coughing up phlegm - but my temperature had fallen to a normal 36.7°c. Sunday the 19th May was day 21, and the last day of the sixth and final cycle. I was delighted, but still had the co-amoxiclav course to complete, and to persevere with the enoxaparin injections.

In summary, the sixth cycle of chemotherapy had turned out to be very much like the fourth and the fifth, all three involving infusions of docetaxel but, in the case of the sixth, I was convinced that I had experienced far greater feelings of exhaustion and fatigue, and slept for longer periods. The sixth cycle, however, had ended quite differently, with my catching a very bad cold, most of whose symptoms mimicked those of the life-threatening neutropenic sepsis. As a consequence, I had learned at first-hand what happens when the Febrile Neutropenia Care Pathway is invoked and followed without waver. Even after I completed the course of co-amoxiclav antibiotic, the cold took an inordinately long time to clear up, and I was still congested, coughing up phlegm, and feeling distinctly under the weather on the 1st June, 12 days after the end of the sixth cycle.

Could I have misread the persistent symptoms of a bad cold for the onset of my seasonal hay fever which, for me, normally commences like clockwork in the last week of May? My eyes were itchy and sore, my nose ran, but the prolonged sneezing fits - the certain perennial indicator of my hay fever - had not yet occurred. My daughter and fellow hay fever sufferer, Toussaint, who had already manifested all of the usual complaints, attributed my failure at sneezing to the fact that my immune system had been compromised by the chemotherapy drugs. Just in case the congestion was due to the hay fever, I began to take my antihistamine cetirizine hydrochloride tablets.

One side effect of the chemotherapy that I had not noticed before, was the white and pink striping of my finger nails. It reminded me of the seasonal growth rings on a cross-section of a tree trunk. As there were six stripes per finger nail, I assumed that each stripe corresponded to a chemo session, the drugs having damaged on each occasion the rapidly-growing finger-nail cells. It was reassuring to know that the stripes would soon be replaced by regular pink nails and, together with the hairs on my head and face, my normal appearance would soon be restored. Indeed, once the chemo was over, to my great satisfaction, a thin covering of downy hairs appeared on my pate. They continued to sprout at a rate of about one and a half millimetres a week.

Shortly after I completed my sixth cycle of chemotherapy, a report was presented to a meeting of the American Society of Clinical Oncology meeting in Chicago, on a study of women with early oestrogen-receptor-positive but node-negative breast cancer, showing that those assessed in the range 0 to 25 on a scale of seriousness from 0 to 100 (that is, 69 per cent of all women diagnosed with breast cancer of that type) did not benefit nor need to undergo chemotherapy, and could in future be spared its punishing side effects. As my breast cancer had been axillary node positive, I guessed that, in my case, this exemption would not have applied. Nevertheless, of the 23,000 women diagnosed with that kind of breast cancer, 69 per cent. or 15,870, would no longer have to undergo chemotherapy. Good news indeed![2]

Twelfth line care on Durnall

We returned to Durnall on the 24th May for my twelfth line care, which was administered promptly and efficiently by *Nurse Heather Dean*, in the presence of two student nurses from the University of Wolverhampton, who observed the procedure attentively. On learning that there were plans afoot to remove my Hickman line,

Heather thought it best to take blood samples in preparation for what would be a minor operation. Afterwards, we went to the desk to finalise date for the remaining line care appointments, and for the line removal, which was booked to be performed by *Dr Narayani* at 3.00 pm on Friday, the 15th June. I queried the time in the belief that I might be undergoing radiotherapy on the same day, but was reassured that that had been booked for a midday slot.

Thirteenth and fourteenth line care sessions

One week later on the 31st May, *Nurse Heather Dean*, once more with student nurses watching and helping, administered my thirteenth line care, explaining in some detail to the students and me the constituent parts of the line, the cleansing process, and what I might expect when the line came to be removed in two weeks' time. The ever-helpful, amiable and attentive *Nurse Dean* certainly knew her stuff. On the 7th June, Mel and I returned to Durnall for my fourteenth line care, dealt with promptly and carefully by *Nurse Sandra Higgins*.

Fifteenth and final line-care appointment.

While billed as line care, my appointment on Durnall on Thursday 14th June did not turn out as expected. *Nurse Saiju Channar* told me that, as the Hickman line was due to be taken out the following day, her job was not to clean, flush, or take blood from it, but to take blood samples from my arm in preparation for the line-removal procedure. She tightened a tourniquet round the vein in my right arm, inserted a needle and tried to draw blood, but no blood was forthcoming, despite further manoeuvring. *Saiju* called for help from *Nurse Michelle Mc Lean*, whom we were delighted to see, having made her acquaintance on the Snowdrop Suite. But *Michelle* had only a little more success than *Saiju* in drawing blood from my arm and was forced to turn to my wrist, before they agreed that they had drawn off enough of the red stuff to fill the three sample bottles. *Saiju* stuck two little round plasters over the punctures in my arm and taped gauze to cover the cut to my wrist. (That little hiccup in drawing blood resulted in two brown bruise marks that took two weeks to fade.) Afterwards, I put on my shirt and tie. Mel and I then walked over to Deanesly for my Thursday radiotherapy session.

Line removal

We returned to Durnall at 3.00 pm on Friday 15th June for the removal of my Hickman line. It had been in place for 14 weeks, since the 8th March and had become part of my body, but not sufficiently integral to permit me to take a daily shower. (Instead I had had to flannel my head, face, arms and torso to avoid wetting the line, and use the shower head for washing my bottom half. I was very much looking forward to resuming a full-body daily shower.)

As soon as we entered the ward, *Amber Hepworth*, the clerical officer, presented me with a form and directed us to the Outpatients' Department to have my finger pricked for a blood coagulation test. My blood from the previous day had coagulated before it had reached the lab. The phlebotomist smeared the drop onto a tiny pallet and used a hand-held machine to conduct the test. She wrote '1.0' onto my form and reassured me my coagulation reading was normal. We took the result back to Durnall.

Shortly afterwards, Mel and I were led by a student nurse to a room with a bed, where we met *Dr Haripriya Narayani*, who explained the procedure she was about to perform, and sought reassurance that I was no longer on anti-coagulant injections. Once briefed, I removed my shirt to expose my chest and line and lay on the bed. She then asked me, referring to Mel, "who is she"?

After explaining to me the procedure she was about to perform on me, *Dr Narayani* turned to Mel and, following an argument about her being in the room, asked her to leave, explaining that a young companion of another of her patients had fainted during a similar session. Mel said that she had been a nurse and would not faint and wanted to stay with her husband, who would prefer her to be present. *Dr Narayani* insisted she leave, as she could not guarantee that Mel would not faint. She emphasised that that was the hospital rule, which she was entitled to enforce. Reluctantly, Mel withdrew from the room. She later asked for a copy of the hospital regulation requiring her to do so. (As to be expected, Mel pursued her quest for evidence of the rule in writing, but Senior Nurse Manager, *Mary McGrath*, was unable to locate.)

I sensed that *Dr Narayani* and the student nurse were troubled by the incident, as indeed was I, but once Mel had left, the procedure went ahead. My chest was cleaned with antiseptic, and a local anaesthetic injected around the area next to my line. The doctor began cutting around the cuff of the line, which took time as the skin had become firmly attached to it. Once loosened, the tube was withdrawn and the incision stitched up and covered with a dressing. In total, the procedure lasted for about half an hour. I was required to stay lying down for a further five minutes to avoid the risk of bleeding. My memory of that occasion is not of the sensation of the scalpel cutting my flesh, nor of the catheter being withdrawn, but of the spectacle of Mel being obliged under protest to leave the room. I would have preferred her to be present. Afterwards, Mel told me how upset she was. We walked over to Deanesly for my radiotherapy session, stopping for a welcome cappuccino en route.

Mel was still annoyed and upset at being barred from the room for no good reason.

On a couple of occasions before bedtime, I took paracetamol to control the dull pain left by the line removal and, knowing that the stitches to my wound had to be removed after seven days, made an appointment to see a practice nurse at the Castlecroft Medical Practice. On Thursday 21st June, *Nurse Lindsay Hurst*, who over many years had given us injections for flu and travel, told me that the wound had healed satisfactorily and took out the stitches in under three minutes. I would be able to shower and bath as normal again when the dressing was removed in three days' time.

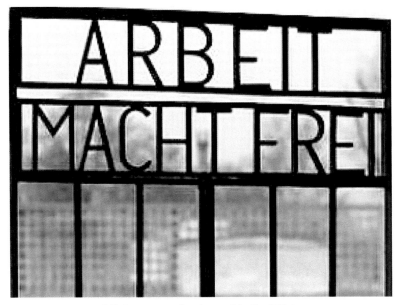

Nightmare on the Acute Medical Unit

Chapter 14

Pursuing the febrile neutropenia care pathway

On Monday the 14th May 2018, day 15 of my sixth chemotherapy cycle, I felt distinctly ill, with a cough, severe congestion, running eyes and nose, and a raised temperature. On Mel's advice, I phoned the Castlecroft Medical Practice at 8.30 am to make an emergency appointment to see a GP, but found myself in a call queue. I told the receptionist that I was undergoing chemotherapy, that I had little resistance to disease, and pleaded my 'neutropenic sepsis' patient status to secure an appointment with *Dr Monica Bianchi*, but was not slotted in to see her until 5.10 pm that evening.

The surgery's electronic registration system failed to register me when we arrived, and my name had not been flashed up and called by 5.30 pm, at which point my mobile phone began ringing. It was a Castlecroft receptionist inquiring as to why I had failed to attend. I told her I had been sitting in the waiting room since 5.00 pm. A few minutes later, we were with *Dr Bianchi*, explaining my symptoms. She was already aware from my electronic record of my chemotherapy treatment and susceptibility to infection and, having measured my temperature at 37.8°c, took my case very seriously indeed. She was disappointed that I had not been given priority with an earlier appointment time. She said she had no alternative but to send me straight away to the Emergency Department at New Cross, and wrote a letter explaining how urgent it was that I receive immediate attention.

Investigating the possibility of neutropenic sepsis

The letter read: 'Francis Reeves, aged 73 years, is currently receiving chemotherapy for breast cancer. He is pyrexial at 37.8°c, flushed and tachycardic, BP 130/80, with a slight cough and congestion. I feel he requires urgent FBC - neutropenic sepsis? Yours sincerely, *Dr M Bianchi*'. As Mel drove me to the hospital emergency department, I took from my wallet a card that I had been given by the Oncology Department to keep on my person from the time my chemotherapy began. On one side it told me that should I become unwell and experienced any of the following:

a temperature of 37.5°c or above,

shivers/fever, flu-like symptoms,

diarrhoea,

sore mouth and/or sore gums,

I should call an emergency number. I had, indeed, all of those symptoms, apart from the diarrhoea.

The other side of the card was more concerning. It read: 'I am currently receiving chemotherapy treatment...I am at high risk of developing **neutropenic sepsis**. This is a potentially life-threatening condition and requires urgent medical attention. Please instigate the Febrile Neutropenia Care Pathway immediately!

"Mel, what exactly is neutropenic sepsis?" I asked.

"It's a serious infection of your blood caused by a fall off in your neutrophil count and, if it isn't treated immediately, it can kill you." She sounded grave and looked anxious. I was shaken. I knew my neutrophils had been low on two previous occasions.

"What's caused it?" I wanted to know.

"It could have a bacterial, fungal, or viral cause," she replied. "It might be just your body's inability to deal with the bad cold or flu you've been having."

At 7.15 pm, when we walked into the New Cross Emergency Department, Mel headed to the sign over the reception desk marked, 'If your condition is life-threatening please report here'. We showed the receptionist the card and *Dr Bianchi*'s letter. She located my name on the screen in front of her and asked me to confirm my date of birth and contact details, before directing me to stand outside the door of the triage nurse. After standing there for about five minutes, I told Mel that I felt weak and went to sit in the waiting room, leaving Mel to stand in my place and call when the nurse emerged. At 7.30 pm, we were called in to see the triage nurse, who asked about my symptoms, took my temperature and blood pressure, and glanced at the doctor's letter.

Admission to the New Cross Emergency Department

About ten minutes later, she led us to an inner room of the Emergency Department and told us to sit on the chairs. After she left, a porter pushed a trolley bed into the room and told me to take off my upper clothes and put on a hospital gown. Once the porter had left, a phlebotomist came in, approached my left arm, and announced she was going to take blood. I told her that I had a Hickman line for taking blood, had had a lymph node clearance from my left armpit, and was at risk of developing a lymphoedema if blood was taken from my left arm. She moved over to my right arm. I explained that that was the arm in which I had had phlebitis, and the reason for having a Hickman line. Frustrated in her purpose, she left the room abruptly.

At around 7.50 pm, a doctor came to tell us that I must allow his staff to take bloods for blood counts and for culture. I told him that that was not a problem, but that I wanted them taken through my Hickman line, a request he seemed reluctant to countenance. He said he would also require a swab from my throat and a sample of urine and to send me for an x-ray of my lungs. (The request for a urine sample was never pursued.) I was asked repeatedly whether I had diarrhoea and vomiting, and I replied repeatedly that I had not. The doctor once more insisted on the urgent need to insert a cannula to administer intravenous antibiotics and fluids, in accordance, I assumed, with the protocol of the neutropenia care pathway. The team had to begin straightaway and could not await the results of the blood tests. A nurse took my blood pressure and temperature once again. A second doctor came in to ask questions about my medical history, and the first doctor left. She asked once again about my bowels and diarrhoea, listened to my chest through her stethoscope, and pressed her hands on my stomach. She looked quizzical and asked if there was anything else I should like to tell her. There was not.

Difficulty in using my Hickman line

Mel and I persisted in asking the doctors and nurses to make use of the Hickman line, but they were clearly reluctant to do so. It emerged that there was only one nurse on the unit - the triage nurse, *Dionne Summer* - who was trained in the care of a central line. At 8.30 pm, she was permitted to return and take blood through my line, but encountered a difficulty. There was a clot in the connector She went to find a replacement part before returning at 8.50 pm, first, to take the much-needed bloods, and then, to connect my line to a drip stand to feed an intravenous antibiotic into my system. By 10.12 pm, the bag of antibiotic had emptied and was replaced by a 1,000 ml bag of sodium lactate compound (Hartmann's solution).

I was pleased that the bloods had at last been taken via my line, until the first doctor came in to tell me that he would still have to use my arm - left or right - it didn't matter as it was an emergency - to take bloods from a 'peripheral site'. This time, he was insistent and determined, meeting my reluctance with logic, explaining that he had to rule out the possibility that the source of the neutropenia was infection in the Hickman line itself, and the only way of doing this was to grow a comparative culture from blood taken from a 'peripheral site', and that the only 'peripheral' place that could be readily accessed was a vein in my arm. Lower limbs were rejected as inaccessible and unsuitable. Befuddled as I was with my illness, I could not quite grasp why what had started as a straightforward choice between a diagnosis of neutropenic sepsis or severe bad cold had suddenly been complicated by a consideration of an infected Hickman line. Why bring that into it? Was I being bamboozled?

The first doctor left me with the impression that I was viewed already as an uncooperative patient, contributing through my stubbornness and ignorance to my crisis. Shortly afterwards, I permitted a phlebotomist to insert a cannula with two connections into the vein in the right arm where I had had phlebitis, and to draw off blood, which she injected into two further bottles for culture. At 10.27 pm, a porter arrived to roll me and my trolley to a nearby x-ray room, where a plate was placed on my chest and an x-ray shot. A swab of my throat was taken and put in a bottle. At 11.27 pm, my pulse and temperature were measured again.

I was told that my temperature had fallen to 37.2°c., my blood count result showed my neutrophil level to be at the highest it had been for months, the x-ray result revealed no shadow, and the stethoscope discovered no sound on the chest. No evidence of neutropenia, after all! As it was now 12.00 midnight, could we go home and return to Durnall Oncology Day Unit for further treatment the following morning? Shortly afterwards, a snatch team arrived to push my trolley to Ward 58, the Acute Medical Unit, where it had been determined I should stay overnight.

Enforcement of the neutropenia care protocol

It began to dawn on Mel and me that I was in the vice-like grip of the immutable neutropenia care pathway and that there was now no means of escape. I refused the initial attempt at transfer, which had come as a surprise and with no communication or explanation from on high. It transpired that the medical team that we had first had dealings with had now been replaced with another shift. I also

250

realised that at 12.45 am, after the first 1,000 ml of Hartmann's solution had been pumped into me, I had been hooked up by my Hickman line to another 1,000 ml bag of the same fluid which, at a scheduled flow rate of 125 ml an hour, would take another 8 hours to pass into my system.

At last, a different, more conciliatory and compassionate doctor entered the room to talk to us directly - not as before via the nurses, phlebotomists and porters. He conceded that the blood results and temperature readings were a good sign, but that I still needed to be kept under observation. At this stage, he was unwilling to risk sending me home. I should consider myself fortunate that, despite stiff competition, I had been found a bed on the Acute Medical Unit, where I would be in capable hands. He was persuasive and made it sound like a privilege I couldn't refuse, like winning a weekend break at a luxury spa! Most people must prefer their own bed at home to a short overnight stay in a hospital, but, from previous experience, I could already predict that my detention would have little to do with clinical need and be extended ad infinitum, or at least until the doctors got round to discharging me, thus boring me to the core and wasting my day.[1]

It was apparent to me that my two lines of self-defence had been well and truly breached: firstly, my earlier insistence that blood should only be taken through my Hickman line, and secondly, that I should be discharged and allowed to return in the morning (since my temperature had fallen, my neutrophil count was sufficient, and my condition was no longer thought life-threatening). It was now 3.00 am on Tuesday and I had exhausted what little energy I had left after chemo and cold. With reluctance, I surrendered to the inevitable. Concerned about Mel, I persuaded her to leave and drive home. Reluctantly, she agreed, but only after she had seen me safely to the overnight ward.

Night on the Acute Medical Unit

A porter came to transfer me to a room in A58, the Acute Medical Unit, situated above the Emergency Department. The trolley, the porter, Mel, and I travelled upwards on a large mirrored lift, accompanied by a nurse carrying my drip pump and bag of Hartmann's solution. Refusing assistance, I climbed off the trolley and onto the bed. I was greeted by Richard, the nurse, who would look after me for the rest of the night on the unit.

Richard found me some pyjamas and went through the routine check-in procedure, including recording my possessions, money, mobile phone, etc. I showed him the cannula, with its twin tubes left dangling from my right arm, and asked whether he could remove it. He obliged straight away.. He turned down the light and told me to expect a visit from the doctor before I went off to sleep.

A little while later, *Dr Hii* entered the room. Polite and unassuming, he sought to reassure me that my temperature was normal, my neutrophil levels had risen (probably as a result of the infection), and my chest x-ray had been clear, which meant that, although I had an infection, it was not the life-threatening neutropenic sepsis originally feared. He would prescribe a course of oral antibiotics to start in the morning, which I would be able to take home with me.

After *Dr Hii* left, I did my best to settle down for the remainder of the night but, despite my tiredness, I found it difficult to sleep with the constant whir of the drip pump. Not until 8.00 am, when all the fluid had gone through, did I have the immense satisfaction of turning off the machine myself. Shortly afterwards Michael, my nurse on the day shift, detached me from the pump and *Sister Neshele Denktash* came in to clean and tape up my Hickman line.

I had hoped to be discharged shortly afterwards but, as always, had to wait on the doctors, whose round, I guessed, began around 9 am. I waited until 11 am, and approached the desk. I was told that I had been seen the night before by a doctor. The doctors' priority was to visit patients recently admitted to the unit.

The floral decor of the Acute Medical Unit

By now very bored with the waiting, I began to examine the decor of my room and the corridors of the Acute Medical Unit, plainly recently built, newly painted and decorated. The walls of my room were in blue and grey, with grey vinyl floor, grey bed and grey bedspread. Other furniture included a high upright chair next to a lower more comfortable-looking chair, a cantilever table, a bedside cabinet with blue doors, a sink, and separate receptacles for domestic and clinical waste. A door led to an en-suite bathroom.

Hung on the wall, was a large picture of a giant 50cm-diameter yellow buttercup, silhouetted against a powder-blue background. (Enlarged to that extent, it may well have been a marsh marigold.) So, I had stayed the night on 'buttercup'! I now noticed other rooms, each themed with its own floral display: blue bell, dahlia, rose, speedwell, and others. An association of images occurs when they become bound together in the mind, a technique often used by therapists to dissipate unpleasant memories and replace them with happier ones. Nevertheless, after my night on the Acute Medical Unit, my imaginary walk along buttercup lane led on inexorably to a gloomy neutropenia care pathway shaded by trees bearing fruit full to bursting with Hartmann's solution.

A registrar, *Dr Salma Abbassi*, came to my room around noon, impressing me with both her pleasant approachable manner and her knowledge of my case history. She told me that I had indeed had an infection, not yet identified, but unrelated to neutropenic sepsis. From what she knew of my blood count and my recent body temperature, she was confident that the worst was over and I would be discharged as soon as possible with a course of antibiotics - co-amoxiclav tablets. As there was a pharmacist present on the unit, I would be given the antibiotics - not a prescription. A good half-an-hour later, I inquired at the desk about progress and was directed to talk to the pharmacist, who went to talk to the registrar, only to report that the prescription was awaiting the consultant's action. Knowing what was expected of patients, I returned to my room to wait.

The Acute Oncology Specialist Nurse

I was visited there by *Nurse Eleanor Hart*, who introduced herself as the Acute Oncology Specialist Nurse. I assumed she had contacted me as a consequence of the neutropenic sepsis alert. *Eleanor* wanted to know how I had ended up in the Acute Medical Unit. It seemed to me and Mel, I explained, that, leaving aside the diarrhoea and vomiting, the listed signs of neutropenia were identical to those of the flu. When I came to think of it, why had I been given 2,000 ml of Hartmann's solution, when I had shown no symptoms of vomiting, diarrhoea or dehydration?

We had a detailed discussion of my experiences to date and what I might expect next from radiotherapy and the course of tamoxifen. She offered to find out, or firm up, some of the treatment dates about which I was vague, and telephone. Sure enough, she phoned me at home the very next day to clarify arrangements for radiotherapy and the tamoxifen course, giving me a provisional start date of the 4th June for the radiotherapy and the 30th May to begin taking the tamoxifen tablets. It was the first time I had met *Eleanor* and become aware of her existence or role. She was warm, personable and compassionate and extremely well informed about the benefits and side effects of the adjuvant cancer therapies. As we spoke, a nurse brought in my antibiotics and cut the tracking device from my wrist.

On Friday the 18th May, *Eleanor* contacted me again, this time by post, sending me information on various courses for cancer patients, organised by the Macmillan Midlands Learning and Development Team. There was a 'Strive and Thrive Recovery Programme' on coping with the consequences of cancer treatment and undertaking physical exercise. Other courses were on nutrition, fatigue, anxiety, and breathlessness, and 'supported self-management' - the last dealing with ways 'to solve problems, enable self-discovery, set goals, use resources, and share the best ways to live well with cancer'. None of these courses interested me particularly, but that may have been because my severe bad cold was still making me miserable and withdrawn from the world. In hindsight, I think it was because my life was already well managed, if not by me, then by Mel.

Discharged on Tuesday the 15th May at around 1.00 pm from the hospital, I phoned Mel, who told me that Philip would come to collect me in his car. Mel was delighted to welcome me home and cooked me an elegant meal of lamb steak, potatoes and Savoy cabbage, which she justified in terms of the red meat potential for boosting my haemoglobin level and the vegetable fibre for keeping an active bowel. With neither Mel nor me getting much rest on Monday night, both of us went to bed early and slept like logs, despite our persistent colds, congestion, and coughing.

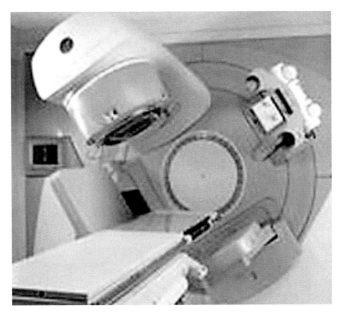

Linac machine, Electa

Chapter 15

Radiotherapy

An appointment to plan my radiotherapy treatment

On Monday 23rd April, following my meeting with *Dr Hetu Charitha Gupta* and towards the end of my fifth chemotherapy cycle, I was asked to attend the radiotherapy department at the Deanesly Centre for a CT scan of my chest, in preparation for the course of radiotherapy which was set to follow my chemotherapy. Five minutes before my 9.15 am appointment, a young woman called out my name and led me and Mel from the general waiting area to a side room equipped with changing cubicles. Her name tag informed us that she was *Waliyah Raza*, a 'therapy radiographer' in the radiotherapy department. She asked me my address and date of birth to make sure of my identity, went through a list of questions (Did I have a pace maker?), and briefed us about the procedure that the therapeutic radiographers were about to conduct. I was directed to the cubicle to remove my upper-body clothing and to cover my chest with a surgical gown, while Mel was left to sit in the adjacent waiting area.

Suitably dressed in my belt, navy blue trousers, shoes, and a surgical smock hanging down to my knees, I was led into the room containing a long narrow couch and the polo-mint-shaped CT scanner. *Waliyah*, *Elaine*, and another therapeutic radiographer assisted me in positioning myself on the couch, before helping me remove the surgical gown concealing my chest and getting me to bend my legs over a knee rest and place my arms on arm rests above my head. I was told that I needed to feel comfortable because the details of my position would be recorded electronically and I would be required to lie in the same position on a similar couch throughout all my subsequent radiotherapy sessions.

At this point, the radiographers retreated behind a screen and the couch propelled me into the polo-shaped cylinder. I could see a rotating plate and hear a whirring sound and what sounded like an extractor fan. The information from the x-ray scan was fed into the computer and used by the radiotherapists to decide on the precise area of my chest to be irradiated and the dose of radiation required.

Three tattoos

Once the couch had emerged from the cylinder, the radiographers highlighted points on my chest with a marker and then stuck on tags. I was warned to expect a little discomfort. I felt what could only be described as three bee stings, as my chest was tattooed in three places to ensure the planned radiation was accurately directed.

The three tattoos - the first and only tattoos I had ever had - were permanent but barely visible - all three being the size of pin heads. They would assist the radiographers to position me accurately and consistently during the fifteen separate occasions of radiotherapy I was scheduled to undergo.[1]

The radiographers helped me to dismount from the couch and to veil my chest with the surgical gown. I was given an information brochure on radiotherapy and a prescription for Zero AQS emollient cream to apply to my chest three times a day during the course of the treatment.

I joined Mel in the side room before entering the changing cubicle to put on my shirt, tie, cardigan and jacket. As we left Deanesly, I told Mel about the 'bee stings' I'd had. She had not realised that the tattoos were real and came with a life-time guarantee.

Radiotherapy and lymphoedema consultation

On Thursday 10th May, Mel and I returned to the Deanesly Centre for an 11 am appointment with *Peter Harrington*, an Advanced Practitioner, Radiotherapy, who met us on time and showed us to his office in Deanesly's extensive radiography wing. Informative, convivial and polite, *Pete* had the dual task of explaining to us in detail the course of the radiotherapy treatment that the radiographers were planning for me, and of providing advice on how best to reduce the post-operative risk of developing lymphoedema (a build-up of lymph fluid under the skin, resulting in swollen limbs, see glossary of terms). Despite being interrupted with a barrage of questions from me and Mel, *Pete* managed to offer us a remarkably lucid account of what to expect from radiotherapy and of how to avoid lymphoedema.

Following my sixth cycle of chemotherapy, I would be given on fifteen successive days, fifteen sessions or 'fractions' of x-ray radiation targeted at my chest wall nearest the sites of my mastectomy and lymphadenectomy. The precise intensity and angle of the beams to be used would be calculated by a computer, using coordinates matched to laser lights aligned to my carefully-positioned tattooed torso. *Pete* brought up a picture on his computer of the kind of radiotherapy machine that would be used and demonstrated its side-to-side movements with the help of a small plastic model on his desk. I would be allocated to Linac 3 - linear accelerator number 3, a substantial 12-year-old IMRT (intensity-modulated radiotherapy) machine, named a 'Varian', and imported from the United States. (I was allocated eventually to Linac 4, an 'Electa', made, I was told, in Denmark).

I would be positioned on the couch under the machine's collimator, or 'head', attached to a gantry, which would be swung from left to right to administer a 20-second dose of radiation on both sides of my chest, but at an angle that avoided exposing my heart and my lung to the x-rays. The aim was to avoid the rays penetrating beyond the rib cage, but some lung tissue nearest to the breast might still be affected, causing minor damage and fibrosis in the longer term.[2] The radiographers did their best to reduce the collateral damage.

With regard to other side effects, *Pete* drew attention, in particular, to tiredness and skin reactions. Not everyone became fatigued: some people sprang up from their couch and went back to work, and most patients thought the tiredness brought about by chemotherapy to be far worse. In regard to the skin, in the area exposed, it should be massaged at least twice a day with an emollient cream both before and after radiotherapy treatment. *Pete* thought that many of the other side effects listed in the brochures, such as hair loss, sickness and sore throat, could occur after certain types of radiotherapy, but were most unlikely after my specifically-targeted treatment for breast cancer.

Post- operative risk of lymphoedema

Pete turned his attention to the post-operative risks of lymphoedema, which, he said, I had a 1 in 4 chance of developing, usually during the first two years after my lymphadenectomy. It was important to check every week for the signs of lymphoedema by comparing the arm from shoulder to fingers on the left side of the body (from where the nodes had been removed) with my right arm, and looking for differences in the form of swelling, sensitivity, or feelings of heaviness. I should never wear tight-fitting clothes on my left arm. The risks of developing lymphoedema in that arm were worse because I was left-handed and made use of that side of my body more often and more actively and energetically.[3]

Other factors that might lead to a lymphoedema were damage to the skin of the arms, wrists and hands, brought about by cuts, hot water, or over-use. The skin should be protected by wearing protective clothing and gloves, using moisturising and antiseptic cream, and undertaking regular 'muscle pump' activity. *Pete* demonstrated an exercise for the arms to be undertaken before and during an aeroplane flight.

The reader may wonder why this detailed lymphoedema advice should appear in the chapter on radiotherapy, to which the answer is that the consultation on lymphoedema was provided by a radiographer in the context of a discussion of the side effects of radiotherapy which took place more than six months after the lymph-node clearance operation. Mel was of the view that this was a repetition of information we had previously been given by the breast cancer nursing team. That may have been true, but not in the same detailed, specific, expert, and practical way as Pete provided on this occasion..

Difficulty in confirming the dates of my radiotherapy

We inquired as to when the radiotherapy was likely to begin. A provisional date of the 22nd May had been written onto the Deanesly Centre Appointment Card, but *Pete* thought that that was a little too soon after the end of the sixth chemotherapy cycle. The radiotherapy regime would be carefully planned and the department would phone me to tell me when the three week course was due to begin.

Two weeks later, following a visit to Durnall for my routine line care on the 24th May, Mel and I decided to call in at the Deanesly Centre to seek confirmation of the start date for my radiotherapy. We had gathered from what the specialist oncology nurse had found out for us, and from entries we had seen in my patient record, that my course had been provisionally booked to begin on the 4th June. We had read in Breast Cancer Care's booklet, *Radiotherapy for primary breast cancer*, that there were national guidelines in England recommending that radiotherapy should begin no later than 31 days after the completion of chemotherapy, although delay could be incurred for a number of reasons.[4] Provisionally booked for the 4th June, my radiotherapy was scheduled to begin exactly 15 days after the completion of the sixth and final 21-day chemotherapy cycle and half-way through the maximum recommended waiting time.

In the knowledge that the radiotherapy was imminent but had not yet been confirmed, and that I would be expected to attend the hospital every day without fail for three weeks, I was encountering great difficulty in committing myself to attend meetings, respond to invitations, or meet social obligations. For example, I had been unable to agree to speak at a conference, confirm my presence at a relative's funeral in Grimsby, or book a rail ticket to an award ceremony Mel was expected to attend in Manchester. To fulfil my commitments and maintain my social itinerary, I felt obliged to firm up the times and dates of my hospital appointments as quickly as possible.

I spoke to one of the receptionists at the desk on Deanesly, explaining that I understood my radiotherapy had been planned and that I would find it helpful to have the dates confirmed. She asked me whether I had received a phone call from the radiotherapy department to tell me the time and date. I told her I had not. Then I must wait, she said, until I was called. I was not satisfied with this response and asked to speak to someone in radiotherapy to provide me with a definitive answer. She told me that this would be pointless but agreed, nevertheless, to make the call.

After five minutes, a senior therapy radiographer came out to tell us that her department was still in the process of planning my radiotherapy and that I would receive a telephone call to let me know the date and time when it had been finalised. I tried to explain why I needed to know in advance, only to be told that I clearly did not appreciate that they were dealing here with radiation and that, for my own sake, my treatment had to be planned meticulously, and signed off by my consultant oncologist. I suggested that it might be helpful for her to involve me in planning the dates and times of my treatment. Surely, one factor relevant to their arrangements was the patient's availability to attend hospital on fifteen successive days? My intervention was not welcomed, but met with the assertion that she was a senior radiographer with many years of experience, and that they would be contacting me (not the other way round) when the process had been finalised.[5] (In the context of what was to follow in the form of the allocation of appointment times on a random daily basis, it never occurred to me that my request to be consulted on the planning of my radiotherapy treatment schedule was subversive of the current system, indeed revolutionary.)

The futility of the impasse upset me. Why could she not have told me the provisional dates that had already been entered onto my patient record, while reaffirming the fact that they might be subject to change at short notice? Not until one week later on the afternoon of the 31st May, and only one-and-a-half working days before my treatment was due to begin, did we receive a telephone call from the radiotherapy department confirming the 4th June start date. We found the radiotherapy department's response to our quite legitimate inquiry about the start date unhelpful, unnecessary, discourteous and, quite frankly, perplexing. Surely, such a short notice period was unnecessary and avoidable in the course of an otherwise well-planned and structured six-month-long adjuvant therapy programme?

First treatment session (Monday 4th June 2018)

On Monday 4th June, Mel and I arrived at the Deanesly Oncology Centre for my 12.20 pm appointment and sat in the waiting room with around twenty other patients and their companions until 12.50 pm, when a radiographer called my name. She led us down a corridor into a spacious radiography suite, where Mel was directed to another crowded waiting area, and I was shown to a changing cubicle. I was instructed to take off my jacket, shirt, tie and wrist watch from my upper body and place them into a basket, and put on an open-backed hospital gown.

I sat on the bench in the little changing cubicle for a further fifteen minutes, before concluding that I must have been forgotten, and venturing out into the corridor next to the suite housing the grandly-named Linac 4 (linear accelerator number 4) - not Linac 3, as *Pete* had first told us. Eventually, a passing radiographer spotted me in my gown, loitering with a basket of clothes, and asked whether she could help. I explained my business, she checked my name, and took me directly into the room containing the Linac.

Checking my identity once more, she and another radiographer got me to sit, and then lie on a couch next to the white linear accelerator, distinguished with the brand tag, 'Electa'. I was required to remove the gown and edge myself up and down the couch while placing my knees over the leg rest and my arms above my head in the arm rests. The radiographers took time to align the pin-point tattoos on my torso with the green laser beams from the machine, while calling out coordinating numbers to one another. They raised the couch and shifted it from side to side, and, when satisfied that I was correctly positioned, attached what they called a 'jelly pad' over my mastectomy scar. (In the information leaflet given to breast cancer patients receiving radiotherapy, the pad is referred to as a 'bolus' - a special pad placed over the chest to concentrate the radiation dose on the surface of the skin and acting as a tissue equivalent, compensating for missing tissue.[6])

265

Above me I could see a circular structure (called a 'collimator'), possibly a metre in diameter, inset with a 40 cm metallic plate, attached to a 2.5-metre mechanical arm (or gantry). One of the radiographers explained that they would first take an x-ray to make sure I was correctly positioned. Then my chest would be targeted with four beams of radiation, two from the left and (once the gantry had swung to the other side of my body), two from the right. The staff retired from the room, reassuring me that they would be monitoring me on a video screen. The collimator began to click and whine, changing position a couple of times, before the radiographers re-entered the room to reposition the jelly-pad on the right of my chest, before departing again. Deprived of my wrist watch (which on this first and only occasion I was told to remove), I estimated that the procedure, from start to finish, lasted for between ten and fifteen minutes.

Once I had received my daily radiation dose and had been thanked by the radiographers for lying still, I attempted to dismount from the couch, not realising that it had been raised to around 1.5 metres above the floor, whereupon a radiographer made haste to lower it, remarking that at this stage in my treatment it would be a pity to break a leg. In future, she said, I should wait for them to hand me my gown. I had completed my first radiotherapy session. It had been completely painless: no heat, no scorching, no rawness, no burning sensation, just the click, whir and whine of a Linac machine.

One of the radiographers went to a computer screen to book me an appointment for the following day, returning with a 4.10 pm date scribbled onto an appointment card. I asked whether for my convenience it would be possible to book all 14 subsequent appointments at the same time each day, but was told that a patient's appointments were made on an individual daily basis after each treatment session. If on any particular day, I had difficulty with the timing, then they would do their best to work around my arrangements. I was shown back to the changing cubicle. Mel and I left the hospital at around 2.00 pm.

The alienation of the machine

I found my first session of radiotherapy different from the cancer treatment that had gone before, not, of course, in respect of the seemingly unpredictable waiting time and delay, but in its more impersonal, solitary and automated aspects. In the short time I had contact with them, the radiographers were friendly and courteous, but self-evidently busy and engaged in their job of measuring and positioning my body on the couch beneath the Linac machine. Although they wore name tags, I was not offered an opportunity to read the name tags, address them by name, involve them in conversation, or ask questions, but merely to respond to their instructions and position my body accordingly. Once I was in place and ready for irradiation, they withdrew to their haven, leaving me alone with the machine.

It put me in mind of a factory job I had undertaken many years ago in the school holidays. I was detailed to mind a complex piece of machinery, at one end ensuring it was fed with materials, and at the other stacking its products, a repetitive and endless process, in the course of which I learned the meaning of the expression 'the alienation of the machine'. Without companions, all by myself, alone in my solitude, the machine became an all-powerful, all-controlling, all-consuming monster, assuming a significance out of all proportion to its essentially labour-saving and benevolent function. Likewise, I sensed the Linac 4 machine controlled me, not I the machine. The human dimension to the radiotherapy treatment was reduced still further by the pressure on the radiographers' time, the preoccupation with 'setting up', the daily variation in staffing rosters and patients' attendance slots, and the fact that radiographers and patients were in contact for very brief periods. Inevitably, the radiographers appeared to bond more with their impressive machines than with their often bewildered and elderly patients.

Second treatment session (Tuesday 5ᵗʰ June 2018)

Tuesday's 4.10 pm radiotherapy appointment meant that Mel was unable to accompany me. I arrived at Deanesly Centre in good time at 3.55 pm, but had to sit in the waiting room until 5.27 pm for my name to be called - one hour and seventeen minutes after the appointment time. I asked the smiling radiographer, *Zafirah*, who came to fetch me, the reason for the delay. She explained apologetically that they usually ended up running late because frail or vulnerable patients took longer to treat than they had allowed for. To be fair, the electronic display screen in the waiting room that day read "Welcome to Deanesly Centre...LA 4 is running 45 minutes behind...We apologise for the delay."

Zafirah showed me to the changing room next to the outer door of the LA 4 suite, where I quickly removed my upper garments and put on the hospital gown. To avoid further delay, I decided this time to wait in full sight in the main corridor next to the LA 4 suite. *Zafirah* soon came to conduct me through the doors and along the passage to the Linac 4 machine.

I took off the gown and placed it in my clothes basket before mounting the couch. On this occasion, and for all subsequent sessions, I was not asked to remove my watch, and began to anticipate proceedings by discarding my hospital gown before mounting the couch. It dawned on me that the hospital gowns were being provided routinely for women in order to hide their breasts and to provide them with privacy on the short journey from the changing room to the Linac couch. Surely, for men, the gown was superfluous and should have been optional?

The two radiographers worked fast to position me, telling me politely, but firmly, to save any questions I might have until they had completed my treatment. They read out a series of numbers while aligning my tattoos with the laser beams, attached the bolus to my chest, and then retreated as the giant machine whirred into action. From entering the room to dismounting from the couch, the procedure lasted no longer than ten minutes. *Zafirah* then gave me the time of my next appointment. Much to my surprise, it was an evening session, fixed for 7.20 pm on Wednesday 6th June. I was left to find my own way from the Linac suite to the changing room.

My failure to knock on the door

As I buttoned my shirt, it occurred to me that the Deanesly reception where patients registered their attendance might be closed at that time in the evening, and that I would need to check how I would notify the radiography department of my arrival on Wednesday. There were no staff in sight to ask, and so I pushed the button to open the door into the Linac suite from which I had just emerged. Leading off to the left was another door into the radiographers' office, where three members of staff were in conversation, including *Zafirah*, who had just given me the 7.20 pm appointment time. I attempted to ask her my question about access, only to be interrupted by her older companion, who told me sternly that I had entered a restricted and private area and should

Breast Cancer Man

have knocked on the door before entering. I had to understand that the staff were entitled to privacy. I was surprised by the vehemence of her comments, particularly as there was no notice on the outer door with instructions to knock, and the door to the side office had been left wide open. Courteously, and without any further fuss, *Zafirah*, who had given me the appointment, clarified evening access arrangements.

My normal reaction would have been to ignore such a petty and unnecessary reprimand, but I remained upset and distressed for the rest of the evening, feelings I put down to my vulnerability as a first-time radiotherapy patient. In regard to the requirement to knock on the door, this was another sure sign of a prevailing status insecurity, first revealed in our encounter with the senior therapy radiographer with 'many years of experience'. Perhaps, unlike doctors and nurses, who were celebrated and seen as paradigms of people-centredness, radiographers were perceived by their patients primarily as technicians ministering to machines, with all that that entailed for their standing in society: alienated by the Linacs they served and constantly needing to be reassured as to their social importance and usefulness.

A few days later, while scanning *The Economist* (9.6.2018), I came across an article on the impact of artificial intelligence on the future of the workforce. It argued that computers' ability to recognise objects in pictures would put many white-collar jobs at risk, citing the example of radiology - the analysis of medical images. One expert in artificial intelligence was quoted as saying, "It's quite obvious that we should stop training radiologists".[7] If radiologists, at the summit of the diagnostic-imaging profession, were in danger of being put out of business by discerning decision-making machines, then the same technology would doubly

Radiotherapy

underscore radiographers' lowly technician status, unless they radically redefined their role and refocused on interpersonal and people-centred skills.

Third treatment session (Wednesday 6th June 2018)

Recognising my distress following the second visit to the radiotherapy department, Mel was determined to accompany me to the third session, and to obtain some guarantee that future treatment times would take into account our commitments, particularly our need to stay overnight in Manchester for the combined 70th anniversary celebration of the foundation of the NHS and the arrival of the ship, the Empire Windrush, which had carried some of the UK's first black-Caribbean migrants. Mel had read in the hospital's radiotherapy leaflet that patients were expected to give plenty of warning if they wanted a specific appointment time.

I had been assigned Wednesday's appointment at 7.20 pm, but we arrived at the hospital at 7.05 pm, and, as previously instructed, made our way to the waiting area, near to the Linac 4 rooms. Almost as soon as we sat down at around 7.10 pm, a radiographer called my name. As the three of us walked along the corridor, Mel informed her of our invitation to the celebratory dinner in Manchester and our need to stay overnight. She acknowledged that we were providing adequate notice and said she would make a note of our request on my record. She escorted me to the changing room, gave me a moment to remove my upper garments, and then led me without further delay to the Linac machine.

The human face of radiography

She introduced herself as *Krystyna*, pausing to allow me to read her name badge, *'Krystyna Kowalczyk'*, which predisposed me towards

271

her. *Krystyna* and her companion positioned me on the couch, read off my numbers, placed the bolus on my chest, and administered the radiation as planned, completing the session by 7.25 pm. *Krystyna* then listened carefully to my request to forward-plan three of my future sessions and entered new times onto my computerised treatment schedule, even drawing my attention to my Thursday morning appointment for line care on Durnall, and suggesting I come to Deanesly immediately afterwards for radiotherapy (which had been previously booked for 11.20 am). Compared with my previous experiences, she could not have been more helpful and accommodating.

Fourth treatment session (Thursday 7th June 2018)

As soon as my line care had been completed on Durnall, Mel and I walked over to Deanesly for my radiotherapy session, and made our way to the Linac 4 waiting area. *Sean*, a male radiographer, with a calm and reassuring voice, came out to tell us he could slot me in after he had dealt with two other patients at the front of the queue. I was admitted to the Linac 4 suite by 9.35 am and my treatment completed by 9.50 am. *Sean* stood out for explaining the details of my radiotherapy programme and how the bolus worked, and for his willingness to answer my questions.

After the friendly and accommodating patient-centred experience of the third and fourth sessions, I was inclined to revise my generalised observations on the status-insecurity and alienation of radiographers which had, after all, been based at the time on a selective sample of only two radiographers. Nevertheless, at this stage, I was only four days into my fifteen-day course of treatment.

Fifth treatment session (Friday 8th June 2018)

Friday's radiotherapy had been scheduled for 9.30 am, so I set out early to allow for the morning traffic and arrived on the car park for 9.20 am. My name was called out bang on time and I had removed my jacket, shirt and tie by 9.35 am, when I was led once more to Linac 4. *Krystyna* and another radiographer were on duty. They very quickly got me to lie on the treatment couch, where they aligned my tattoos with the green laser lights. They retired to their office to switch on the x-rays, leaving me alone with the bolus on my chest and a collimator buzzing, first to the right, and then to the left, of my body. By now, on the fifth day, I knew what to expect and the time passed quickly - between ten and fifteen minutes. Aware of my request to timetable treatment around the Manchester event, *Krystyna* then wrote the times of my Monday, Tuesday and Wednesday appointments onto my appointment card, relieving my anxiety and earning my gratitude. I was dressed and walking out of Deanesly by 9.50 am, the shortest radiotherapy session so far.

First week of radiotherapy

Family and friends inquired how I had found my first week of radiotherapy. What were the side effects? Was I feeling tired and exhausted? I had been feeling unduly tired and exhausted on and off since January and was not sure whether to attribute the symptoms to the current radiotherapy, the aftermath of the six cycles of chemotherapy, the tamoxifen tablets (that I had started to take on the 30th May), or, indeed, at that time of the year, my hay-fever medication. The same went for my sore throat which had persisted for three days, and was listed as a recognised side effect in the Breast Cancer Care booklet on radiotherapy[8] but, in my case, might well have been a symptom of hay fever, as in previous years.

Since January, I had retired for a short afternoon nap roughly three times a week, and had not noticed any change or extension to that routine. Similarly, the diminution in my strength and stamina and occasional breathlessness had been discernible since the start of the chemotherapy, although I believed I was now showing signs of recovery. Likewise, the hairs on my head and chin were beginning to grow, but not yet enough to disguise my baldness or restore my beard. Hair loss was also a recognised side effect of radiotherapy but only to the treatment area, that is, to my chest.[9]

Since my radiotherapy began, I believed that I had experienced an occasional pang of pain or burning sensation in my left breast[10] but, when I stopped to examine the area, I felt and saw nothing further. Mel, too, had looked but had not noticed anything out of the ordinary. The hospital's information leaflet on radiotherapy warned of the possibility of shooting pains, aches and twinges,[11] but almost ten months since surgery, and after one week of radiotherapy, I had little to complain about.

Other commonly-mentioned side effects were redness and dryness to the skin in the area irradiated, and soreness and swelling of the arm. I was already applying the prescribed Zero AQS emollient cream to the chest area next to my mastectomy scar, as well as to both arms and, so far, had witnessed no reddening, dryness, or soreness. Overall, I was comforted by the absence of side effects but still perturbed by the daily variation in treatment times and my inability to plan my itinerary more than one day at a time. Over the last week alone, appointments for treatment had been at 12.20 pm, 4.10 pm, 7.20 pm, 8.30 am, and 9.30 am and, on one occasion, I had to wait 1 hour 17 minutes before my name was called. When I read over this comment some time later, I was inclined to delete it as somewhat trivial in the grand scheme of adjuvant therapy, but preserved it in situ as representative of the irritation and anxiety I felt at the time.

I welcomed the two-day weekend break in the 15-day cycle, noting my radiotherapy course was due to begin again at 18.45 pm on Monday 11th June - indeed calculated in hours, an interlude of over 80 hours, or 3 days 7 hours. If they could miss three days without impacting on the treatment's efficacy, couldn't I miss a day? I noticed the Saturday and Sunday breaks in treatment were presented in the literature as patient recovery time, but a suspicion crossed my mind that, in reality, it was because the day centre did not open at the weekend, and the concentration of treatment into intense-five-day blocks arose from the industrial scale of the process and the need to maintain and measure a regular throughput.

Second week of radiotherapy

In the second week, I lay under the white Linac 4 machine for roughly ten minutes each day with my tattoos aligned with the green laser beams, in the same way as I had in the first, but no longer with a bolus resting on my chest. On Monday 11th June, my name was called at the appointment time of 6.45 pm, but I was left to wait in a hospital gown for a quarter of an hour in the changing room. My mood improved when I realised *Krystyna* and her companion were conducting the session.

On Tuesday 12th June, my appointment time was 8.30 am, with my name called at 9 am. Once again, my two favourite radiographers, *Krystyna* and *Sean*, were present. As per routine, they positioned me efficiently, leaving the room as the Linac clicked, whirred and whined into action. Mel and I had left the hospital by 9.25 am, with plenty of time to spare before catching the train to Manchester.

The NHS Windrush Award Celebration

Mel had been invited to the 12th June 2018 NHS Windrush Awards, celebrating the contribution of black and minority ethnic staff to the 70-year history of the National Health Service. The founding of the NHS at Trafford Hospital in Manchester on the 5th July 1948 coincided closely with the arrival of the ship, the Empire Windrush, at Tilbury Docks on the 22nd June 1948, bringing 492 West Indian migrants to work in the United Kingdom. Mel and I had a very enjoyable dinner attended by well over 500 people at Manchester Central Conference Centre, with speeches by Yvonne Coghill and Professor Jane Cummings of NHS England, and Andy Burnham, the mayor of Greater Manchester, followed by presentations to NHS Windrush Award winners, and the introduction of the guest of honour, Alford Gardner, born in Jamaica in 1926 and one of the few surviving passengers who arrived on the Empire Windrush in June 1948. Guests were presented with a supplement produced by *The Voice* (June 2018) containing profiles of senior and successful contributors to the NHS from black and minority ethnic backgrounds.[12] A half-page article was devoted to Mel's career. Having had a good time at the event, where Mel met old friends, we were both very tired by the time we returned to our hotel. Quite frankly, I felt so exhausted I was scarcely able to take off my clothes and climb into bed. I put this down to the fact that I was now half way through the radiotherapy course and was suffering from its most widely-acknowledged side effect - fatigue.

We had breakfast at Manchester Piccadilly Station before boarding the train back to Wolverhampton. I had time for an afternoon nap in my own bed before my Wednesday radiotherapy session, which had been deliberately arranged for 8.00 pm in the evening. We arrived at the Deanesly Centre early and made our way to the Linac

4 waiting area. My name was called early at 7.50 pm by someone familiar: I recognised *Waliyah Raza*, the radiographer who had helped in the initial planning of my treatment in April, almost eight weeks previously. More to the point, she recognised me. The second radiographer was the ever-helpful and courteous *Krystyna*. By 8.05 pm my treatment was completed and, soon after, Mel and I left the hospital and were on our way home via our favourite Chapel Ash kebab shop.

On Thursday 14th June, we had to visit the Durnall Day Unit for blood samples to be taken prior to the the removal of my Hickman line on the following day. Afterwards, as instructed, we made our way to the Deanesly Outpatients Department and were told to wait in the Linac 5 waiting area. (We were told Linac 4 was being serviced.) There, we waited from 9.10 am to 10.25 am, as the busy radiographers did their best to slot me into the patient queue. When the time came, *Zafirah* took me to the Linac 5 changing room suite and then to the Linac 5 machine itself, where she and another radiographer put me into position and administered the radiation. To my untutored eyes, Linac 5 looked identical to Linac 4, but was housed in a more modern and spacious suite of rooms. By 10.45 am, I had completed my treatment for the day and Mel and I were ready to leave the hospital. We were not, however, able to secure an appointment time before 3 pm on Friday, prior to the removal of my Hickman line, and faced the prospect of walking over from Durnall after the procedure to wait for a 6.00 pm radiotherapy slot.

My Hickman line was removed to plan on the afternoon of 15th June, We left Durnall at 4.35 pm and, feeling in need of a pick-me-up, went for cappuccinos at the hospital coffee bar. Knowing that we might have to wait two hours for my radiotherapy appointment, we drank it in a leisurely fashion before strolling to register our presence at Deanesly. Just on time, we made our way to the Linac 4 waiting area to see *Krystyna's* welcoming face. She showed me to the changing room and, a moment or two later at 5.15 pm, I was positioned and given my requisite x-ray dose. With my treatment for the week completed by 5.35 pm, Mel and I left the hospital, both of us greatly relieved.

In the second week, treatment had been scheduled early and late in the day, sometimes at my request to suit me, but usually to fit the needs of the radiotherapy department (6.45 pm, 9.00 am, 8.00 pm, 10.30 am, 6.00 pm). The good news was that, on two occasions, I had been treated early, well before the designated appointment time.

Third week of radiotherapy

After ten 'fractions' of radiotherapy, I was becoming used to the routine, each daily session lasting around ten minutes from the initial setting up to being given the next appointment. I was led into the Linac room, where I took off my gown to lay bare my chest. I lay on the couch, with my knees bent over a rest and my arms supported above my head. The radiographers manipulated me into position with the aid of my tattoos, the green laser lights, and a series of numbers they called as they adjusted the angles of the Linac machine. Once they had retreated from the room, the radiation doses - two from the right and two from the left - were administered automatically. When they came back in, they praised me for keeping still, lowered the couch, helped me to dismount, and gave me the time of my next appointment. After thanking them for my treatment, I took up my clothes basket containing the discarded hospital gown and, starkly bare-chested, left via the corridor to return to the changing room, where I put on my shirt and jacket, and deposited the gown in the laundry bag.

I must have watched too many films or television programmes about the death penalty in the United States, for every time I tried to visualise my radiotherapy treatment, the first image that entered my mind was of a prisoner strapped to a gurney, surrounded by men in white lab coats, who gave him a lethal injection, before retreating to a separate chamber to observe him from behind a glass partition. Radiotherapy wasn't like that at all, but I did not seem able to control that particular image. At least, US prisoners on death row - barring last-minute reprieves - were given a definitive execution time and date and, only on very exceptional occasions, did they return for a further appointment.

After the first ten sessions, I began to memorise the numbers called by the radiographers, and finally asked *Krystyna* to confirm them by writing them down. They read: 21.1/22.0/89.0/10.0/9.0.

What were never routine or readily remembered were the appointment times. They were given out after each session for the following day, without any opportunity for the patient to express a preference, although I presumed a time would be altered if the patient found it impossible to attend. My times varied wildly from day to day: early morning, around lunch, and evening. On Monday the 18th June, my appointment time was at 6.15 pm. *Krystyna* called me at 6.30 pm, the radiotherapy took place a few minutes later and by 6.45 pm I was on my way out of the hospital. My appointment on Tuesday was at 1.15 pm. I was called at 1.25 pm. My mood improved when I realised that the radiographers on duty were *Krystyna* and *Zafirah* who, by now, were able to position me routinely and rapidly under the Linac 4. By 1.40 pm, I was dressed and ready to leave. On Wednesday, my appointment was at 6.40 pm, and on Thursday at 1.05 pm (but my name was called early at 12.50 pm and Mel and I had already left Deanesly by the officially-scheduled time). My fifteenth and final radiotherapy session, on Friday the 22nd June, was memorable not only for being the last in the series and cause for celebration, but for being timetabled at 7.15 am in the morning.

Even at this early hour, *Krystyna* was in attendance with another of her colleagues, both of them equally bright and alert, and dressed in white morning-clean uniform. The procedure went like clockwork and afterwards, realising it was my final visit, *Krystyna* found time to inquire about my health and the way I had responded to radiotherapy. She presented me with the Oncology Directorate's completion-of-radiotherapy form, which listed the ongoing side effects I should look out for over the following weeks, and gave the likely date and place of the follow-up appointment with my oncologist (six weeks' time at New Cross). I was provided with a telephone number to call if I experienced particularly acute red, dry, itchy, moist, sore, or broken skin in the area of the breast/chest that had been treated, and advised to drink more water to deal with any pronounced symptoms of fatigue.

Mel and I drove home to Blue Roof, pleased that the radiotherapy and, indeed, all the hospital-based adjuvant treatment was complete, and sat down to a celebratory breakfast of cereals and tea. I was still apprehensive about late side effects, having felt sensitivity and soreness in the vicinity of my mastectomy scar - fleeting spasms of pain, which Mel sought to treat with the ZeroAQS emollient cream.

Twice a day, Mel helped me in massaging the irradiated area with the emollient cream, with the aim of soothing any remaining inflammation and reducing the ruddy-brown appearance of my chest. Despite regular treatment, it still displayed the distinctive telltale 20cm x 25cm rectangular brown mark for many weeks after the radiotherapy had come to an end, although it never felt sensitive or sore.

Breast Cancer Man

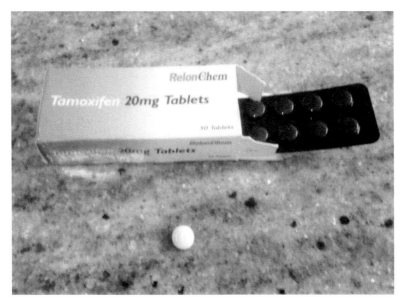

Tamoxifen tablets

Chapter 16

Hormone therapy with tamoxifen

The benefits of tamoxifen

On the 30th May 2018, shortly before my radiotherapy treatment was due to begin, I started on the course of tamoxifen that *Dr Hetu Charitha Gupta* had prescribed for me six weeks earlier on the 16th April. I had been under the misapprehension that the three adjuvant therapies followed on from one another, like the coaches of a train, until *Dr Gupta* explained that the sooner I began on tamoxifen the better. Research showed that the efficacy of the anti-oestrogen drug was not impaired by radiotherapy treatment.

The tamoxifen 20mg tablets were produced by RelonChem and came in a box of 30, one tablet to be taken orally at the same time every day for the next five years[1] - and then possibly for a further five years beyond that date. My GP at Castlecroft Medical Practice would be responsible for prescribing all future tamoxifen tablets.

Dr Gupta made clear the benefits of taking tamoxifen for patients with oestrogen receptor positive (ER+) breast cancer. It reduced the risk of the old breast cancer recurring or of a new breast cancer developing, by reducing the level of oestrogen in the body and preventing it from attaching to the cancer cells. I, along with 9 out of 10 men who had breast cancer, had the oestrogen-receptor-positive form of the disease.[2]

Preferable to castration

The tamoxifen hormonal therapy was essential for preventing the return of my cancer. It was important that I went on taking the tablets consistently. I knew this to be true, but was incentivised, not so much by *Dr Gupta's* pep talk, but by information I acquired many years previously on genital mutilation. While participating in a research project on that subject, I learned of the horrific prospect of orchiectomy (effectively, castration), the surgical removal of the testicles as a means of reducing androgens (male hormones). As androgens could convert into oestrogens, the performance of an orchiectomy provided a way of treating male breast cancer before the widespread availability and prescription of tamoxifen.

Tamoxifen's intolerable effect on Victoria Derbyshire

Unhesitating in my preference for tamoxifen and acknowledging its effectiveness in reducing the risk of my cancer returning, I remembered Victoria Derbyshire's account of its intolerable side effects:

'When I wake in the morning and get out of bed, walking those first few steps is awkwardly painful - my muscles around the tops of my legs ache and click as I try to get them going again. And then all day I can feel a dull ache around my abdomen, like constant period pain....I'm not sure I can do this for ten years.'[3]

Twelve days later she decided to take control and stop taking it for a while.[4] Before starting my course and in consideration of her experience, I studied the Breast Cancer Care booklet on what tamoxifen is, how it works, and its side effects.[5] I also reread the section on hormonal therapy in Macmillan's *Understanding Breast Cancer in Men*.[6]

Most accounts state that tamoxifen affects those who take it in different ways, some experiencing more side effects than others and others not noticing any side effects at all. The most common side effects, described as 'menopausal symptoms', are hot flushes, night sweats, sleep disturbance, vaginal irritation. loss of libido and mood changes,[7] and appear to be listed with women in mind. However, Macmillan's *Understanding Breast Cancer in Men*, makes clear that hot flushes and sweats, loss of libido and mood swings can also be experienced by men, alongside erectile dysfunction.[8] Other recognised side effects affecting both men and women are headaches, light headedness, unsteadiness, dizziness, nausea, fluid retention, tiredness, leg cramps, and muscle pain.

The box of blister-packed tamoxifen tablets came with a leaflet listing even more serious side effects: symptoms of a blood clot (swelling of the calf or leg, or chest pain), symptoms of a stroke (weakness or paralysis of arms and legs), and symptoms arising from a reduction of the blood supply to the brain (difficulty in breathing, swelling of the face, lips or tongue).[9]   A patient experiencing any of these must stop taking the tablets and seek medical help immediately.

My first tamoxifen tablet

With this information in mind, and alerted to the many other possible side effects, I took my first tamoxifen tablet at 8.30 am on Wednesday 30th May 2018.   I swallowed it cautiously with a mouthful of water, accompanied by a breakfast consisting of a bowl of oats porridge with honey and dates.   In accordance with advice, I deliberately downed my tablet with food, in the hope that I might avoid any feeling of sickness or nausea.[10]   This being the first time, too, that I had taken tamoxifen, I decided as a precaution to refrain for the day from my hay fever medication.

Afterwards, I cleaned my teeth, read the newspaper and worked on the computer until 11 am, before making Mel and myself a welcome cup of cappuccino.   Realising that, so far, I felt surprisingly normal, I decided to follow my regular Wednesday routine, and drove to B&Q to buy slabs and plants for the garden. Still no discernible side effects!

I took the second tamoxifen tablet with breakfast on Thursday and spent much of the morning in the garden trimming the box hedges. Feeling drowsy, I sat on the bench and drank coffee with Mel while watching the bees flying from flower to flower.   Annoyed with my idleness, I stood up and made my way indoors, only to be overcome by a feeling of dizziness, which forced me to sink to my knees on the step.   My unexpected light-headedness was soon overcome and I arose and went on with my business, thinking no more of the matter.   It was only much later that evening that I realised that my dizzy spell may have been connected to taking the tamoxifen tablets.[11]

I was distracted that afternoon by the onset of hay fever symptoms, a prolonged bout of sneezing and itching eyes - the consequence of stopping my anti-histamine on the previous day. From then on, I took my tamoxifen with breakfast and my cetirizine with supper. I purposely refrained from telling anyone about the dizziness because I knew family and friends would insist that I stop driving the car and perhaps even mowing the lawn. The feeling of fatigue continued. It may have been due to the lingering effect of the chemotherapy or exacerbated by the course of tamoxifen. In any case, I no longer fought the exhaustion during the day, but capitulated on a regular basis to an afternoon nap.

By the fifth tamoxifen tablet on Sunday 3rd June, I had experienced one solitary instance of dizziness and was strongly disposed to an afternoon nap, but otherwise I seemed to have settled into a steady and uneventful pill-popping routine., taking the tamoxifen at breakfast to keep the cancer at bay, and the cetirizine at supper to fend off my seasonal hay fever.

By the tenth tamoxifen tablet on Friday the 8th June, and after my first five fractions of radiotherapy, I began to relax on the assumption that, if I were going to experience any major adverse side effects, they would by now have made themselves apparent. At this stage, at least, I did not appear to be among the 20 per cent of men who stopped taking the drug (either of their own accord or on the advice of a doctor) because of its unacceptable side effects.[12]

Securing a regular supply of tablets

In recognition that I was in for the long haul - was it for five or ten years on the pill? - I resolved to visit the Castlecroft Medical Practice to secure a repeat prescription. (Only the first 30 tablets were provided on prescription by the hospital.)

Carol, the clerk responsible for the operation of the prescription service, listened to my request, found the letter on my medical record from *Dr Gupta* at the hospital to *Dr Shakeshaft*, head of the Castlecroft Medical Practice, and organised a repeat prescription for tamoxifen there and then, with a facility for monthly reordering. Obtaining the drug for the foreseeable future could not have been simpler. Just as impressive, the tamoxifen course came at no charge to me, as I was 60 years of age or over and therefore entitled to free NHS prescriptions. What a marvellous arrangement for elderly cancer suffers like me, and one more personal reason for supporting the National Health Service's founding principles!

The threat and fear of sexual dysfunction

By the 28th June, I had consumed my first box of tamoxifen - thirty tablets in all, and was beginning to believe that I could manage the next 4 years 11 months without any difficulty. Was it possible that I had escaped the side effects unscathed? The package leaflet listed plenty of side effects that applied only to women. Tamoxifen worked on my oestrogen-receptor positive breast cancer by blocking the effects of oestrogen, the primary female sex hormone. (It was an 'anti-oestrogen'.) But what of all those men I had read about who chose to stop taking tamoxifen? Could the tablets be affecting me in more subtle ways that I had yet to discover?

Could my virility be under threat? By now, I had read that about 1 in 5 men taking tamoxifen experienced sexual dysfunction.[13] The possibility that, for the duration of the tamoxifen course, I might not be able to get an erection or experience sexual desire, even at 73 years of age, was, for me, the most daunting of the recognised side effects, only made tolerable in the knowledge that the drug I was taking prevented breast cancer returning and was undoubtedly preferable to the unthinkable alternative, the orchiectomy, hopefully a thing of the past. So far, so good! To date, I'd not noticed any discernible change to my sex drive.

I had read that an orchiectomy could result in weight gain and increase of fatty tissue on hips and chest, as portrayed in the stereotypical depiction of eunuchs. Likewise, weight gain was a well-recognised side effect of tamoxifen.[14] I had noticed, too, that, while hair was visibly returning to my head, the whiskers on my chin were not growing so profusely (no sign of a beard as yet), and my pubic hairs were sparser than ever. Very worrying, indeed! Would tamoxifen allow me to return to my former masculine hairy self? Only time would tell. After all, it was barely a month since the sixth chemo-cycle came to an end. (Some time later, *Dr Grigoryev* advised me that the sluggish growth of my hair on parts of my body was more likely to be an after-effect of chemotherapy, and that the tamoxifen, being an anti-oestrogen, should not affect my testosterone level, or the gradual return of my hairiness.)

New Cross Hospital Site

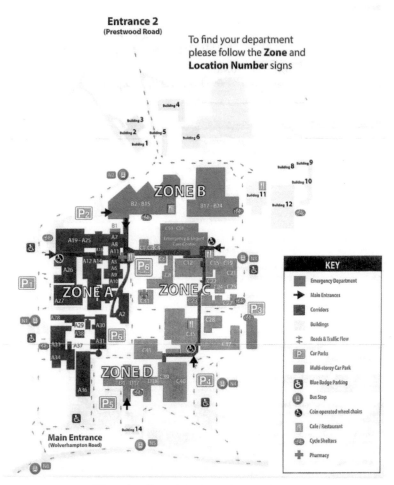

The sprawling New Cross Hospital site

Chapter 17

My time at the hospital

After the GP's initial referral of my case to the consultant, *Mr Venkatramanan*, the New Cross Hospital site of the Royal Wolverhampton NHS Trust became the focal point of my diagnosis, surgery, and subsequent adjuvant therapies. From the 23rd August 2017 to the 22nd June 2018 – a period of ten months - I visited the hospital on 69 occasions. Consultations, operations, procedures and therapies involved morning, afternoon, or whole-day visits to the out-patients department, or to the Appleby Suite for day surgery. On two occasions I was required to stay in a hospital ward overnight, the first for observation after surgery, and the second when the febrile neutropenia care pathway was invoked as a precaution. Thus, while my diagnoses and treatments were initiated and administered on the hospital site, most of my time was spent at home, where I took my prescribed medicines (capsules, tablets, creams and subcutaneous injections), lived with the after-effects, and recuperated from the hospital-based medical interventions, in particular the six 21-day cycles of chemotherapy and the fifteen daily fractions of radiotherapy.

Hospital images that stayed with me

Nevertheless, the numerous hospital visits, and the hospital setting in which the treatment took place, shaped and coloured my experience in such a profound and lasting way that my memories of having had breast cancer are frequently accompanied by images of wards full of patients, encounters with consultants and nurses, the drawing of blood, interminable chemo injections, drip stands and radiography/radiotherapy apparatus (particularly the Linacs), as well as, more prosaically, car-parking pay machines, crowded waiting rooms, electronic display boards (flashing up waiting times), orange receptacles for clinical waste, and vast expanses of blue or beige vinyl flooring.

In 2017, most of my visits were to New Cross Hospital's Outpatients Department to meet the consultant or the breast cancer nurses, to the Appleby Suite for day surgery, and to the Imaging Department and other technical facilities for x-rays, scans and biopsies. In 2018, when the emphasis switched to adjuvant therapies, I spent time in the Deanesly Centre Snowdrop chemotherapy day unit and the radiotherapy Linac suites, and in the Durnall Day Unit run by the hospital's Clinical Oncology and Haematology Directorate. The nightmares I occasionally experience are populated by *The Brides of Dracula* in lab coats drawing my blood with giant syringes, porcupines covered in cannula spines, drip stands pumping me up like Michelin Man, and mighty Linac machines marching menacingly in my direction like the tripodal heat-ray machines in Wells's *The War Of the Worlds*. And why did I always imagine the neutropenia care pathway in shades of grey, leading on through wrought-iron gates, under the sign 'arbeit macht frei'?

The extent of the hospital site

New Cross Hospital is situated on a 40-hectare (100-acre) site to the north of the Wolverhampton Road, between Heath Town and Wednesfield, approximately one-and-a-half miles to the north-east of Wolverhampton City centre. Encircled by car parks, with spaces for nearly 3,000 cars, the hospital buildings cover a central area of 23.6 hectares, The blocks vary immensely in size, scale, construction, function, condition and age, and have had to be connected by a complex web of covered passageways or corridors, the chief among them running south and north, and east and west from main entrances on the south, east and west of the site. The scale, spread and complexity of the slowly-accumulating brick, concrete, steel and glass building agglomeration is referred to, aptly, as 'a medley' in a Wolverhampton City Council report.[1] As a consequence of the layout, distances from one side of the complex to the other are considerable. From the surrounding car parks, it takes time to reach treatment locations, specialist departments, different wards and the various social facilities.

I measured the distance from the east entrance to the west entrance to be 338 metres (370 yards), and from the south entrance to the Heart and Lung Centre to be 418 metres (458 yards). Mel and I kept fit walking between the hospital's two centres of cancer treatment, Deanesley and Durnall, a work-out of 467 metres (510 yards), or just under half a kilometre. The main access corridors carry a constant stream of visitors, patients and staff on foot, and of porters pulling or pushing wheelie bins, driving electric scooters, buggy trains or tugs, or moving patients on trolley-beds or wheel chairs to and from operating theatres and diagnostic radiology and imaging departments. Elderly, frail and infirm day patients and visitors must find walking distances and times particularly onerous, even when assisted by the buggy train service.

Despite its modern and improved facilities, New Cross has never enjoyed the same local pride and affection as the old Royal Hospital, not least because it was a former workhouse and is situated well out of town and, in marked contrast to the Royal's majestic architecture, has developed haphazardly and untidily, acquiring a unique, but unendearing, higgledy-piggledy style

Currently, the Royal Wolverhampton Hospital NHS Trust provides around 800 beds on the New Cross site (including intensive care beds and neo-natal-care cots) and employs more than 8,000 staff. In 2015/16, it performed nearly 59,000 day care operations. No doubt, day operation statistics for 2017/18 include the three procedures – mastectomy, lymph node clearance, and insertion of a Hickman Line – performed on me. A large teaching hospital, New Cross takes medical students from the University of Birmingham and student nurses from the University of Wolverhampton, who were often present in the course of my treatment. The hospital budget in 2015/16 stood at more than £500 million.

Getting to the hospital

Mel and I live in Tettenhall to the west of Wolverhampton, 4.6 miles away from the New Cross Hospital site near Wednesfield to the east. We can access the hospital by using public transport (two buses), phoning for a private hire car service, or driving our own car there.

It might be assumed that, as old age pensioners with free bus passes, the cheapest and most convenient way of us making our way to the hospital would be by bus, but other considerations have to be borne in mind. Our nearest bus stop for the number 1 into the city is 1,190 metres away (almost three quarters of a mile, or a 16-minute walk. The number 1 takes us into the city centre, where a second bus, the number 59 has to be caught along the Wednesfield and Wolverhampton Roads, to a bus stop, 400 metres away from the hospital proper. The hospital is well served by the 59 service (Centro claims that 17 buses an hour, in each direction, pass by the hospital on the Wolverhampton Road), but the number 1 runs less frequently (at intervals between 15 and 30 minutes depending on the time of day – slackening off around midday).[2]

From our home in Tettenhall, we have to allow between 1½ and 2 hours for travel to be sure of arriving at the hospital on time for an appointment, bearing in mind walking time, bus frequency, traffic levels, and other possible delays For patients who have undergone hospital treatment, particularly chemotherapy, or daily radiotherapy, a return journey by bus is a daunting prospect, best avoided, especially when, as in my case, it involves relatively long walks to, from, and between bus stops.

Another practical, comfortable and relatively inexpensive way of getting to the hospital is to phone beforehand for a private car hire service to take us from our door to one of the hospital entrances, and then arrange a return journey home again. In April 2018, Go Cars charged me £8 for the 4.6 miles one-way journey from home to the hospital. The drawback was the worry over how long the car-hire driver would take to turn up (especially at peak times, such as during the school run).

For me, Mel, and probably a majority of people, the most convenient way to get to the hospital on time and without relying on others is by private car, as evidenced by New Cross's busy and crowded car parks. The drawback for frequent and regular visitors, however, is the car park charge, paid by patients, patients' visitors, and also by hospital staff.

Car parking considerations

Consistent with my life-time habit of making notes, recording events, and collecting memorabilia, I kept a diary of my and Mel's car journeys to the hospital, from the initial referral to the consultant breast surgeon on the 23rd August 2017 to the 22nd June 2018. In that time, I visited the hospital on 69 separate occasions, Mel possibly slightly more, as she came to visit me when I stayed for a day-long procedure, or was kept in overnight. Over that ten-month period, my accumulated standard hospital car parking charges would have totalled £268.00, averaging £3.88 a visit, had it not been for the discounted provision for oncology patients.

Concessionary car-parking charges for oncology patients

In recognition of the burden imposed on day patients with serious conditions that require regular treatment, the hospital offers concessions to oncology patients undergoing chemo- or radiotherapy, as well as to those on renal dialysis.

Try as I might, I could never get a clear statement from the Patient Information Centre or staff on Deanesly as to whether the concessionary charge of £1.50 per visit applied to any treatment other than my appointments for the six sessions of chemotherapy, the fifteen sessions of radiotherapy, and the fifteen sessions of line care. The Patient Information Centre tried to access the information I asked for online, but ended up giving me the telephone number for the Car Parking and Security Control Centre, despite my pointing out that the car-parking tokens were issued at reception on the oncology wards. Only at the Durnall and Deanesly reception desks, as I booked in for line care or radiotherapy, was I regularly asked whether I had travelled by car and would be requiring a car-parking token.

Should the reduced charge have applied to all visits for phlebotomy, oncology appointments and chemotherapy reviews? The oncology nurses advised me that the £1.50 charge only applied to hospital visits for chemotherapy, radiotherapy, and line care, but pointed out that, now that I had a Hickman line, all my phlebotomy sessions would have to be done on oncology wards, thus entitling me to the same reduced charge as for line care. As for appointments and reviews with the oncology doctors, the reduced charge did not apply, unless, of course, I was seen by the doctor in the course of my treatment on the Durnall Unit.

However, the precise terms of the policy were never made clear and the car parking tokens were available only when reception staff were present, which ruled out concessions for early morning or evening appointments. (It was only in June 2018 when, in conversation with parking-wise patients, we learned of other ways of dealing with the out-of-office-hours issue.) Taking into account the reduced parking charge of £1.50 for my chemotherapy, radiotherapy and line care sessions, the total concession for oncology came to £85.60p, meaning that, overall, I paid £182.40p in car parking charges for my ten-month-long cancer treatment, constituting a discount of almost a third.

Car parking charges compared

How did New Cross Hospital's car parking charges compare with those of the local authority? Wolverhampton City Council varied its charges in different city districts: for example, in Bilston and much of Wednesfield, car parking was free. In the sixteen or so Council-run city centre car parks, charges for two hours varied from £1.20 to £3.60, half (8) at £1.20, 3 at £2, 4 at £3, and only 1 at £3.60. Charges at the City Council's Fold Street car park, where Mel and I usually parked when visiting the city centre, were 70p for up to 1 hour, £1.20 for up to 2 hours, £2.50 for up to 3 hours, and £4.00 for 4 hours, etc.

An important difference between New Cross and the city-centre Fold Street car park was that New Cross was a 'pay on exit' system, with the charge calculated, displayed, and then paid at a booth before exiting, whereas Fold Street was a 'pay and display' on arrival, with a standard fine imposed for an overstay. The difference reflected a crucial difference between visiting New Cross and visiting the city centre. Most patients attending the hospital were unable to calculate the length of their stay, as they had no control over hospital waiting times. On a number of occasions, I visited the hospital expecting to be there for no more than an hour, but ended up staying for three hours or more. The hospital banding system, coupled with the exit charge, meant that any stay beyond the few minutes of grace time allowed over the hour incurred a charge for a full further hour. In contrast, when visiting the city centre, Mel and I were normally able to judge the length of time we intended to spend on shopping, drinking coffee, or visiting the art gallery.

Bearing in mind these considerations, I compared the normal parking charges for ten occasions that I had spent visiting the hospital, with the cost of staying for the same length of time on ten occasions at the Fold Street car park. The extent of the difference surprised me. It was 60 per cent cheaper to stay in the local authority's Fold Street city centre car park in normal office hours, than at the hospital, and even cheaper out of office hours.

The insidious effects of the car parking charges

With both of us in receipt of adequate occupational pensions, Mel and I could well afford the hospital car parking charges. We viewed them, however, as an unnecessary levy on the sick and, especially, the elderly and infirm, undermining the principle that the National Health Service should be available to everyone, free at the point of delivery, and based on clinical need, not on the ability to pay. In addition, most people wanted and, indeed, felt morally obliged, to attend their family members and friends in hospital, often driving there for the twice-daily visiting times, and sitting at their relatives' bedsides for long periods following their serious operations, or when they were terminally ill. Could it be right for a hospital to be making a charge on compassion?

The overall impact of car-parking charges on patients and relatives, however, was more insidious than implied by these abstract ethical considerations. Most people's lives are spent balancing hard-won income against expenditure, and guarding against unnecessary costs. From an early age, we are taught that 'every penny counts', 'to waste not and want not' and, with the burden of mortgages, fuel bills, and the upkeep of children, are drilled into the discipline of fiscal restraint. As hospital patients and visitors wait - as they must in hospital waiting areas - they not only worry about their symptoms of illness, their diagnoses and the medical procedures they face, but about the length of their wait and the open-ended bill on the car park, over which they have no control – thus contributing still further to their anxiety levels. Worse still, the longer day patients have to wait for their appointments, the more money the hospital makes out of them, a perverse counter-incentive to the drive to cut hospital waiting times.

False stereotypes of a hospital

As a 73-year-old man, I have had a life-time's experience of hospitals, from childhood to adulthood, sometimes as a patient, sometimes as a tutor to medical staff, sometimes as a visitor to sick relatives and friends, and sometimes as an attendant at the bedside of a dying parent or aunt. In common with others of my age, I have been in the care of the NHS since its creation in 1948, and am inclined to take for granted the daily appearance and routines of the hospital, making it hard to discern and describe their distinctive features and the impact they have had on me over the last few months. Nevertheless, my recent experience as a breast cancer patient who has undergone surgery and various adjuvant therapies has given me much to digest, categorise and appraise.

My stereotype of a hospital as a health spa, or hotel, where sick patients lay in bed for days, weeks and months to recover, was quickly dispelled. Along with thousands of others, I have been a walk-in day-patient who made use of only two nights of the full board and restaurant service, spending most of my time in recovery mode at home. Consultations, diagnostic tests, surgery, and adjuvant therapies were conducted at hospital to a strict hourly schedule on a daily basis, largely without any overnight stays. In this way, the health service was able to offer medical treatment on an industrial scale to many thousands of people.

I was perfectly aware that hospitals employed not only doctors and nurses but clerks, clinical assistants (who looked after wards), dieticians, medical assistants, patient services assistants (who provided, for example, drinks and meals), pharmacists, porters, technicians, technologists, and a range of therapists, plus many others. But I went on assuming in a common-sense way that the organisation was run to support the surgeons and physicians, who spent their time respectively in operating on patients or treating them with a variety of medications. The hospital, I thought, was entirely geared up to surgery and medicine.

My hospital attendance experience soon taught me otherwise. Instead, I began to recognise the scale and extent of the parallel and supportive diagnostic and monitoring activity that preceded, accompanied, and succeeded almost all in-patient and out-patient care. Much of the hospital provision, guiding doctors and nurses alike, depended on systems for testing, screening and scanning to determine the cause of patients' illnesses and the appropriate courses of treatment. Patients were being continually sent for blood counts, colonoscopies, CAT (computer axial tomography) scans, echocardiograms, electrocardiograms, magnetic resonance imaging, mammograms, PSA (prostate specific antigen) tests, and other diagnostic investigations. Even after discharge, patients were expected to return periodically for further tests and reviews of their state of health.

Crowd control

The sheer scale of the provision made the hospital site a crowded, busy and bustling place, similar in many ways to an airport terminal and, likewise, involving preparing and processing large numbers of people, and crowd control, included controlling access to limited facilities, the use of gathering rooms, queuing systems, and waiting times. For many people, including myself, the dominant hospital experience was of waiting to see a consultant, a doctor, a nurse, a radiographer, a pharmacist, and other personnel, in order to be admitted, to be treated, to be discharged, or to have a prescription made up. If it were not for the patients' apprehension, anxiety, and distress, then boredom and dullness would dominate. For much of the time I spent waiting, I found it difficult to contain my impatience. The tedium could only by be partially relieved by reading *The Guardian*, immersing myself in a gripping book, or aimlessly pacing long hospital corridors. I tried on many occasions to discover the reasons for the waits, eventually coming to the simple conclusion that the demand for medical attention as expressed by the sheer number of patients outstripped the ability and availability of hospital staff to supply medical services. When I asked of the nurses why I had had to wait for so long, they invariably replied that they were short-staffed.

Social inclusiveness

Another feature of a National Health Service hospital which people either tolerate, love or hate, is its social inclusiveness. By virtue of its principle of being available to all, gratis, in accordance with clinical need - that is, irrespective of the ability to pay – it is, by definition, a socially-classless place, where rich and poor, those of high and low status, people in professional occupations, manual workers and the unemployed, persons from different ethnic and racial groups and nationalities, and the young and old, must sit, queue and wait together for their treatment. Of course, it is to avoid this commonality of experience and treatment, or to get treatment more quickly, that some pay to go private.

The unique socially-inclusive environment of the National Health Service can come as shock to those used to paying for and mixing in more exclusive environments. Work places, residential estates, shops and shopping malls, theatres, schools, universities, leisure centres, restaurants, etc., are far more socially segregated than a National Health Service general hospital.

I recalled my time on the Beynon Ward amongst elderly demented men, a broken-jawed prisoner in chains, and a supporter of far-right political views. Interesting times, but I would never have selected such company! Nor did I enjoy sitting in waiting rooms with malodorous people who, perhaps for no fault of their own, had clearly not washed themselves for many days or weeks. Yet in a medical context in which damaged tissues, fluids and odours are often disclosed, surely this was a small price to pay for such comprehensive and inclusive health provision? After my post-operative incontinence and urinary tract infection, what right had I to complain?

I regard the National Health Service's high-quality care, free to all at the point of delivery, as operational proof of the success of the welfare state. The size of one's pocket should never be allowed to determine the quality of care, or one's place on the waiting list.

Organisational complexity

Functioning in factory mode, New Cross just about managed to cope with the number and diversity of its patients, even when it missed its targets and time lines. A highly complex organisation, it was compartmentalised into specialist units, each carefully coordinated with others to avoid silo working – helped by the persistent focus on patients' multiple needs and the integrated electronic patient record (IEPR), rapidly transmitting personal data to the staff who needed to access it. Analysis of blood samples, so essential to diagnosis, could be entered quickly onto the system, allowing the consultants to make immediate evidence-based decisions.

I was impressed by the operation and industrial scale of the phlebotomy service, not having realised that a hospital is dependent on blood, much like the Aztec cosmology of constant blood sacrifice to the sun god, Huitzilopochtli. The phlebotomists, working as a team, take blood samples from the arms of patients who have been directed to the hospital's various phlebotomy hubs and sampling booths. On taking a numbered ticket from a dispensing machine, I saw my number flashed up almost immediately on an electronic display board which directed me to go to one of the booths. My blood sample was expertly extracted by a friendly fast-working phlebotomist, who checked that it was labelled correctly, and despatched it to the laboratory. The oncologist was soon able to access the result from my on-line medical record.

Multi-ethnic environment

As a black and white couple ourselves, with three mixed-race children, Mel and I could not help noticing and appreciating the hospital as an harmonious multi-ethnic environment, where workforce, patients and visitors successfully intermingled and related to one another in the routine of their daily lives. Before her retirement, Mel had been the Dean of the University of Wolverhampton's School of Health and responsible for nurse education, and so we were well aware of the National Health Service's dependency on doctors and nurses from ethnic minority backgrounds and overseas. Mel herself was born in Jamaica and had come to the UK to train as a nurse, a midwife, and a health visitor, and to work for the NHS.

As my chemotherapy progressed, the press and the BBC did much to promote the 20th April 2018 as the fiftieth anniversary of Enoch Powell's notorious anti-immigration 'river of blood' speech, in which he warned of the disastrous effects that Commonwealth immigrants and their descendants would have on British society. The MP, who represented the Wolverhampton South West constituency where we lived, had been Minister for Health between 1960 and 1963 in Harold Macmillan's cabinet, and was well aware of, if not responsible for, the contribution that Indian doctors and

Caribbean nurses were making at that time to the NHS. This had not stopped him describing Commonwealth immigration as: "like watching a nation busily engaged in heaping up its own funeral pyre…As I look ahead, I am filled with foreboding; like the Roman I seem to see the river Tiber foaming with much blood" (20th April 1968).

In Wolverhampton fifty years later, the attempt to revive interest in Powell's views had provoked a public debate on the merits of his speech – had he been right after all? News coverage had resulted in a campaign in the city to display a blue plaque in honour of 'the great man' – with an opinion poll of *Express & Star* readers showing a majority supporting the gesture. Mel and I, who had lived with the consequences of his speech and the tangible damage and distress it had caused at the time, were appalled. Nevertheless, what struck us forcibly as we visited New Cross, was that, although the hospital ran with blood (drawn by the phlebotomy department) like the Tiber, it provided conclusive proof that Powell's dystopian vision was entirely without foundation.

In regard to my own recent breast cancer experience, nearly every medical practitioner I had encountered, either at the Castlecroft Medical Practice, or in the hospital, was either from an ethnic minority background, or had been born and brought up overseas, often in a Commonwealth country, or in Eastern Europe. New Cross was not untypical of the NHS as a whole. Approximately 30 per cent of the NHS workforce of nurses and doctors is drawn from ethnic minority backgrounds, with 30 per cent of doctors and 40 per cent of nurses born outside of the UK.[3]

As my diagnosis and treatment progressed, I became entirely reliant on the medical staff's professional and intelligent judgement and self-evident concern and compassion for my personal welfare. In my view, and allowing for the demand on limited resources, they had done their utmost, without exception, and irrespective of their ethnic background or country of birth, to afford me a first-rate service. I winced at the thought of the impact that any residual Powell-inspired racism might still have on their personal or professional lives.

Scientific medicine

In addition to the extensive use of blood analysis in the diagnostic process, there was evidence throughout the hospital of the systematic application of science and technology to medical practice and health care, the most simple and obvious being the measures for infection control. At hospital entrances, and before entering wards, all patients and visitors were expected to make use of hand gel dispensers. All toilet facilities carried instructions to wash hands with soap and water, advising those with symptoms of diarrhoea and vomiting to stay at home and to avoid visiting their relatives in hospital. The systems in place to control and prevent infections, such as MRSA (methicillin resistant staphylococcus aureus – which is resistant to several antibiotics) were pronounced, extensive, and well used and, judging by the hospital's *2016-2017 Infection Prevention Annual Report*, extremely effective in reducing incidents of these kinds of disease.

In regard to my own diagnosis and treatment, I was impressed by the widespread use of medical technology, particularly the diagnostic equipment in the form of imaging machines, such as the MRI (magnetic resonance imaging), the ultrasound sonography, and CT (computed tomography) scanners. I had received my radiotherapy in fifteen separate 'fractions' from a Linac (linear accelerator). All were big and impressive machines, improved by being coupled to the latest computer technology. In my case, the various scans had come back clear, showing no sign of metastases, thus contributing directly to my and our family's relief and happiness at Christmas.

I was also aware that the so-called adjuvant therapies were dependent on the pharmaceutical industry. With my daughter employed as a senior clinical trials manager, the rigour and sophistication of the scientific tests involved in selecting and developing these drugs came as no surprise. Apart from the FEC-T chemotherapy infusions, so carefully measured and administered, a veritable cornucopia of tablets, capsules, pills and syringes were available to control the adverse side effects – most affording some measure of relief.

A friendly and welcoming place?

Normally, people enter a hospital for one of three reasons. They work, train or volunteer on the site. They are patients with medical problems who go or are sent there for treatment. They are relatives, friends, or companions, accompanying, assisting, advocating for, or visiting patients. Of the three groups, only the first turns up month after month on a regular and systematic basis and forms part of the organisation, committed to realising its aims and providing a service to patients. The patients are there to be treated, in order to improve, stabilise, or ameliorate their condition, with the hope of returning home in the shortest possible time in a better state of health than when they entered the place. Patients attend hospital reluctantly, and cease their visits when their health improves, or when nothing more can be done to assist them. Family and friends continue to care for their sick relatives, but believe they have fulfilled their visiting duties once the individual is discharged, or dies.

It follows that only the regular workforce is in a position to sustain the hospital's organisation, services, culture and ethos. Patients and visitors may be long-standing and regular in attendance, but they remain transient, a trend encouraged by constant economic pressure to accelerate throughput, cut waiting times, and increase the number of out-patients and instances of day surgery. For example in the year 2016 to 2017, the number of day care operations increased at New Cross by 15 per cent.

As in any large institution, the work force at New Cross was divided into different departments and specialisms which were coordinated with others to provide a tailor-made service for patients' individual needs. In my case I was allocated initially to the breast cancer team of consultant surgeon, registrars and breast cancer nurses, in the Outpatients' Department, before being transferred into the care of the oncology directorate, currently accommodated in New Cross's Deanesly Outpatients' Department, the Snowdrop Millennium Suite chemotherapy unit, and the Durnall Day Unit.

The breast cancer team

The first people I came to know by name were the breast cancer team – *Mr Venkatramanan*, *Sister Carys Jevons* and *Nurse Donna Dobson* at the Outpatients' Department who, at all times, treated me and Mel in a most professional, courteous and friendly manner. It was obvious to us that the doctors and nurses got on well together, relayed and reinforced a supportive message to their patients, and coordinated their work, popping in and out of each other's rooms to ensure they were in agreement as to the best way to treat me. In the first dark days of being diagnosed with cancer, I remember with gratitude their friendly smiling faces and reassuring remarks. Mel and I were always seen as a pair by the nursing staff who soon realised that she, like they, was a trained nurse and professional, which helped to lubricate the bonhomie and friendship still further.

It helped that we engaged on an almost weekly basis in the common task of expressing my seroma and helping my breast to heal. As might be expected in this context of confidentiality, we had almost no contact or conversation with other breast cancer patients visiting the clinic. In any case, as far as I was aware, I was the only man there with breast cancer. All the rest were woman. In hindsight, I judged the care I received at the Outpatients' Department, albeit constrained by the circumstances, to be compassionate, competent and effective.

The oncology team

In January 2018, I commenced the six 21-day cycles of chemotherapy, under the auspices of the oncology directorate, staffed by a different set of doctors and nurses. Once more, it took time to get to know the medical staff and familiarise myself with the locations, expectations, routines and practices involved. We met the mild *Dr Grigoryev* and his team of registrars and nurses, in particular, the conscientious *Dr Gupta*, with her almost saintly calm and benevolent manner. Over the many weeks of assessment and pre-assessment, I formed the impression that my pain relief, welfare, progress, and recovery, mattered to them. When I developed phlebitis, I was surprised and delighted to discover that *Dr Grigoryev* was personally monitoring my progress and had intervened to ensure his registrars dealt with my condition.

Perforce, meetings with consultants and registrars were limited, but I was convinced that they took an active interest in the welfare of their patients and were doing their best to adapt the adjuvant therapies to my personal circumstances.

Over a period of four months Mel and I attended the hospital's oncology facilities for weekly or twice-weekly appointments, most usually for chemo-infusions and blood samples at the Snowdrop Millennium Suite, or for line dressing, care and blood samples on the Durnall Day Unit, where most oncology patients, who developed complications, such as phlebitis, ended up.

Chemotherapy and line care

On every occasion we visited the Snowdrop Suite, we found it a busy and crowded place, as evidenced by the 20 minutes to 1 hour we were usually kept waiting after our appointment time. Generally, procedures and protocols were followed liked clockwork, but I sensed that things did not always run to plan, and there was scope for even tighter conformity with professional standards and quality control.

Accompanied by Mel, I would be taken onto the U-shaped ward and allocated a chair for the duration of my stay. I would then be connected to a succession of bags of fluid suspended from a drip stand, and the chemotherapy would begin, a procedure which, if uninterrupted, would last between 2 and 2½ hours. During this time, the oncology nurses would talk amiably – I suspect with distractive therapy in mind – as they inserted a cannula, linked me up to the drugs, or emptied syringes into my veins. Over the course of the cycles, we got to know the names of the nurses – for example, *Jemima Holyoak*, *Michelle McLean* and *Cassia Mainwaring* – and came to respect and admire their professional competence. Attentive to their patients' sensations, moods and anxieties, they would inquire how they felt at regular intervals, drawing attention to the button alarm. Patients', visitors' and practitioners' seating arrangements restrained the opportunity to converse with fellow recipients of the chemo drugs.

A friendly gesture, or smile exchanged with the patient or family member sitting opposite was the most that could be achieved, unless treatments commenced or concluded simultaneously. Then conversation based on a common chemo-encounter could occur:

"Didn't we see you on Durnall last week?"

"What cycle are you on?"

"Was that docetaxel? How are you finding it? Pretty grim?"

"I've been okay, since the line was inserted."

In reality, there was little opportunity on the Snowdrop Suite to share experiences with fellow patients. A reluctance to contravene the privacy of others prevailed.

I found the Durnall Day Unit for oncology and haematology patients more relaxing and sociable, at the queue at reception, among the gossiping crowd in the waiting space, and as the patients lined up in the side wards. I attributed this to the frequency and familiarity of our visits for line care, bloods, and emergencies, when we met patients and friends scheduled like us each week in the same time slots, as well as to the continuity of nursing care.

Sister Natalie Edmunds, *Nurse Samantha Coburn*, *Nurse Liza Warmington*, and *Nurse Rosie Puttock* treated me on a regular basis, and we grew to know and trust them, inquiring after their welfare in their absence. Durnall was a surprisingly friendly and welcoming place, given the normal reasons for going there. Were there lessons to be learned? Given patient numbers and the shortage of nurses, was there any scope for pairing nurses and patients to develop still further continuity of care, personalised caring relationships, and a greater degree of trust? What is commonly referred to as 'relationship continuity of care' is acknowledged to improve early diagnosis and to encourage patients to act more readily on their doctor's advice but in NHS General Practice this practice is in steady decline. I suspect the frequency with which hospital patients are seen and treated by the same nurses and doctors during the course of their hospital treatment is decreasing, too.[4]

Radiotherapy

My conflicted views of the radiotherapy I received have already been set out in Chapter 15. While I underwent the fifteen-day course of consecutive treatment sessions without disruption, I found the way my radiotherapy was organised annoying and stressful, an experience mitigated only by the kind and thoughtful manner of individual radiographers who, unlike others, were prepared to look beyond the body on the couch and to spend a moment or two conversing with and reassuring their patients. To me, the repetitive job of setting up patients under a linear accelerator and then retiring from the room for a while, before coming back in to cover them up and send them away, could not have been fun. After intercourse with a giant machine for the duration of a shift, I, too, would find it hard to relate normally to my fellow human beings.

New Cross's quality of care ratings in relation to my surgery, cancer treatment and nursing care

In comparison with other NHS Trusts, how did New Cross Hospital rate? The Care Quality Commission's report on its inspection in June 2015 found that overall the quality of care required improvement, and gave it an amber light. In regard to the areas of care that I encountered, the report stated that:

- good services were provided by surgical services, care was delivered within national guidance, and the Trust was largely meeting the 18-week referral-to-treatment target.
- the Trust was meeting cancer access targets and the 18-week referral-to-treatment times in outpatients and in many of its surgical specialities.
- there was largely good and compassionate care within the hospital and the staff were focussed on patient care.
- there was good compliance with hand hygiene and the Trust's 'bare below the elbow' policy.[5]

New Cross Hospital
Pay on exit car park

Tariff

Set Down / Pick Up Maximum 15 Minutes			£0.00
Up to 1 hour	£2.40	Up to 6 hours	£5.80
Up to 2 hours	£3.40	Up to 7 hours	£6.40
Up to 3 hours	£3.70	Up to 8 hours	£6.60
Up to 4 hours	£4.80	Up to 9 hours	£7.20
Up to 5 hours	£5.10	Up to 24 hours	£7.30

Concessions Weekly (7 consecutive days) £16.50
Oncology Patients £1.50
(Chemo / Radio Therapies)
Renal Dialysis Patients £0.00

Concession Charges Please contact the Car Parking and Security Control Centre
on 01902 695344 or visit the office (location B20) for further information

Remember your registration number
Please note:
You need to have your vehicle registration number
when you pay at the pay station.

Car parking charges at New Cross, 23rd February 2018

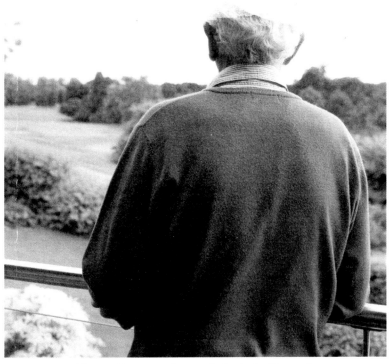

A practical guide to living with and after cancer

HOW ARE YOU FEELING?
THE EMOTIONAL EFFECTS OF CANCER

Macmillan guidance on the psychological effects of cancer

Chapter 18

After hospital treatment finishes

Once a cancer patient, always a cancer patient

Every morning I take a 20mg tablet of tamoxifen with my cereals and will continue to do so for the next five or ten years. The hormone therapy for my breast cancer is long term. However, I am immensely relieved to have completed the courses of chemotherapy and radiotherapy. They have dominated my time and my thoughts for the last six months and, before that, there was the mastectomy and lymph node clearance. What happens next?

When first diagnosed with breast cancer, I read Lisa Lynch's *The C-Word* and found the following comment particularly telling:

'Once you've had cancer, no medical professional will ever say the word 'cancer free' to you. You're too much of a risk, and they'd be opening themselves up to a world of trouble if it turned out that the cancer was sneakily plotting a return, as it often does...There's a lifetime of tablets, appointments, tests, scans, mammograms. And while it's hugely comforting that the NHS doesn't just spit you back out as soon as you've had the necessary treatment, it does seem like a case of once a cancer patient, always a cancer patient.'[1]

John Diamond's *C* was of the same opinion: 'Once you've had that diagnosis it stays with you for good'.[2]

It is obvious that regular medical check-ups will be needed, whether a person has responded well to treatment and shows no sign of further illness, or continues to live with and manage a cancer on an ongoing basis. *Sister Carys Jevons* had caused us confusion in 2017 by making an appointment for me at a nurse-led breast review clinic a year in advance on the 13th November 2018. My consultant breast cancer surgeon, *Mr Venkatramanan*, was already getting into his stride by making me an appointment on the 24th August 2018 at the New Cross Hospital Breast Imaging Department to have a mammogram taken of my remaining breast.

There is also a prevailing belief, no doubt grounded on practical experience, that once diagnosed with breast cancer, a person's life will never be quite the same as it was before the condition was first detected.

Macmillan practical guides to life after cancer treatment

It is widely assumed that the disruption to daily routine caused by the so-called adjuvant therapies will be so drastic that patients will need guidance and advice on what to do when their treatment has finished, hence Macmillan's booklets, *Life after cancer treatment,*[3] and *What to do after cancer treatment ends: top tips*,[4] which share common themes.

The advice offered seems to be premised on the assumption that cancer treatment will almost always have a negative effect on patients' physical fitness, emotional equilibrium, social relationships, and ability to work, earn a living, and travel, and that they will need to take action if they wish to re-establish the lifestyle choices and autonomy they experienced before their cancer was diagnosed.

Both booklets make clear that after hospital day-care treatment has ended, patients should feel free to seek advice and assistance at any time from their designated key worker (nurse, doctor, health-care professional), or other relevant persons and organisations, such as Citizens Advice. (As a trustee of Citizens Advice, I found it comforting to note that Citizens Advice was mentioned.[5]) Patients are also reminded to keep scheduled hospital appointments and participate in routine health tests and monitoring.[6]

Planning of follow-up care

The booklets begin by describing the practicalities of finishing treatment, the importance of looking out for the side-effects that might be experienced afterwards, the follow-up care that might be expected, and the means of accessing it. The guidance says that on completion of their treatment, patients will be given the opportunity to discuss their needs with their cancer team and to agree a plan of care that takes into account their physical and mental health, their work, and family requirements.

Care plans will vary from place to place, but are likely to have the following features:

- a treatment summary, describing the treatment that a patient has received and what is to be expected once treatment is completed (for example, possible late side effects and follow-up appointments)
- a 'holistic needs assessment' summarising the patient's various and diverse needs, both medical and personal.
- any recommendations for further action, care, support, or referral.[7]

When and how will the patient care plan be drawn up, and issued to the patient? To what extent will patients participate in the planning of their follow-up care? The Macmillan guidance makes clear that not all hospitals provide Holistic Needs Assessments, care plans, and treatment summaries.[8] When my hospital treatment came to an end on Friday 22nd June, the Deanesly-based radiotherapy unit gave me a form telling me that I would be contacted within six weeks for an oncology appointment. Eight days later on the 30th June, I received a letter notifying me of an appointment with *Dr Grozdan Grigoryev*, my consultant oncologist on the 1st August 2018, the contact and appointment well within the promised time schedule, demonstrating that the hospital was effectively tracking the progress of patients riding its cancer treatment conveyor belt.

It occurred to me, nevertheless, that if the health professionals were sincere in developing a patient-centred breast cancer after-care service, then they would have issued a draft or preliminary care plan long before the hospital-based treatment phase came to an end. It was now the 30th June, one week after my last radiotherapy session, and thirty tablets into my five-year tamoxifen course, and I was none the wiser as to whether or when I would receive a written care plan or a treatment summary, or indeed, whether I would receive any help whatsoever in preparing for what Macmillan variously referred to as 'the end of treatment', or 'improving the quality of life after treatment'[9] . I do not consider myself to be an anxious person, but if I were, this failure to discuss or consult in good time about 'life after treatment' would certainly contribute to my anxiety level. When I eventually asked when I was likely to receive my after-care plan and/or treatment summary, I was told that it was not the practice of that hospital trust to issue them as, henceforth, my health would be monitored and I would be kept informed of any significant changes to my condition.

Dealing with the physical after-effects of treatment

The Macmillan end-of-treatment guidance acknowledges that it is common for people to worry about their cancer recurring and for them to think that every ache and pain they experience is cancer-related.[10] If, in August 2018, well after my hospital treatment had ended, my breast surgeon considered it necessary to have my right breast checked for lumps, then surely it was only to be expected that I, too, would be concerned about the possibility of my cancer returning. After-effects may be imaginary (a product of fear), but are frequently real (the recognised consequences of surgery, treatment, medication and, yes, signs that the treatment has failed). Patients should be on the look-out for tiredness, fatigue, pain, peripheral neuropathy, lymphoedema, loss of libido, and other physical ailments (including lumps).[11]

Physically, how had I fared to date (30th June 2018)? When I glanced in the mirror, I saw a cockled, haggard, and hairless 73-year-old man. I was told by family and friends that, to their eyes I looked surprisingly well, but this might have been because, in the knowledge of my cancer, they had come to believe that I had knocked on death's door, and only recently returned from the call. I had a good ruddy colour in my cheeks and no longer had reason to proffer a grimace. While I had managed to sprout 4ml of dark hair on my head and my chin was in shadow, I still had a predominantly hairless and glabrous demeanour, with much-diminished eyebrows and lashes.

Those parts of my body concealed by my clothes - my chest, armpits, thighs and pubic area - were still largely bereft of new hair growth. My bare chest revealed a horizontal 15cm (6 ins) mastectomy scar extending into the pit of my arm on the left-hand side. Around it, a rectangle of skin was no longer bright red and inflamed from the radiotherapy, but had turned a ruddy brown, following weeks of massage with ZeroAQS emollient cream. On the right of my chest, 4cm below my shoulder blade, was a short vertical 1.5cm scar with a tiny 0.5cm horizontal mark just below it, configured like an inverted T. Scarcely scabbed over, these little scars were all that remained of my Hickman line. Bruising to the crook of my right arm, where the nurses had struggled to take blood two weeks ago, was now barely visible. Each of my finger and toe nails revealed a series of six distinct growth rings, the consequence of successive cycles of chemotherapy.

The most ubiquitous physical sensation and after-effect that I recognised was tiredness, but I concluded that the fatigue I was experiencing was far less severe one week after the end of radiotherapy, than it had been after a 21-day cycle of chemotherapy. Whereas I had taken an afternoon nap almost every day during chemotherapy, I had slept only twice at that hour in the last week (of June). Undoubtedly, I felt more tired during the day, than I had before my treatment began, and had not fully recovered, but I was now considerably less fatigued than during the chemotherapy. I was unaware as to whether the tiredness attributed to radiotherapy was one of its late side effects (which I believed I was yet to encounter). It was true that I tired much more easily now after physical exercise, such as walking, gardening or hedge-cutting, than I had before the treatment began, and found my lack of stamina in the course of a self-set task a source of great frustration - possibly the most annoying so far of all side effects.

Tiredness was linked to the risk of pain, lymphoedema, and peripheral neuropathy. In recent weeks, following a short spell of hedge clipping, I had felt pain in my chest over the area of my mastectomy scar (and, of course, near to my heart) and had stopped work immediately. Perversely, I stopped, not because of the pain, nor the fear of a heart attack, nor to avoid exacerbating the effects of the radiotherapy, but because I was aware of the risk of developing a lymphoedema which, to my mind, would have brought my long-term prospect of cutting hedges to a painful and permanent end.

To check whether I was developing lymphoedema, I raised my arms to shoulder level every morning (as *Pete* from radiotherapy had taught me), comparing the left arm closely with the right for signs of swelling and fluid retention. The threat of developing lymphoedema made me hesitant to test whether the strength in my arms and upper body was returning. Apart from numbness in my fingers immediately after surgery, I had not experienced the tingling sensation of peripheral neuropathy. Nevertheless, the operations seemed to have damaged the nerves in my left arm, which remained very numb underneath, from armpit to elbow, and was unresponsive to regular applications of emollient cream. I have come to think of the numbness as a permanent affair - collateral damage, along with the mastectomy scar. As for loss of libido, I was not sure at my age what to expect but, if it referred to an inability to get an erection, then, unless I was dreaming, I had yet to encounter a problem.

Dealing with the effects of cancer on mental health

Physical appearance and performance aside, I was asked repeatedly "How do you feel in yourself?"

"Oh, I'm fine, now that the chemo's behind me," I told them, but found it more difficult to provide an answer that satisfied me. They were asking about my feelings, which were constantly changing, like the colours of a chameleon. They formed and faded as a response to the circumstances in which I found myself, for example, as I lay under a Linac machine while it beamed radiation at my chest, or played with my grandchild, or sat wasting my hours in a hospital waiting room. I recognised, nevertheless, that the prolonged cancer treatment had had a profound effect on my state of mind, my psychology, and my mental health (terms that I suspect I am using interchangeably).

The Macmillan booklets make clear that cancer treatment is likely to affect patients' ongoing mental health. Individuals may experience heightened feelings of fear, anxiety, uncertainty, loneliness, guilt, anger, sadness, or depression. Not only do those feelings impact on their ability to lead their own lives in a normal fashion, but on the way they relate to those closest to them and, in turn, are related to.[12] Recognising the profound impact of cancer on the mind, Macmillan has produced a guide dedicated to cancer's emotional effects, entitled *How are you feeling?*, containing tips on how the patient might deal with those feelings, or go about seeking help.[13]

As the reader will be aware from earlier chapters, I found the chemotherapy drugs deeply unsettling and, at times, became very emotional, bursting into tears, without good reason (or so it appeared to me). Now that my hospital treatment had come to an end, I tried once again to set down in print my current moods and emotional states.

Fear and anxiety

Was I living in fear, especially of the cancer returning, this time, perhaps, to the right side of my chest, or of it metastasising elsewhere in my body? My attitude throughout the course of my treatment and now after it, was one of resignation. There was little I could do about my current situation, apart from making the most of the scientific evidence, medical expertise, and NHS facilities currently available.[14]

As one of the few men, compared with the considerable number of women who caught breast cancer in the UK, Europe, the USA, or worldwide, I had been a statistical aberration from the start. I knew that there was no satisfactory explanation as to why some people - including women - caught my type of breast cancer, and others did not, and that there was no reliable or informed advice on how to prevent it occurring again in me. I was aware that the three adjuvant therapies I had received gave a statistically-significant group of recipients an 87 per cent chance of breast cancer survival over a five-year period. But given the long odds of a man developing breast cancer in the first place, what reassurance was I to draw from that statistic? I might be among the 13 per cent for whom it came back. The statistic applied to the group, not to the individual, and I was never a gambling man - believing in the arbitrariness of chance, not luck.

Our inability to foretell our future, especially in regard to matters of health, is something we all must live with on a daily basis. I knew there was nothing practical that I could do to prevent my cancer returning. In that context, fear or anxiety are pointless. One might as well live the whole of one's life in fear of death. Similarly, in that nobody had a clue as to why I had developed breast cancer, I experienced no guilt or anger. Unlike lung cancer caused by cigarette smoking, I could not blame myself, or those around me, for smoking, neither did I feel angry or resentful with those around me for just happening to be healthy and well.[15]

It occurred to me that the acceptance of one's powerlessness might after all be the appeal of the currently-popular mindfulness - a subliminal message of living in the moment without expending unnecessary emotional energy on trying to fix an unpredictable future. Now, with hospital treatment at an end, I was far less fearful and anxious, than when it began.

Uncertainty

I have already expressed my views on uncertainty. I prefer to do what is within my power to control and manage my immediate itinerary and social environment. I don't think I am unusual in that aspiration. Macmillan guidance suggests that fear and anxiety are natural reactions to uncertain situations [16] - such as not knowing whether cancer will come back. Allowing for that particular exception, for me and many other cancer patients, uncertainty is exacerbated by procedures that fail to take into account the patients' opinions, that tolerate unpredictable waiting times, that insist on giving minimal notice of treatment, that plan a fifteen-day course of radiotherapy on a day-to-day basis, and that delay issuing, or fail to provide, care plans or treatment summaries until well after hospital treatment has ended. Some other NHS institutions and health practitioners have already succeeded in giving patients greater control over the way their treatment is conducted, and organising their procedures differently, thus removing unnecessary sources of anxiety and stress.

Loneliness

Macmillan guidance observes that it is common for people affected by cancer to feel lonely or isolated, and recommends talking or connecting to others as the solution, as 'connecting with other people can help you feel less alone and help you manage your emotions'.[17] In my case, I was supported from the start by my wife, family and friends, and learned very quickly that it was in my best interests to tell them about my cancer, rather than to keep it secret.

I cannot emphasise sufficiently the importance of my wife, Mel's support and advocacy. She accompanied me to the hospital on almost every occasion, never allowing me to become lonely.

The Macmillan message of talking or connecting with others[18] is not explored in the context of a hospital environment. For me, as a patient, who visited the hospital in the course of ten months, the courteous, respectful, attentive and welcoming attitudes of hospital staff were crucial to my coping with the intrusive features of the treatment they provided. A kindly quip from a nurse, a smile or reassuring remark from a doctor, or radiographer, meant the world to an apprehensive patient. Encouragement of that kind was not always forthcoming. I am convinced that the quality of human intercourse between patients and hospital staff contributes significantly to the efficacy of treatment, improving patient morale, confidence, resilience and outcome.

During my treatment, I became aware of the friendliness, warmth, and solidarity of my fellow cancer patients, and realised the central role that group therapy, self-help, and cancer support groups, have to play in maintaining the morale of those under treatment, particularly during extended periods of chemotherapy. Whereas I enjoyed sharing experiences with other cancer patients, I had a long-established circle of close friends and family members to share my experiences with, of whom some had already been treated for cancer, or had attended on relatives, and were aware of what I was going through. No doubt, I would have enjoyed meeting members of the Wolverhampton and District Breast Cancer Action Group, and might well have joined them if the coffee morning had not clashed with line care treatment or other already-established commitments of mine. But, given my fatigue, and the existing circle of friends I mixed with, I hadn't much extra energy at the time for further contacts, camaraderie, coffee mornings, or campaigns. Once hospital treatment concluded, my former pattern of social commitments resumed with a vengeance, leaving few gaps to fill in a busy itinerary. I was pleased that everyone had coped well in my absence. The aphorism: 'The graveyards are full of indispensable people' came readily to mind. Indeed, still tiring easily, I sensed just how dispensable I had become.

Depression

The Macmillan practical guides advise that patients with cancer can become very sad and depressed, but draw a distinction between being in an understandably low mood as a result of the disease and its consequences, and the more serious diagnosis of clinical depression. Symptoms of the clinical form of depression include:

- feeling in a miserable mood for a prolonged period,
- weeping uncontrollably,
- lacking energy and motivation,
- finding it difficult to concentrate or make a decision,
- showing impatience and irritability without good cause and,
- avoiding the company of others.[19]

I have never in my life (not even in the last ten months) suffered from a clinical form of depression but, during my treatment, there were occasions when I showed one or more of the symptoms listed above. For example, I broke into tears in front of my children - an outburst I attributed to the chemo drugs. The pain and discomfort of a urinary infection (developed after my mastectomy operation) made me feel extremely miserable but, once on the road to recovery, my mood soon changed for the better.

Unlike people with clinical depression, my moods during treatment responded almost exactly to circumstance. I was sad when I was in a sad situation, and happy when I judged matters to be going well for me. To date, my response to my treatment has been predictable. I became apprehensive before every session of chemotherapy and relieved once the injections had been given. When I was feeling especially weak and vulnerable, I was able to turn to my wife, my children, and friends for comfort and support. Currently, I am pleased to have completed my hospital treatment and look forward to a cancer-free future with optimism.

The social impact of cancer treatment

Macmillan's *Life after cancer treatment* emphasises that an individual's cancer may have a profound impact on family life, social relationships, and the wider context, work, employment and income.[20] Advice is given on maintaining, strengthening, and broadening relationships with partner, children, family, friends, and other people. There is information on returning to work, employment rights, managing finances, and travelling (including travel and holiday insurance).

The importance of family and friends

I have already mentioned the role of my wife, children, family members, and friends in helping me cope with my cancer treatment. They rallied round from the start without prompting or encouragement, each lending strength to a collective effort to see me through the ordeal and along the road to recovery.

At weekends, my children would travel from London to stay with their parents in Wolverhampton, giving domestic and emotional support to me and Mel, and bringing my grandchildren to visit me. I soon came to realise my grandchildren's immense therapeutic benefits: young lives adding value, energy, and joy to their grandparents' currently restricted activities. My friends, too, were proactive in offering to come to the house and give me practical help as and when needed, plus a series of meals they brought round for us, offers of transport, help with the bins, jobs in the garden, sorting out snags on the p.c., etc. I counted myself lucky that my social network was robust and effective - no need to seek out new contacts or interests.

Work, employment, and income

In its practical guide, *Work and Cancer*, Macmillan recognises the importance of work and that having cancer and undergoing treatment can result in patients having to stop or curtail their working activities.[21] For most people of working age, work is important for giving purpose and routine to their lives and enabling them to earn money to provide for themselves and their families. Any interruption to normal working relations can lead to worry about losing pay, promotion, prospects, colleagues, friendship and respect, and even the job itself.

Cancer and cancer treatment affect individuals in radically different ways. On learning that I was undergoing chemotherapy, Sue, a director of human resources and former colleague of mine, told me how she found it impossible to predict the impact that chemotherapy would have on the working lives of colleagues: some would insist on working throughout their treatment, even coming in on days that the chemo drugs were administered, while others were clearly incapable of sustained activity, confined to a bed or chair, and remaining at home for the three-month duration.

How had it affected me? I told her that I might have been able to cope for one week at work out of each of the six three-week cycles, but wasn't sure whether my performance would have been up to scratch. I pointed out that apart from individual variations in response, patients suffered from different types and stages of cancer and were on diverse treatment regimes.

Sue reminded me that employees who had cancer were defined in law as disabled and protected by the Equality Act 2010. They were entitled to ask for reasonable adjustments to help them carry on working, or to return to work. They could not be treated less favourably than others at work, because of their cancer.[22]. I should have been aware of the legal status of employees with cancer, given my previous role as an equality officer. That relevant provision in employment law had slipped off my radar, I suspect, precisely because I was no longer in employment.

Long retired, I, unlike million of others, did not have to concern myself with how much time I could take off from work before having my pay docked, or the financial implications of being so ill that I could no longer hold down a job. I had been fortunate, too, in always being able to earn my living in occupations that gave me satisfaction and stimulated me mentally, to such a degree that I had come to define work as purposeful activity - something that I was not able to do without. In that sense, retirement had not affected my working life. As a pensioner, I continued at full throttle to engage in activities and projects that interested and stimulated me, such as researching, campaigning, writing, preparing manuscripts for printing, painting, gardening, serving on charitable trusts, and organising social events. Knowing that I was now well into my 70s and on the last lap, I pursued my pet projects with a greater intensity than in my younger years, but possibly to less effect, as age made me tire more easily. Nevertheless, I still considered myself to be in work in the sense of expending effort in setting, planning and completing systematically tasks that I set for myself. Without any warning, my newly-discovered breast cancer disrupted the long-established work routines of my retirement.

Ten months elapsed between my breast cancer diagnosis and the completion of my chemotherapy and radiotherapy courses, a period that became crowded with operations, recovery, aftercare, blood tests, monitoring, hospital appointments, receiving treatment, dealing with crises and side effects, and generally feeling ill, sick, and sorry for myself. Ten months of my life were dominated by my cancer: its physical removal, the treatment to prevent its recurrence, the planning and participation in the treatment regime, the search for information, and speculation about the prognosis.

I became the focal point of a profound physical, social and psychological turbulence, the all-seeing eye, so to speak, of a hurricane, hovering above a devastated domestic landscape, threatening to disrupt or destroy all my customary expectations, habits, routines, itineraries and friendship patterns. Cancer was physically and mentally time-consuming, largely displacing other concerns. The thought of it, and what needed to be done about it, occupied the mind constantly, to the exclusion of everything else - even eating and sleeping.

(I might add as an aside that many of the recommended psychological and complementary therapies aimed at dealing with the side effects are conceived as a means of relieving the anxiety, stress, and depression of cancer sufferers, by distracting them from the effects of the disease, for example, by persuading them to participate in gentle physical exercise, discussion groups, or psychological techniques, such as visualising pleasurable past occasions, or focusing selectively on the immediate sensations of the present moment - as long as it isn't the moment the nurse empties a syringe of chemo drugs into the arm. But it is not just the thought of cancer and its consequences that is so concerning, but the amount of time and energy spent in treating it, which leaves the cancer patient with little opportunity for doing anything else.)

Thinking about cancer may preoccupy the mind but, also, in regard to the body, the practical measures undertaken to treat the condition gradually replace former activities, pursuits, social engagements and commitments, if not in their entirety, then in the priority given to them. A scheduled appointment with a consultant, a surgical procedure, or a chemotherapy injection, always outrank the trustee board, celebratory lunch, or holiday arrangement. In this respect, only when cancer treatment finishes can the routines of a previous existence return to normal. But for most breast cancer patients, including me, a full ten months of treatment is a long time to endure. What was the best way to deal with my on-going cancer treatment, while simultaneously attempting to lead a normal existence? How was I going to cope?

In common with me and everyone else in the know, Toussaint, my daughter, was shocked and surprised by my breast cancer diagnosis. As a senior clinical trials manager working for a large pharmaceutical company, she did her homework and, like me, was quick to recognise the statistical oddity of a man developing breast cancer . We discussed my diagnosis, the proposed course of treatment, and the prognosis, before she said: "Dad, you enjoy writing. Why don't you write an account of your experience? It might help you learn more about BCIM." I did not need much encouragement, having already produced a record of my visits to the hospital outpatients' department. Some weeks later, once I had embarked upon the project, I found further encouragement in a Macmillan guide, which read: 'Some people find it helpful to keep a diary, journal, or online blog, where they can write down all their thoughts, feelings and frustrations...Creative writing may also help you to relax and express your feelings'.[23]

It was obvious. My work project, occupying my time and energy, would have to be a study of breast cancer in men, drawing on my own common-or-garden experiences of being diagnosed with and treated for breast cancer. The more physically and mentally time-consuming the process became, the more subject matter I would have to write about. I could continue working throughout my treatment, but would have to work harder the more demanding and intense the treatment became. A perfect project and a perfect therapy! Indeed, an ethnographical no-brainer! And so writing continued until the 30th June 2018, well after hospital treatment had come to an end. The time-consuming job of correcting, amending, editing, marketing, and publishing, was to follow. But in pursuing a stimulating project throughout the ten-month period, my business before, during, and after treatment, had been business as usual, sustaining and supporting me mentally.

As I have remarked before, the worst aspect of life after treatment was the realisation that I was weaker, more easily tired, and less resilient, than I was before I began. I was still attempting to pursue my various projects, but my ability to sustain my efforts without let-up was greatly reduced. I found that very frustrating, more so, in the knowledge that there was a danger that, should I exert myself unduly, I stood the risk of developing a lymphoedema. Fortunately, the weakness and fatigue seemed more closely associated with my physical exertions. My mental agility, alertness, and powers of concentration remained unimpeded (or so I chose to believe).

Travel and cancer

For ten months, from September 2017 to June 2018, the need to visit the hospital on a regular basis, as well as the debilitating effects of the cancer treatment, obliged me to stay near to home, making even day excursions to Birmingham or London impossibly arduous. For ten months, we were unable to drive to our house in Wales, and Mel went by herself on two occasions to visit her grandchildren in London. Being confined to base made me yearn for a holiday away from it all once my hospital treatment had come to an end. Planning the end-of-treatment holiday became in itself a therapeutic exercise. But when would I be sufficiently recovered from the side effects of the adjuvant therapies to travel?

I looked for advice in the Macmillan guide, *Travel and Cancer*[24], which spelled out the way cancer and its treatment could affect a person's ability to travel. Still experiencing fatigue, I understood immediately that, while extreme tiredness would not stop me from travelling, it might limit the length of my journey time and the activities I undertook. I was also reminded that my immune system had been affected by the chemotherapy, increasing my risk of infection. I knew I had to be careful about insect bites, as they were prone to becoming infected. I had already inquired about the impact of chemotherapy on my immunity to diseases for which I had been vaccinated (especially when going abroad), but the answers I received were never definitive. Long-distance air travel also carried the risks of lymphoedema, or blood clots (deep-vein thrombosis), developing. Both conditions were exacerbated by breast surgery, chemotherapy and hormonal therapy drugs, such as tamoxifen.

If I were going to take a holiday after my treatment, it was probably safer to stay in the United Kingdom, or in countries nearby, so that in case of a medical emergency, I could make a rapid return. With this reasoning in mind, in February 2018, during my third chemotherapy cycle, I began to plan a post-treatment holiday in Ireland for September which, I guessed, would allow me two months of recovery time.

Meanwhile, our daughter, Spartaca, who was living in Kenya, informed us that she and her husband were having a baby, with a delivery date estimated for early October 2018. Spartaca was keen for Mel, her mother, to visit and support her when the baby arrived, and invited us both to fly over to Kenya and stay for a while. Mel was not only Spartaca's mother, but had trained as a midwife and health visitor. All family members agreed that it was essential for Mel to be with her daughter and baby after the birth. I might serve as a travelling companion and enthusiastic grandfather but, while I would have liked to visit my daughter and grandchild, my health status conspired against me.

The invitation to Kenya came during my fifth chemotherapy cycle, when I was not feeling at my best, and had a sixth cycle and a course of radiotherapy to follow. Would I be fit enough to travel by then? We had no way of telling. Feeling unwell, conscious of the risk of infection in Kenya, unsure of the protection provided by previous holiday vaccinations, and aware of the post-operative risks attendant on long-distance flights, we came to the conclusion reluctantly that Mel would have to travel to Kenya on her own.

It was afterwards that I became conscious that cancer patients experienced difficulty in obtaining reasonably-priced travel insurance, whether their cancer was current, waiting on test results, or a thing of the past. Insurance providers treated cancer as a pre-existing condition, along with heart complaints, or respiratory disease, meaning that they might choose not to offer insurance cover, or charge more for it if they did. If I failed to let them know about my condition, my policy could be invalidated. One consequence of life after cancer, then, is that travel insurance is harder to come by and more expensive.[25]

Has cancer changed my outlook on life?

I read in the Macmillan guide, *Life after cancer treatment*, that my cancer experience might change my outlook on life and make me 'think about things differently' from the time before my diagnosis.[26] Patients who had finished their treatment were quoted as saying, "My whole outlook on life has changed"[27], or "For me, finishing treatment means appreciating the small things in life - the sunshine on my face, a delicious meal, or a hug from my daughters"[28].

A belief in the transformative nature of the cancer experience is widespread. Former breast cancer patients I have spoken to, claim that they are now different and see the world differently. As I, too, have been treated for cancer, they assume that I share their revelatory vision. I have an inkling of what they are trying to say. I sense that my ten-month-long ordeal from first diagnosis to completion of hospital treatment has had a profound and permanent effect on me, but I find that episode of my life complex to analyse and hard to express in words. Has its undisputed impact on my life been a result specifically of cancer treatment, or would any prolonged trauma, crisis, tragedy, or other life-threatening disease, have had the same or similar effect? I imagined that being captured, imprisoned, or caught in a terrorist attack might lead to the same result. I sensed intuitively, nevertheless, that my outlook had indeed changed. I have done my best to encapsulate those elusive features of my current state of mind below.

Selective perception of breast cancer matters

Ten months ago, I knew about breast cancer, felt sympathy for its sufferers, and had raised money for breast cancer charities. Since then, I have been initiated through diagnosis, surgery, and the ordeals of chemo and radiotherapy into the fraternity of those who have experienced and survived their breast cancer treatment. It is not just that I have become a member of a very special group, but that I have become sensitised, sensitive, and fully participative in a parallel breast cancer universe. No longer do I merely listen to a conversation about breast cancer. I am now, and forever will be, the subject of that conversation. At a cognitive level it is different, too. Just as one picks out a particular make of car on the road when seeking to purchase that make, so, too, do I notice the slightest reference, printed or oral, to breast cancer.

Awareness of physical transformation and limitations

My physical appearance has changed, with the scars left from the mastectomy and Hickman line removal, although these are hidden beneath my clothes. The hairs on my head and face have yet to grow back to their former length, but are on course to do so. Nevertheless, I cannot forget the shock of that alien, Mr Hyde, staring back from the mirror, an image so vivid that, whenever I see my reflection, the menace of mortality springs to my mind. I have contemplated the looming prospect of dying, and re-evaluated the time that remains. Henceforth, I am resolved to live my life with a greater purpose and focussed intensity.

I am more conscious than ever of physical health and the decline in my stamina and strength, due both to my age and my cancer treatment. I have become more measured, cautious and careful in my movements, in recognition of my limitations and the risk to my health of cuts, scratches, and infections. Reluctantly, I was forced to concede only yesterday that I no longer had the energy to cut down a dead tree in the garden - a severe disappointment. Will I be able to resume my gym membership and go swimming by August, without provoking infection or lymphoedema on my left-hand side? While I am told that my strength will eventually return, my life has already been changed by an inhibiting caution.

Cancer at my age

My diagnosis at 72 years of age, with 71 being the age at which breast cancer is most frequently diagnosed in men, has made me acutely conscious that cancer is a feature of the ageing process, as evidenced by the statistical data and the appearance of fellow hospital patients who, in most instances, look to be my age or older. With life expectancy now exceeding 80 years in developed countries, cancer is affecting more and more of the older age group: 43 per cent of men and 38 per cent of women develop an invasive cancer during their lifetime, and 23 per cent of men and 19 per cent of women die from it. [29]

My breast cancer has alerted me more than ever to my advancing age and the unavoidable consequences of the ageing process, spurring me on to make the most of the limited years I have left and to consider myself fortunate in having already survived in good health for over 70 years. At the same time, it has made me more conscious and accepting of, and resigned to the inescapable cycle of life: birth, childhood, maturation, sexual coupling, parenthood, ageing, and death. That cycle will soon roll forward without me, an insight I gain anew each time my children and grandchildren pay me a visit, or I them. Just being a grandfather in itself gives me hope and optimism for the future, and strengthens my purpose for living.

My long-suffering body and I are inseparable

For ten months now I have been preoccupied with breast cancer: my response to learning that my lump was cancerous, my decision to have it removed and prevent the cancer spreading, and my determination to undergo all the available treatments, however unpalatable, to prevent its recurrence. That intense and prolonged experience affected my physical and mental state in a most profound way. It confirmed that my individuality, and my unique means of expressing it as me, were inextricably linked to my body. The mastectomy removed my lump, but left both a scar on my chest and an indelible memory. I am now and will always be a person who has had breast cancer. I am breast cancer man! My bodily experiences - my physical sensations through time - make me what I am. My long-suffering body and I are inseparable. Throughout the course of my cancer experience, what I felt, sensed or suffered, my perception, awareness, and reasoning, were combined, inextricably. When my senses fail and my body dies, there will be no thinking sentient part of me - no self, no ego, no me, at all. My breast cancer has confirmed for me, once and for ever, that immutable truth.

The increased importance of family members

Cancer treatment has increased immeasurably the value I attach to my relationships with family members - wife, children, daughter- and sons-in-law, grandchildren, sisters, brothers-in-law, cousins, etc, which was already substantial. Once they knew of my illness, I received a constant stream of phone calls. texts, emails, WhatsApps, get-well cards, letters, presents, and visits from relatives, by blood or marriage, living close by, or in other parts of the country, or abroad. When my son learned of my sore gums and painful eating, he despatched immediately a powerful Ninja Auto IQ blending machine to process my meals.

My son and daughters soon discovered the power of grandchild therapy, applying it during chemotherapy cycles to lighten my distress. Maxi, Genevieve, and Baby Caio might not have been aware of their therapeutic value, but their visits to Blue Roof succeeded beyond expectation in lightening my moods and making life tolerable. My cancer treatment took place in a happy, informed and supportive family environment, which contributed to both my physical and psychological health, and transformed for ever my appreciation of the warm family blanket of love and care.

The immense value of friends

I value more than I could have possibly imagined the attitude and behaviour of my friends, who, once they were told of my cancer, rallied round and did what they could, or thought best, to give comfort and care. The reader will find ample evidence in earlier chapters of their ingenuity in providing me with support. I have learned from my cancer ordeal who my friends are and appreciate them now in the brightest of lights. A further subsidiary lesson, forever learned, is to trust friends and acquaintances with the knowledge of one's illness: of its cancerous nature and type, and whether it is potentially life-threatening. If they are not told and find out further down the road, they will feel that their friendship is of no consequence, or guilty that their response to date has been inadequate. The reality of cancer needs to be communicated, not hidden.

'Cancertified' for life in the cancer club

Another salient change to my outlook has been to recognise and identify almost viscerally with the pain and suffering of others - not only patients with cancer, or breast cancer, but all fellow human beings experiencing discomfort, hurt, distress, sickness, disease, and misery. Sitting in the Snowdrop Chemotherapy Suite, watching others with far more advanced cancers than I, undergoing simultaneously the same or similar infusions of chemo drugs, brought home to me that I was one among many sharing a common plight. To reduce or prevent our cancers, we were participating in chemotherapy on a mass industrial scale, attached through cannulas to our drip stands, each hoping for a successful outcome, not only for ourselves, but for those sentient beings sitting next to us. All were, to coin an expression, 'cancertified' for life as members of a world-wide cancer club.

I have now to find a way of contributing to the cancer care cause. I was impressed by Rod, who volunteered to drive a buggy around the hospital, and Veronica, who raised money for the Breast Cancer Action Group. In the vast sprawl of the hospital complex, Rod had understood the need for additional internal transport to help the elderly and frail, including patients affected, like him, by their cancer treatment, while Veronica had recognised the morale-boosting power of like-minded others working together for a common cause.[30]

Breast cancer is asexual but gendered by the infrequency of its occurrence in men

That esprit de corps among patients, the feeling of being at one with my fellow cancer sufferers, of sensing their pain as well as my own, so to speak, carries with it the implication that we are all of the same flesh. The differences between us in gender, age, race, ethnicity, religion and belief, or sexual orientation, ceased to exist in the face of our common plight. And in that alternative world of the cancer patient, it mattered not one jot whether we were being treated for breast, prostate, lung, bowel, skin, or other forms of cancer. To prolong our survival rate, we were all the willing recipients of those generally unpleasant adjuvant therapies, so liberally prescribed by the helpful oncologists.

The revelation that my fellow patients were receiving similar treatments, experiencing many of the same side effects, and expressing and exhibiting pain, anxiety and distress in common with me, confirmed what I had suspected from the time I was first diagnosed. Individuals developed breast cancer, women in far greater numbers than men, but the breast cancer itself was asexual. So-called 'male breast cancer' and its binary, 'female breast cancer', were social constructs in their entirety, existing in name only, as partially recognised in recent efforts to replace those terms simply with 'breast cancer', yet still distinguishing between the sexes by adding 'in men', or 'in women'. Breast cancers in men and breast cancers in women are detected, diagnosed and treated in the same way, while breast cancer patients, irrespective of their sex, respond to their tumours, diagnoses and treatment in self-same fashion.

Mastectomy, chemo- and radio-therapy are never attractive propositions, whatever one's age or sex.

Breast Cancer Man, the title of the book, is a social invention, reliant for the curiosity it may provoke on the infrequency of breast cancer's occurrence among men, as compared with its incidence among women. The single most significant risk factor for developing breast cancer, of course, is being a woman. However, in this respect, too, my personal experience of cancer has changed my outlook on life, for I am convinced, more than ever I was, that the breast cancer I experienced was the same, or almost the same, as the experience encountered by women. The reader of this book, nevertheless, is likely to conclude that my story is told from a man's point of view drawing, as it does, on my exclusive personal knowledge of living for 73 years as a man. But what I had experienced was not a breast cancer specific to men, but a breast cancer common to both sexes, while playing the gendered role of a man. It is only my interpretation of the experience, not the experience itself, that is gendered.

Angry for a just cause

At some point in a book about the treatment of a patient in the UK, a tribute will be paid to the National Health Service's doctors, nurses, and health professionals. Previous chapters describe in detail the personal attention I received and my gratitude for the kindness of staff. Undoubtedly, their treatment of me, and my experience of hospital life, have had a lasting impact on my outlook and opinions, yet I have come away from the hospital, angry, furious and frustrated. These emotions have nothing to do with the treatment I received from the staff who, in the main, were struggling to do their best in the impossible conditions under which they were forced to work. My problem was with the hospital facilities, which were everywhere crowded and overused, with queues for the car park, long waits for treatment, and inexplicable delays. Even under such pressure, staff strove to befriend the vast numbers of patients in transit and put them at their ease. In hindsight, what was extraordinary was the patients' politely passive acceptance of the poor level of service, and their reluctance to complain. Quite right not to turn on the staff! The blame lay with those in government who, despite the demographics of an ageing population, refused to fund a health service at a level and to a standard that could make it the best in the world. Oh! I came away angry, indeed.

Frank Reeves

Saturday 30th June 2018.

After hospital treatment finishes

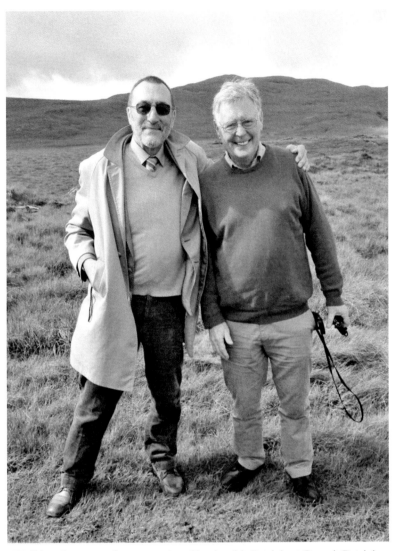

Holiday therapy and recuperation, Frank with Patrick at Croagh Patrick,
Co Mayo, 13th September 2018

Postscript: update after one year

August appointment with the oncology consultant

Mel and I returned to the Deanesly Outpatients Department at the hospital on Wednesday 1st August 2018 for an appointment with *Dr Grigoryev,* my oncology consultant. *Dr Grigoryev* asked me how I had found the radiotherapy course and wanted to know how I was responding to the tamoxifen tablets. I told him that I still had a rectangular brown mark around my left breast which I was massaging twice daily with the prescribed ZeroAQS emollient cream but, apart from the discoloration, had noticed no other after-effects from the radiotherapy. Likewise, I was taking the tamoxifen tablets on a daily basis without any apparent reaction. I felt my life was returning to normal, but I had not as yet regained my former fitness, enthusiasm for life, and energy levels.

Dr Grigoryev asked me to remove my shirt and examined my chest, palpating the tissue of my remaining right breast and along the line of my mastectomy scar. He assured me that the area that had been irradiated was recovering nicely, and that I should continue to apply the emollient cream. He found no further lumps, but urged me from then on to examine my chest regularly in like fashion on a monthly basis. He and *Mr Venkatramanan* would monitor my progress over the long term, and I would be invited for regular check-ups. They had begun the process by arranging for me to undergo a mammogram of my right breast as a precautionary measure. Thereafter, they would recommend for me to be x-rayed at regular intervals, although currently the protocol did not allow for follow-up mammograms for male breast cancer patients. They would have to receive authorisation from the appropriate body. If it were to be agreed, I would be setting a precedent.

346

Return to the gym

I asked whether it was now time for me to resume my membership of the gym. *Dr Grigoryev* confirmed that I could return to my former activities provided I took them on gradually and paced myself. With that, I resumed paying my gym subscription which I had put on hold for the year. On Sunday morning, the 5th August 2018, I went to the gym to swim, restricting myself to a distance of twenty lengths. Changing into my trunks, I became conscious that I would be exposing my mastectomy scar, but nobody in the changing room, gym, or swimming pool gave me - or my chest - a second glance. I was, after all, a quite unremarkable 73-year-old man. From then on, I, too, was oblivious to my disfigurement, in much the same way as I had been blind to my breasts before I discovered my lump.

I experienced a little stiffness in my shoulders and arms as I propelled myself slowly along the pool, but soon loosened up and climbed out feeling fresh and exhilarated. By the afternoon, however, I had become very tired and went to lie down, falling soundly asleep for at least two hours. The next week, I swam thirty lengths and resolved to build my performance over time to pre-cancerous distances.

Dr Grigoryev's report summarising concisely my diagnosis and treatment

On the 5th September, a month after my meeting with *Dr Grigoryev* at the hospital oncology clinic, I received a copy of the report he wrote to *Dr Shakeshaft* at the Castlecroft Medical Practice, describing my diagnosis, the treatment I was given, and his observations after his most recent examination of me. I was most impressed by the concision of this short document and decided to reproduce it here as a fitting summary of what had befallen me over the last twelve months.

Dear *Dr Shakeshaft*,

'**Diagnosis**: Left breast, grade 2, ductal carcinoma NST, pT1c, 13.5 mms (whole tumour size with DCIS 14.2, pN1a, 3/20 lymph nodes positive, 1 sentinel lymph node plus 2 from axillary dissection), ER, Q8, HER-2 negative, surgical margins clear, NPI 4.27.

Treatment received: Left breast mastectomy, sentinel lymph node biopsy on 22 September 2017 followed up by left axillary dissection on the 20 October 2017. Completed FEC-T chemotherapy May 2018, followed by adjuvant radiotherapy left chest wall completed 22nd June 2018.

Current treatment: Tamoxifen. I reviewed Dr Reeves in the oncology clinic today. He tolerated radiotherapy well with minimum side effects.

Clinical examination: No palpable locoregional lymph nodes. No sign of recurrence left chest wall, right breast normal. I noted that Dr Reeves has been booked for a right mammogram. I explained to him that I will check at the next Breast MDT if the protocol has been changed. Previously I was told that we do not do follow-up mammograms for breast male patients.

Plan: To be seen by the surgical team in November. To come back in June. Baseline bloods including CA 15-3 and CEA to be taken today.

The patient has written a book about his experience and would like to have some feedback from our Department. I will inform the management.

Dr Grigoryev

Locum Consultant Clinical Oncologist.'

(I would indeed have liked some feed-back prior to proceeding to press, but the deadline for modifying the manuscript had long since passed. But perhaps *Dr Grigoryev* had in mind an official response by the hospital management after the book had been published? Only at this point did I begin to appreciate that I had been naive and unreasonable to think that medical staff, as NHS hospital trust employees, could have responded individually and informally to my request for suggestion and comment.)

Return to the hairdresser

A reassuring sign of my return to full health was the re-growth of the hair on my head and my face. By mid-August it had become so long, thick and plentiful, that I was able to visit the hairdresser and ask for a regular haircut. Having stayed away for at least eight months, I was surprised at the changes to the saloon that had occurred in my absence, with old familiar hairdressers leaving and younger ones taking their place. I was so pleased with the smartness of my appearance after the trim, that I caught my reflection deliberately in the windows of shops as I walked back to the car.

Another mammogram

On the 24th August 2018, one year and one day after the original mammogram and biopsy detected my breast cancer, I returned to New Cross Hospital's imaging department for a second chest x-ray. I was reassured that this was an entirely precautionary measure to rule out the possibility of the growth of further tumours in the

349

tissue of my right breast. When Mel and I entered the reception area, we approached the counter together and I handed the appointment letter to the clerk while mentioning my name. She looked down into her document basket, spotted the name and then looked up quizzically. "Which one of you is Francis?"she asked.

"I'm Fran**cis**, not Fran**ces**!" I said, quickly, adding my date of birth.

I did not have to wait long. Almost immediately, the radiographer, *Karen Storey*, led me along a corridor, past a waiting area where two elderly women sat wrapped in surgical gowns, and into the room containing the x-ray machine. I was asked to take off my shirt and my tie and stand next to the glass panel in front of the machine - from its trade mark, a 'Siemens'. She positioned me in such a way that the tissue of my right breast was squeezed between two facets of the machine, although there wasn't much flesh to squeeze. She then retired behind a glass panel, activated the x-ray, looked at the resultant image, and emerged to reposition me and my chest at a different angle. The same process was repeated. After that I was asked to put on my shirt and tie, and led back, past the waiting women, to the reception area, where Mel was startled by my rapid reappearance. In total, we had spent no more than seven minutes in the imaging department.

One week later, I was much relieved when I received a letter from *Mr Venkatramanan* informing me that the mammogram had not shown any worrying features. I was glad he had not been worried by what he had seen, and assumed that meant that he had found no sign of any further lump or tumour in my remaining right breast. Nevertheless, the receipt of the letter reminded me the next day to palpate with great care both sides of my chest, as *Dr Grigoryev* had shown me. It was now the 1st September, and a month had passed by since the last manual examination of my breast tissue. Henceforth, I determined to examine my breasts to a regular monthly cycle and made entries in my diary to remind me.

Back to normal?

Twelve months on from my breast cancer diagnosis, I tried once again to assess how the course of treatment and year-long patient experience had affected my life. I was aware that I was less physically strong and became tired more easily when engaged in the routines of daily life, but was undecided as to whether to attribute that to the after-effects of surgery and the adjuvant therapies, or simply to the steady march of time. The aches and stiffness I experienced in my dominant left arm following exercise had surely to be a consequence of the surgery. They made me reluctant to press on with the task in hand for fear of provoking a lymphoedema, but I always felt impelled to finish the job.

But the change of which I was most conscious was one of demeanour and attitude. I believed I was more apprehensive, cautious, less prone to express an opinion, or assert myself, join in a debate, or relate in an open, friendly and spontaneous way to others. I had retreated into myself and was much more prepared to accept inconvenience than to resist it. I still interpreted and sought to understand the world around me, but was noticeably less inclined than before to make the effort to change what I found unsatisfactory or unjust. At first, my new and unusual passivity was perceived by family and friends as a symptom of illness and excused on the grounds that, while progress was slow, I would eventually make a full recovery and return to my normal self. As time went on, my quietness and failure to join in family banter and jollity was assumed to be a feature of my senescence. Put simply, I had turned into a grumpy old man, a living embodiment of Victor Meldrew, seen as concerned only in serving my own narrow interests and showing little interest in others. including, I am ashamed to admit, my own adorable grandchildren.

Why, I was asked, didn't I behave like the other grandparents and take a more active role in my grandchildren's care and upbringing? The deficit in my behaviour was obvious even to me, but despite me struggling to make amends, I found myself incapable of investing the necessary effort to maintain the quality of childcare expected of me. Was my behaviour towards family and friends markedly different from how it had been a year ago? And if it were, why had it changed? Was it an after-effect of the breast cancer treatment or a feature of ageing? After careful consideration, I came to the conclusion that the ten-month ordeal of being diagnosed and treated for breast cancer, the ever-present prospect that the cancer might return at any time, and my eagerness to make the most of the rest of my life, had had a more profound effect on my state of mind than I could ever have expected.

Strange feelings

As a prime example, I seemed to have lost interest and any enthusiasm for the social activities that once gave me pleasure, such as conversing with family and friends, or playing with my grandchildren. I loved my grandchildren, but currently found looking after them unusually stressful and utterly exhausting. I was conscious that my reluctance to take on the social responsibilities expected of me might be judged lazy or selfish, and knew that my performance compared unfavourably with others in the family who, unlike me, took great delight in their child care duties.

My behaviour and mindset were as much a mystery to me as they were to my wife and children. It felt like being withdrawn and detached from the family circle, as if I were looking into a brightly-lit room from a doorway or window. More worryingly, I experienced a sense of relief at my lack of involvement and intimacy. It was as if, like Greta Garbo, I wanted to be left alone, but not to be alone.

Anhedonia

I found this state of mind so unusual and out of character for me that I began to investigate whether it had ever been recorded before. Surely, I could not be the only person to have felt detached and aloof from the reality of my immediate social circumstances? Indeed, I was not. A psychiatric condition known as 'anhedonia' - an inability to gain satisfaction from normal social intercourse - has long been recognised, and identified, together with depression, as a side effect of diagnosis and treatment for cancer. People at risk are those who have recently experienced trauma or stress. It occurred to me there and then that there might be a medical basis to my grumpy-old-man reputation. I was by no means clinically depressed, but I had noticed that in the past two months my mood had become uncharacteristically pessimistic, sombre, dark, anxious and bleak. In more metaphorical terms, I was seeing the world not in the cheerful rainbow colours of my pre-cancerous life, but in increasingly gloomy monochromatic shades of grey. Nevertheless, I remained convinced that my symptoms of anhedonia and non-clinical depression were mild and would soon dissipate, and that I would again come to enjoy to the full the company of my family, grandchildren and friends.

My self-diagnosis of anhedonia was given short shrift by my wife and family. As Mel put it, "You were just as distant, withdrawn and bad-tempered before your cancer was diagnosed. You've worked hard to find a spurious medical label to excuse your anti-social behaviour, but it really won't do. I notice how you perk up suddenly when visitors come to the house." The significance of her assessment did not escape me.

A full recovery

The sympathy and support that had been lavished on me ever since my cancer was first diagnosed was running thin. Those who knew me most intimately had assessed my current state of health and concluded that I had recovered sufficiently from my illness and treatment to resume once again the full mantle of social responsibility. I might seek to cling on to the shield of ill health, mental or physical, but all those around me believed I had made, or was well on the way to making, a full recovery. Anhedonia? What utter tosh! Once family members had cancelled my cancer licence (withdrawn my blue badge disability parking permit, so to speak), my symptoms of mild-depression and social withdrawal faded away, exposing, to everybody's great relief, my normal cantankerous self. Shortly afterwards, I found myself helping to feed and bath a grandchild, and even using my woodworking skills to make him a toy.

Footnotes and references

Introduction: why I came to write this book

1. Macmillan Cancer Support, *Talking About Cancer*, London, February 2015, (7th edition), p. 41.

2. . Macmillan Cancer Support, *Understanding Breast Cancer in Men,* London, June 2015 (3rd edition), p. 1.

3. Derbyshire, Victoria, *Dear Cancer, Love Victoria, A Mum's Diary of Hope*, Trapeze, Orion Publishing, 2017.

 4. Ibid, see for example, pp. 57, 72, 73, 83, 84, and photo captions between pp. 90-91.

5. Macmillan Cancer Support, *Understanding Breast Cancer in Men,* London, June 2015 (3rd edition).

Chapter 1, A lump in the breast

1. www.mybreastsurgeon.org

2. Rudlowski, Christian, 'Male Breast Cancer', in *Breast Care* (Basel), July 2008, 3 (3), pp. 183-189, and Macmillan Cancer Support, *Understanding Breast Cancer in Men*, 2015 (3rd edition), p. 14.

3. Rudlowski, Christian, op. cit.

4. Confirmed in Mr Mylvaganam's letter of 1st September 2017 to Dr P. Wagstaff at the Castlecroft Medical Practice.

5. Ditto.

6. See also Rudlowski, Christian, op. cit.

7. See also Rudlowski, Christian, op. cit.

8. See also 'Risk factors for breast cancer in men', in Macmillan Cancer Support, *Understanding Breast Cancer in Men*, 2015 (3rd edition), pp. 14-17, and Rudlowski, Christian, op. cit.

9. See also Rudlowski, Christian, op. cit.

10. Macmillan Cancer Support, *Understanding Breast Cancer in Men*, London, June 2015 (3rd edition), p. 1.

11. See Cancer Research UK website.

12. Rudlowski, Christian, op. cit.

13. Macmillan Cancer Support, *Understanding Chemotherapy*, London, July 2015 (14th edition), p. 80.

14. Macmillan Cancer Support, *Understanding Breast Cancer in Men,* London, June 2015 (3rd edition), p. 87.

Chapter 2, Mastectomy, lymph node biopsy and clearance

1. Breast Cancer Care (the breast cancer support charity), *Exercises after breast cancer surgery*.

2. Breast Cancer Care, op.cit.

3. Confirmed in Mr Mylvaganam's letter of 11th October 2017 to Dr P. Wagstaff at the Castlecroft Medical Practice.

4. Confirmed in Mr Mylvaganam's letter of 11th October 2017, op.cit.

5. Macmillan Breast Cancer Support, *Understanding Lymphoedema,* London, 2015 (14th edition), pp. 11, 12, 13.

Chapter 3, Biopsies, precautionary scans and adjuvant therapies

1. Macmillan Cancer Support, *Understanding Breast Cancer in Men*, London, June 2015 (3rd edition), p.49.

2. Confirmed in Mr Mylvaganam's letter of 9th November 2017 to Dr P. Wagstaff at the Castlecroft Medical Practice.

3. Confirmed in Mr Mylvaganam's letter of 9th October 2017, op.cit.

4. Confirmed in Mr Mylvaganam's letter of 9th October 2017, op.cit.

5. Chia, S., Bryce. C. and Gelman, K., 'Effects of chemotherapy and hormonal therapy for early breast cancer on recurrence and 15-year survival: an overview of the randomised trials', *The Lancet*, Vol. 365, Issue 9412, 14-20 May 2005, pp. 1663-1744.

6. Chia, S., Bryce, C. and Gelman, K., op.cit.

7. Chia, S., Bryce, C. and Gelman, K., op.cit.

8. Chia, S., Bryce, C. and Gelman, K., op.cit.

9. See Macmillan Cancer Support, *FEC-T chemotherapy*, www.macmillan.org.uk/cancerinformation/cancertreatment/treatme nttypes/chemotherapy.

10. See Macmillan Cancer Support, *FEC-T chemotherapy*, op. cit, pp. 3-8.

11. See Macmillan Cancer Support, *FEC-T chemotherapy*, op. cit, p. 4.

12. Confirmed in Mr Mylvaganam's letter of 13th December 2017 to Dr P. Wagstaff at the Castlecroft Medical Practice.

13. Wolverhampton NHS Trust, *Oncology Patient Emergency 24-hour helpline*, Patient information leaflet for pre-assessment, VI.NE., December 2016.

Chapter 4, Beginning chemotherapy with FEC

1. See Macmillan Cancer Support, *FEC-T chemotherapy*, www.macmillan.org.uk/cancerinformation/cancertreatment/treatme nttypes/chemotherapy,p.1.

2. Macmillan Cancer Support, *Statistics Fact Sheet* (December 2017) p. 4, www.macmillan.org.uk/about-us/what-we-do/evidence/cancer-statistics.

3. Cancer Research UK, *Cancer Risk Statistics*, www.cancerresearchuk.org/health-professional/cancer-statistics/risk.

4. Cancer Research UK, *Cancer Mortality Statistics*, www.cancerresearchuk.org/health-professional/cancer-stastistics/mortality-by-age.

Chapter 5, Second chemotherapy cycle

1. Macmillan Cancer Support, *How are You Feeling? The Emotional Effects of Cancer*, London, March 2017 (4th edition), p. 32.

2. See, for example, Macmillan Cancer Support, *Coping with Hair Loss,* London, August 2017 (9th edition), p. 8.

3. Macmillan Cancer Support, *How are You Feeling? The Emotional Effects of Cancer*, London, March 2017 (4th edition), pp. 6-8.

4. Macmillan Cancer Support, *Understanding Chemotherapy,* London, July 2105 (14th edition), pp. 68-69.

5. Macmillan Cancer Support, *Understanding Chemotherapy*, London, July 2105 (14th edition)*,* p. 71.

6. Humphrys, John, Interview with Sir John Bell, Regius Professor of Medicine, Oxford University, Today Programme, BBC Radio 4, 8th February 2018.

7. Sample, Ian, and Glenza, Jessica, 'Therapy clears woman's late-stage breast cancer', *The Guardian*, 5 June 2018, pp. 1, 7.

Chapter 6, Urological interlude

1. Confirmed in Mr Hariom Sur's letter of 7th February 2018 to Dr. P. Wagstaff at the Castlecroft Medical Practice.

2. Confirmed in Mr Hariom Sur's letter of 7th February 2018 to Dr. P. Wagstaff at the Castlecroft Medical Practice.

3. Confirmed in Mr Hariom Sur's letter of 7th February 2018 to Dr. P. Wagstaff at the Castlecroft Medical Practice.

4. Spencer, B., 'Is this a case of bias against men?' front page headline and article in *Daily Mail*, 2 February 2018.

Chapter 7, Third chemotherapy cycle

1. 'Cyborg' is shoprt for 'cybernetic organism', a term first used in 1960 by Manfred Clynes and Nathan Cline to describe an entity with a combination of organic and mechanical body parts.

2. Wolverhampton NHS Trust, *Oncology Patient Emergency 24-hour Helpline*, patient information leaflet for pre-assessment, VI.NE., December 2016.

Chapter 8, Thrombo-phlebitis and its consequences

(This chapter is without footnotes or references)

Chapter 9, Fourth chemotherapy cycle with T

1. Macmillan Cancer Support, *FEC-T chemotherapy*, www.macmillan.org.uk/cancerinformation/cancertreatment/treatme nttypes/chemotherapy, p. 5.

2. Derbyshire, Victoria, *Dear Cancer, Love Victoria, A Mum's Diary of Hope*, Trapeze, Orion Publishing, 2017, p.183.

3. Derbyshire, Victoria, op. cit. p. 185.

4. Templeton, Sarah-Kate. Health Editor, 'Newsreader George Alagiah: If only I'd had the Scottish cancer test', *The Sunday Times*, 25 March 2018.

5. Rudlowski, Christian, 'Male Breast Cancer', in *Breast Care* (Basel), July 2008, 3 (3), pp. 183-189.

6. Confirmed in Dr H Ghanta's letter, typed 18th April 2018, to Dr Wagstaff at the Castlecroft Medical Practice.

7. Macmillan Cancer Support, *FEC-T chemotherapy*, www.macmillan.org.uk/cancerinformation/cancertreatment/treatme nttypes/chemotherapy, p. 6.

Chapter 10, Chemo-induced thinking on hair loss

1. The Royal Wolverhampton NHS Trust Directorate of Oncology, *Patient Record Book and Advice for cancer patients having chemotherapy treatment,* New Cross Hospital, November 2012.

2. Breast Cancer Care (support charity), *Chemotherapy for Breast Cancer Treatments and Side Effects*, Breast Cancer Care, 2015.

3. Macmillan Cancer Support, *Coping with Hair Loss*, Macmillan Cancer Support, August 2017 (9th edition).

4. See, for example, Lynch, Lisa, *The C-Word*, London, Arrow Books, Random House, 2010, 2015.

5. Derbyshire, Victoria, *Dear Cancer, Love Victoria, A Mum's Diary of Hope*, Trapeze, Orion Publishing, 2017, p. 96.

6. The Macmillan Cancer Support Statistics Fact Sheet, December 2017, p.4, states that there are now 2.5 million people living with cancer in the UK.

7. Look Good Feel Better Services, supporting women with cancer, *Pampering Therapy*, www.lgfb.co.uk.

8. Hansen, Professor Helle Ploug, 'Hair loss induced by chemotherapy: an anthropological study of women, cancer and rehabilitation', in *Anthropology & Medicine*, Vol. 14. 2007, Issue 1, pp. 15-26, published online, 21 February 2007.

Chapter 11, Fifth chemotherapy cycle

1. Savage, Michael, 'Nurses are seeing worst shortage of staff for decades', *The Observer*, 13 May 2018, p. 7.

Chapter 12, Chemo-induced thinking on therapy

1. Names have been changed to ensure patients' anonymity.

2. For criticism of psychotherapy, see for example, Masson, Jeffrey, *Against Therapy* (1988), London, Harper Collins, 1989, 1990, and 1992.

3. Royal Wolverhampton NHS Trust, Directorate of Oncology and Clinical Haematology, *Complementary Therapies, Information for Patients*, November 2009.

4. Monbiot, George, 'A bold medical breakthrough. Experts call it community', Opinion, *The Guardian*, 21 February 2018, p. 4.

5. Wolverhampton and District Breast Cancer Action Group, *Supporting, Liaising, Fundraising* (undated).

6. Monbiot, George, 'I have prostate cancer. But I am happy', *The Guardian*, 13 March 2018.

7. Mental Health Foundation, *Poverty and Mental Health, A review to inform the Joseph Rowntree Foundation's Anti-Poverty Strategy*. Mental Health Foundation, supported by Joseph Rowntree, Policy Review, August 2016.

8.   Macmillan,   www.macmillan.org.uk/information-and-support/coping/complementary-therapies/complementary-therapies-explained/psychological-self-help-therapies.htm/

9.   Cancer   Research   UK,   www.cancerresearch.uk.org/about-cancer/cancer-in-general/treatment/complementary-alternative-therapies/individual-therapies/meditation.

10. Wikipedia, https:/en.wikipedia.org/wiki/Mindfulness.

11. Wikipedia, https:/en.wikipedia.org/wiki/Jon_kabat_Zinn.

12.   Mindspace,   Mindful   Eight-Week   Beginner   Course, https://www.mindspace.org.uk/2011/07/27/meditation-classes-in-tettenhall-wood-wolverhampton.

Chapter 13, Sixth chemotherapy cycle

1. Compare Breast Cancer Action Group (Wolverhampton and District), *Supporting, liaising, fundraising,* two leaflets, both undated.

2. Glenza, Jessica, 'Targeted approach may avoid chemotherapy for breast cancer patients', *The Guardian*, 4 June 2018, p. 4.

Chapter 14, Pursuing the febrile neutropenia care pathway

1. The American sociologist, Erving Goffman (1922-1982), father of symbolic interactionism and dramaturgical analysis, might have described this exchange as 'cooling the mark out', a form of persuasion aimed at helping people accept their loss or failure, described by Goffman, in Goffman, E., 'On cooling the mark out. Some aspects of adaptation to failure,' in *Psychiatry*, November 1955, pp. 451-463.

Chapter 15, Radiotherapy

1. The radiotherapy planning process is described succinctly in the Royal Wolverhampton Trust, Directorate of Oncology and Clinical Haematology, booklet, *Radiotherapy for breast cancer - information for patients*, July 2015, pp. 3-4.

2. See also Breast Cancer Care, *Radiotherapy for primary breast cancer*, January 2017, (7th edition), pp. 14-16.

3. For systematic explanations of lymphoedema and information on reducing risk, see Macmillan Cancer Support, *Understanding Lymphoedema*, December 2015 (14th edition), and Breast Cancer Care, *Reducing the risk of lymphoedema*, March 2014 (5th edition).

4. See Breast Cancer Care, *Radiotherapy for primary breast cancer*, January 2017, (7th edition), p. 11.

5. Name withheld, though freely offered by the senior radiographer.

6. See the Royal Wolverhampton Hospital Trust Directorate of Oncology and Clinical Haematology, booklet, *Radiotherapy for breast cancer - information for patients*, July 2015, p. 5.

7. Leader, 'Images aren't everything. AI, radiology and the future of work,' *The Economist*, 9-15 June, pp. 15-16.

8. Breast Cancer Care, *Radiotherapy for primary breast cancer*, January 2017, (7th edition), p. 19.

9. Ibid, p. 19.

10. Ibid, p. 19.

11. Royal Wolverhampton Hospital Trust, Directorate of Oncology and Clinical Haematology, booklet, *Radiotherapy for breast cancer - information for patients*, July 2015, p. 8.

12. Special supplement, 'NHS 70 Celebrating 70 years 1948-2018, Celebrating Windrush 70. High achievers share their stories', *The Voice*, preview edition June 2018, final edition, 5 July 2018.

Chapter 16, Hormone therapy with tamoxifen

1. RelonChem, Tamoxifen 20mg tablets package leaflet, information for the user.

2. Macmillan Cancer Support, *Understanding Breast Cancer in Men*, section on hormonal therapy, London, June 2015 (3rd edition), pp. 70-73.

3. Derbyshire, Victoria, *Dear Cancer, Love Victoria, A Mum's Diary of Hope*, Trapeze, Orion Publishing, 2017, p.222.

4. Ibid, p.228.

5. Breast Cancer Care, *Tamoxifen*, February 2018 (7th edition).

6. Macmillan Cancer Support, *Understanding Breast Cancer in Men*, London, June 2015 (3rd edition), pp. 70-73.

7. Breast Cancer Care, *Tamoxifen*, February 2018 (7th edition), p. 4.

8. Macmillan Cancer Support, *Understanding Breast Cancer in Men*, London, June 2015 (3rd edition), pp. 72-73.

9. RelonChem, Tamoxifen 20mg tablets package leaflet, information for the user.

10. Macmillan Cancer Support, *Understanding Breast Cancer in Men*, London, June 2015 (3rd edition), p. 73.

11. RelonChem, Tamoxifen 20mg tablets package leaflet, information for the user.

12. Breastcancer.org, 'Many men stop taking tamoxifen', 17 November 2011, on line at www.breastcancer.org/research-news/20111117-2.

13. University of Texas MD Anderson Cancer Center, 'Tamoxifen causes significant side effects in male breast cancer patients', News Review, 16 November 2011, on line at www/mdanderson.org/newsroom/2011/11/tamoxifen-side-effect-in-male-breast-cancer-patients.

14. Ibid.

Chapter 17, My time at the hospital

1. Wolverhampton City Council Planning Committee, Report, 8 January 2008, Regeneration and environment, 7/01112/OUT, Site Description (New Cross Hospital site), p.63.

2. See also Wolverhampton City Council Health and Wellbeing Board, New Cross Hospital Transport Facilities, 3 July 2013.

3. www.history-andpolicy.org/policy-papers/papers/immigration-and-the-national-health-service-putting-history-to-the-forefront.

4. See, for example, 'Health of patients put at risk as fewer get to see their own GPs', *The Guardian*, 9 May 2018, p. 5.

5. Care Quality Commission, The Royal Wolverhampton NHS Trust, *New Cross Hospital Quality Report*, visit 02-05.06.2015, publication 15.12.2016.

Chapter 18, After hospital treatment finishes

1. Lynch, Lisa, *The C-Word*, London, Arrow Books, Random House, 2010, 2015, p. 80.

2. Diamond, John, *C, Because cowards get cancer too...*, London, Vermilion, Penguin Random House, 1999, p.8.

3. Macmillan Cancer Support, *Life After Cancer Treatment*, London, June 2017 (8th edition).

4. Macmillan Cancer Support, *What to do after cancer treatment ends: 10 top tips*, London, May 2017 (3rd edition).

5. Macmillan Cancer Support, *Life After Cancer Treatment*, London, June 2017 (8th edition), pp. 69, 85.

6. Macmillan Cancer Support, *Life After Cancer Treatment*, London, June 2017 (8th edition), p.18; Macmillan Cancer Support, *What to do after cancer treatment ends: 10 top tips*, London, May 2017 (3rd edition), p.14.

7. Macmillan Cancer Support, *Life After Cancer Treatment*, London, June 2017 (8th edition), pp. 6-7; Macmillan Cancer Support, *What to do after cancer treatment ends: 10 top tips*, London, May 2017 (3rd edition), pp. 3-7.

8. Macmillan Cancer Support, *Life After Cancer Treatment*, London, June 2017 (8th edition), p.7.

9. Ibid, p.7.

10. Ibid, pp. 22-24.

11. Ibid, pp. 28-41.

12. Macmillan Cancer Support, *Life After Cancer Treatment*, London, June 2017 (8th edition), pp. 54-59; Macmillan Cancer Support, *What to do after cancer treatment ends: 10 top tips*, London, May 2017 (3rd edition), p. 11.

13. Macmillan Cancer Support, *How are you feeling? The Emotional Effects of Cancer*, London, March 2017 (4th edition).

14. Macmillan Cancer Support, *How are you feeling? The Emotional Effects of Cancer*, London, March 2017 (4th edition), pp. 7, 26-33; Macmillan Cancer Support, *Talking About Cancer*, London, February 2015, (7th edition), p. 34.

15. Macmillan Cancer Support, *How are you feeling? The Emotional Effects of Cancer*, London, March 2017 (4th edition), pp. 7, 8; Macmillan Cancer Support, *Talking About Cancer*, London, February 2015, (7th edition), p. 33.

16. Macmillan Cancer Support, *How are you feeling? The Emotional Effects of Cancer*, London, March 2017 (4th edition), p. 28.

17. Ibid, p.11.

18. Macmillan Cancer Support, *Talking About Cancer*, London, February 2015, (7th edition), pp. 8-10.

19. Macmillan Cancer Support, *How are you feeling? The Emotional Effects of Cancer*, London, March 2017 (4th edition), pp. 36-39.

20. Macmillan Cancer Support, *Life After Cancer Treatment*, London, June 2017 (8th edition), pp. 58-61.

21. Macmillan Cancer Support, *Work and Cancer*, London, November 2016, (6th edition).

22. See ibid, pp.61-66.

23. Macmillan Cancer Support, *Talking About Cancer*, London, February 2015, (7th edition), p. 41.

24. Macmillan Cancer Support, *Travel and Cancer*, London, April 2017, (6th edition).

25. See ibid, pp. 32-48.

26. Macmillan Cancer Support, *Life After Cancer Treatment*, London, June 2017 (8th edition), p. 13.

27. Ibid, p. 13.

28. Ibid, p. 4.

29. Aunan, Jan R, Cho, William C, and Søreide, Kjetil, 'The Biology of Aging and Cancer: A Brief Overview of Shared and Divergent Molecular Hallmarks', in *Aging & Disease*, JKL International LLC, at www.ncbi.nim.nih.gov>articles.

30. Names have been changed to ensure patients' anonymity.

Glossary of terms

The glossary defines and contextualises the medical, pharmaceutical, psychological, technical, and other specialist terms and abbreviations used in this book. In its style guide (nice.org.uk), the National Institute for Health and Care Excellence (NICE) advises that generic names (British Approved Names) should be used for drugs unless a brand name makes more sense in context. Generic names do not take a capital letter. Where possible, generic names have been used for non-branded drugs.

adjuvant therapy

Medical treatment to suppress secondary tumour formation. Examples of adjuvant therapies mentioned in this book are: chemotherapy, chest-wall radiotherapy, and a five-year course of tamoxifen.

allopurinol

A drug used to lower blood uric acid levels in order to prevent gout, or the high uric acid levels that can occur with chemotherapy.

alopecia

See chemically-induced alopecia.

alopecic

An adjective derived from alopecia, see chemically-induced alopecia.

anhedonia

A psychiatric term used to describe an inability to engage in or draw satisfaction from social interaction. Symptoms include social withdrawal, negative feelings towards the self and others, lack of emotion, and a reluctance to engage in conversation.

anti-emetic

A drug that is used to prevent vomiting and nausea and, in my case, prescribed to deal with the side effect of chemotherapy treatment.

aprepitant

One of a group of medicines called neurokinin 1 (NK) that works as 'receptor antagonists', blocking signals to control the area of the brain (the vomiting centre) to reduce feelings of nausea and vomiting. It is marketed as a course of 125mg and 80mg capsules under the brand name, Emend.

arthralgia

Joint pain, in my case, caused by the administration of the docetaxel chemotherapy drug.

audible peristalsis

Sounds produced by the movement of the gastro-intestinal tract's content as it passes through the small intestine or stomach, caused by contractions of the gut, known as peristalsis.

axilla

The area of the body under the shoulder joint, connecting the arm to the shoulder, commonly referred to as the armpit or underarm. **Axillary** is the adjective, meaning 'relating to the armpit'.

BCIM

BCIM is an acronym for 'breast cancer in men', a preferred expression to 'male breast cancer' (acronym, MBC) and used deliberately in the title of the Macmillan practical guide, *Breast Cancer in Men*.

biopsy

The extraction of tissue or cells from the body for examination and testing, to establish the presence or extent of disease.

bolus

In radiography/radiotherapy, a bolus is a special pad placed over the chest of a breast cancer patient to enhance the effect of the radiation on the surface of the skin. It acts as a tissue equivalent, compensating for missing tissue, and helping to concentrate the radiation dose on the surface of the skin. To avoid technical jargon for patients, radiographers sometimes refer to it simply as 'the jelly pad'.

BRCA 1 and BRCA 2 genes

BRCA is an abbreviation for BReast CAncer gene. BRCA 1 and BRCA 2 are genes that have been identified as affecting the chances of developing breast cancer. All people have both BRCA 1 and BRCA 2 genes, which normally help prevent the development of breast cancer by repairing DNA and uncontrolled tumour growth and act, therefore, as tumour suppressor genes. In a small number of people, however, these genes mutate (0.25 per cent of the population) in a way that increases the likelihood of developing breast cancer at a younger age. Persons with a mutated BRCA gene can pass the mutation on to their children.

candidiasis

Usually called thrush, is a fungal infection of the mouth, often revealed by white spots on the tongue or gums.

cannula (plural, cannulae)

More fully, an intravenous cannula, is a tube that is inserted into the body for the delivery or removal of fluid, to administer drugs, or to take blood samples. The word derives from the Latin 'cannula', meaning 'little reed'.

catheter

A thin tube inserted into the body to perform a wide range of medical functions, such as drainage of urine, the administration of chemotherapy drugs, or the insertion of surgical instruments. In most cases a catheter consists of a thin flexible tube, in my case, a constituent part of my Hickman line, inserted underneath the skin of my chest and into the vein draining into my heart.

chemically-induced alopecia

Hair loss caused by the use of chemicals as in chemotherapy and in cosmetic treatments. **Chemotherapy-induced alopecia** is hair loss and baldness caused by the use of anti-cancer (cytotoxic) drugs during chemotherapy. The drugs attack both the cancer cells and hair follicle cells, both of which divide quickly but, unlike the cancer cells, the hair cells recover. During my treatment, the alopecia extended to much of the hair on my head, my beard, my moustache, my eyebrows, and eyelashes, my body and pubic hair.

chemotherapy

Cancer treatment where medication is used to kill cancer cells and stop them reproducing, thus preventing them from growing and spreading. Many different anti-cancer drugs have been developed which can be given in different ways, for example, intravenously, as an infusion administered, in my case, through a Hickman line.

CIA.

See chemically-induced alopecia.

cirrhosis of the liver

A complication of liver disease involving the loss of liver cells and scarring, causing long-term liver damage which can eventually lead to liver failure and death.

co-amoxiclav

Co-amoxiclav, brand name Augmentin, is a medicine containing amoxicillin (an antibiotic) and clavulanic acid, used to treat a range of bacterial conditions, in my case to treat a respiratory tract infection (congestion following a bad cold) after I was discharged from the Acute Medical Unit on the 14th May 2018. I took it orally then in the form of 21 doses of Augmentin 625mg tablets.

Also referred to simply as **amoxicillin, i**t was prescribed for me previously to treat a skin and soft tissue infection.

colchicine

A drug commonly used to treat the onset of gout.

colonoscopy

A medical procedure involving the insertion of a flexible fibre-optic camera into the anus to scan the interior of the colon. A colonoscopy examines all of the colon, whereas a **sigmoidoscopy** is a scan of only the rectum (the lower part of the colon).

complementary therapies

So called because they complement, augment or support other therapies, such as (in the context of this book) chemotherapy, radiotherapy, and hormone therapy, when they are used to boost physical and emotional health, and relieve symptoms and side effects. Macmillan Cancer Support distinguishes complementary therapies from alternative, psychological and self-help therapies. New Cross Hospital Directorate of Oncology and Clinical Haematology provides an information leaflet for patients, *Complementary Therapies*, which lists aromatherapy, reiki, reflexology,, and Indian head massage. The leaflet states that complementary therapies, such as these, aim to make patients feel better in general, improve their quality of sleep, reduce stress, tension, anxiety and depression, relax them, and reduce the symptoms of pain and nausea.

cording

Also known as **axillary web syndrome (AWS)**, cording can be a side effect of the removal of the lymph nodes to prevent the spread of breast cancer. It is a sensation as if a rope is being stretched along the inner arm from the shoulder to the finger tips, thus causing pain and restricting movement.

Corsodyl

The brand name for a mouth wash/oral rinse based on the active ingredient, chlorohexidine, used as a disinfectant and antseptic to prevent yeast infections of the mouth, microorganisms and dental plaque.

CT or CAT scans.

CT or CAT stands for **computerised axial tomography**, involving a barrel-like rotating scanning machine, which uses an x-ray beam to create a three-dimensional image.

CVC

Acronym for **central venous catheter**, an example of which was my Hickman line.

cyclophosphamide

One of the drugs used as an immune suppressor in chemotherapy for breast cancer, in my case, in the first three cycles alongside flurouracil and epirubicin, a combination treatment referred to as FEC. Common side effects include low white blood cell counts, nausea, vomiting and hair loss.

cytotoxic

Being toxic or poisonous to cells. **Cytotoxic drugs** used in chemotherapy are aimed at destroying cancer cells, but have the potential to damage normal healthy tissue as well.

DCIS

In full, **ductal carcinoma in situ**, is a breast cancer. 'Ductal' means that the cancer started in the milk ducts of the breast, 'carcinoma' means that it is a cancer of the tissues lining or covering, internal organs, and 'in situ', that the cancer is situated in its original position or site.

desquamation

Desquamation, or skin flaking or peeling, is the shedding of the outer layer of skin. The word derives from the Latin 'desquamare', meaning to scrape the scales off a fish.

dexamethasone

A steroid (short for corticosteroid) tablet used to reduce inflammation and to suppress the immune system in a variety of contexts, such as when treating breast cancer and in order to prevent nausea and vomiting following chemotherapy. It is marketed in the form of Glensoludex 2mg, 4mg and 8mg soluble tablets.

diabetology

The study of the diagnosis and treatment of **diabetes**, a metabolic disorder in which a person's level of sugar in the blood becomes too high. Type 1 diabetes occurs when the body's immune system destroys insulin-producing cells. Type 2 diabetes occurs when the body does not produce enough insulin, or the body's cells do not respond to insulin.

Difflam

The brand name for a mouth wash or oral rinse based on the active ingredient, benzydamine hydrochloride (which belongs to a group of medicines called non-steroidal ant-inflammatory drugs (NSAIDS), used to prevent pain and inflammation of the mouth and throat, for example, in the form of mouth ulcers or soreness caused by dentures.

Digital rectal examination

Often abbreviated to **DRE**, this a rectal examination, often used to detect a prostate problem or prostate cancer, in which a medical practitioner inserts a finger (digit) into the rectum, or back passage.

docetaxel

A chemotherapy drug used to treat cancer, including breast cancer, prostate cancer, and head and neck cancer. It is administered by injection into a vein. It is often referred to by its brand name initial: 'T', for **Taxotere**. Side effects include, nausea, muscle and joint pains, fatigue, hair loss and low blood cell counts.

domperidone

A medication belonging to a group of medicines known as 'dopamine antagonists'. It is used to treat nausea and vomiting. It should be taken before food to enhance its absorption. It is marketed under the brand name, Motilium.

drip stand

Medical equipment, consisting of a frame, hooks and monitor, on which bags of liquids, such as saline solution, blood, blood plasma, or chemotherapy drugs, can be hung and fed gradually through a tube into a patient's veins, as during the chemotherapy administered in New Cross Hospital's Snowdrop Millennium Suite.

ECG

An acronym for **electrocardiogram**, which is a way of recording the electrical activity of the heart over a period of time with electrodes attached to the skin. An electrocardiogram measures heart rate, heart rhythm and heart pathology.

echocardiogram

An image of heart activity, built up from ultrasound waves, used for monitoring or diagnosing heart problems.

E 45

A non-greasy dermatological body lotion, quickly absorbed, which is used to treat dry and itchy skin, eczema, dermatitis and psoriasis, and is also recommended to deal with the dry skin and scaling caused by chemotherapy.

electrocardiogram (ECG)

A recording in the form of a graph of a person's heart beat produced by placing electrodes on the skin of the chest, see also ECG.

enoxaparin

Enoxaparin, or enoxaparin sodium, is an anti-coagulant, or blood-thinning, medication, derived from heparin and used to treat and prevent deep-vein thrombosis. After I developed thrombo-phlebitis, Mel administered enoxaparin to me through syringes injected on a nightly basis under the skin of my midriff.

epirubicin

A drug with a ruby colour used in chemotherapy, together with flourouracil and cyclophosphamide, to treat breast cancer patients who have had tumours removed (It can be used to treat other cancers too.) It is the 'E' drug of the FEC cycles. Side effects include increased risk of infection, breathlessness, tiredness, weakness, and hair loss. After it is administered, it causes the patient's urine to turn pink or peach in colour.

ER-negative

ER stands for **oestrogen-receptor** (estrogen with an E is the American spelling). **Oestrogen-receptor negative** breast cancer, (unlike oestrogen-receptor positive) is not dependent on hormone receptors and does not respond to hormonal therapies. Most breast cancers (70 per cent) are ER-positive.

ER-positive

ER stands for **oestrogen-receptor** (estrogen with an E is the American spelling). **Oestrogen-receptor positive** breast cancer (70 per cent of all breast cancers) has receptors or proteins for the hormone, oestrogen, and responds well to treatment with hormonal therapies.

FBC

An acronym for **full blood count**, an FBC is a blood test to assess a patient's general state of health. An FBC measures the numbers of red cells (carrying oxygen) and white blood cells (which fight infection), the levels of haemoglobin and hematocrit (the proportion of red blood cells to blood plasma), and the platelet count (which causes blood to clot).

FEC-T chemotherapy

An acronym referring to four drugs: fluorouracil, epirubicin, cyclophosphamide and docetaxel (represented by the T of its brand name, Taxotere), commonly administered, as in my case, in the cycles of chemotherapy used in the treatment of breast cancer.

fibrosis

Scar tissue (excessive fibrous tissue) developed as a response to injury. Pulmonary fibrosis is the build-up of scar tissue in the lungs, which can be caused by the side effects of radiotherapy.

filgrastim

A medication used to treat neutropenia, a side effect of chemotherapy. Filgrastim stimulates the bone marrow to increase the production of neutrophils. It is administered by injection under the skin or into a vein. It is marketed under the brand name, Neupogen.

flucloxacillin

An antibiotic used to treat inflammatory and bacteriological infections.

fluorouracil

A drug used in chemotherapy, together with epirubicin and cyclophosphamide, to treat breast and other cancers. It is the F drug of the FEC cycle. Common side effects include nausea, vomiting, hiccups, diarrhoea, hair loss, and mood changes. In my case, it was injected into a vein.

follicular lymphoma

A type of non-Hodgkin lymphoma where the body produces abnormal B-lymphocytes (white blood cells that fight infection). The lymphoma cells develop in the lymph nodes, leading to swelling in the neck, armpit or groin,

Fucibet cream

The brand name for a cream comprising two ingredients, fusidic acid (a kind of antibiotic) and betamethasone valerate (a kind of steroid). The fusidic acid kills the bacteria causing infection, while the betamethasone valerate reduces swelling, redness or itching of the skin. The cream is used to treat bacterial infection and inflammation of the skin, in my case, between the buttocks.

gastritis

Inflammation of the lining of the stomach, causing nausea, heartburn, vomiting, bloating and upper abdominal pain. In my case, this was a side effect of the chemotherapy drugs.

gout

Inflammatory arthritis of a joint, in my case, the big toe joint of my left foot, which some years ago became red, and swollen and excruciatingly painful when touched . Gout is caused by the build up and crystallisation of uric acid.

haematology

The branch of medicine concerned with the study of the blood, blood formation, and blood diseases. A **haematologist** is a medical specialist who studies the cause, prognosis, treatment, and prevention of diseases related to the blood.

heparin

Medication used as an anticoagulant, or blood thinner, to treat and prevent thrombosis and thrombo embolism, etc. Heparin occurs naturally in bodily tissue, such as the liver.

HER2

An acronym for **human epidermal growth factor receptor 2**, HER2 refers to a gene that can play a part in breast cancer by triggering the development of HER2 receptors or proteins. These are normally healthy but, in a quarter of breast cancers, the HER2 gene malfunctions and causes breast cells to grow faster. These are known as HER2 positive breast cancers. They are more likely to spread and return, compared with HER2 negative breast cancers.

Hickman Line

One form of central venous catheter (see CVC), a Hickman line is a long flexible plastic tube inserted underneath the skin of the chest wall and into the large vein draining directly into the heart. After I was given a Hickman line, it was used to administer my chemotherapy and for taking blood samples. The Hickman line is named after Dr Robert Hickman, a paediatrician who developed it in the course of his work at Seattle Children's Hospital.

histology

The study of the structure, composition, and functions of tissues and cells. **Pathologic histology** is the study of diseased tissues.

hormone

A chemical substance, usually occurring naturally in the body, that controls and regulates the activity of a cell or organ. Specific hormones are secreted by the various glands of the body, for example, the pituitary, thyroid and adrenal glands, pancreas, and kidneys. A hormone is sometimes conceived of as a 'chemical message'.

hydrocortisone cream

A cream that contains steroid (in full, corticosteroid) and is used on the skin to treat swelling, itching and irritation.

hyperuricemia

A condition of having an abnormally high level of uric acid in the blood, caused by various factors, such as over consumption of alcohol, obesity, a genetic disposition, and the administration of chemotherapy drugs.

ibuprofen

A drug used for pain relief, which also has important anti-inflammatory properties.

IEPR

An acronym for the **integrated electronic patient record**, a computerised medical record, used at New Cross Hospital.

Imodium

The brand name for loperamide , a drug used to reduce the frequency of diarrhoea, working by slowing intestinal contractions.

IMRT

An acronym for **intensity modulated radiography**, a way of administering external-beam radiotherapy, in a way that can deliver varying amounts of radiation to different parts of the body, thus reducing the harm done to non-cancerous cells.

Inhixa enoxaparin

See enoxaparin.

intertrigo

Intertrigo, or **intertriginous dermatitis**, is an inflammatory condition of the skin folds, in my case, soreness, itching and ulcers between the buttocks.

isotopes

Isotopes are variants of a particular chemical element, having the same number of protons and electrons, but different numbers of neutrons. Radioactive isotopes are used in medicine for diagnosis and treatment. Radioactive tracers injected into the body emit gamma rays that are detected by a gamma camera, thus allowing an image to be built up. In radiotherapy, rapidly-dividing cancer cells are targeted and destroyed with radiation. Imaging machines using isotopic materials include x-rays, magnetic resonance imaging (MRI) and computerised tomography (CT) scanners. External radiation therapy uses a beam of radiation – x-rays and protons – to zap cancerous cells.

lansoprazole

A drug taken in capsule form to reduce stomach acid and to treat heartburn, indigestion, burping and acid regurgitation caused, in my case, by the chemotherapy drugs. It belongs to a category of medicines called proton pump inhibitors that reduce the levels of stomach acid.

laryngectomy

The surgical removal of the larynx (the air/wind pipe from the mouth to the lungs and containing the voice box). Following the operation, the patient has to breathe through an opening or hole in the neck known as a **stoma**.

linac

An acronym for a **linear accelerator**, a linac is an X-ray machine used in radiotherapy to deliver an external beam through the skin to a part of the body. Sometimes 'linac' is further abbreviated to 'LA'.

lollipops

Or lollipop swabs, are swabs, (absorbent pads used for cleaning wounds), mounted on a plastic shaft or stick, which , in my case, were used to clean around my Hickman line.

lorazepam

A benzodiazepine medication, used to treat anxiety, insomnia, and chemotherapy-induced nausea and vomiting.

lumbar region

Or lumbo-sacral region, refers to the lower back and the area in the vicinity of the lower spine, consisting of the lumbar vertebrae and the sacrum (the five fused bones in the bottom).

lymph nodes

Lymph nodes are small bean-shaped structures, linked by lymph vessels, that are found throughout the body, but mainly in the neck, armpits, groin and abdomen. They filter and breakdown bacteria and other harmful cells from the lymph fluid. Different parts of the body have different numbers of nodes. For example, there are 15 to 30 small nodes in the armpit (Macmillan).

lymphadenectomy

An operation to surgically remove one or more of the lymph nodes, in my case, to prevent the spread of breast cancer.

lymphoedema

A build-up of lymph fluid under the skin, occurring when lymph nodes or lymph vessels are damaged or blocked, or if lymph nodes have been removed by surgery. Lymphoedema results when lymph fluid cannot drain away through nodes or vessels in the normal way. Lymphoedema can develop months or years after surgery to remove lymph nodes.

lymphoma

A cancer of the lymph nodes and lymphatic system, which develops from the lymphocytes (a type of white blood cell).

lymph vessels

Lymph vessels are a network of tubes that connect to groups of lymph nodes throughout the body. The lymph fluid travels through the lymph vessels and drains into the bloodstream (Macmillan).

magnetic resonance imaging

Often referred to by its acronym, **MRI**, magnetic resonance imaging is the creation of images of the inside of the body by using magnets, radio waves, and a computer. Unlike with x-rays and CT scans, MRI does not make use of radiation.

mammogram

An x-ray image of the breast, used to decide whether a breast lump is a gland, cyst, or tumour.

mastectomy

A surgical operation to remove a breast. A **total mastectomy** involves the removal of the entire breast tissue. A **modified radical mastectomy** involves the removal of breast tissue and sentinel lymph nodes for biopsy. A **radical mastectomy** is one in which the breast is removed, along with levels I, II and III of the underarm lymph nodes, and the chest wall muscles under the breast (see Breastcancer.org).

MBC

An acronym for male breast cancer, commonly used as an abbreviation in research literature, but now being deliberately avoided and replaced by the expression 'breast cancer in men' (acronym, BCIM). The adjectival phrase, 'male breast cancer' might be understood wrongly to mean that there is a form of breast cancer specific only to men. My breast cancer was of the oestrogen receptor positive type, common to women as well as men., and the treatment regime was the same for both sexes, hence the preference for the expressions, 'breast cancer in men' and 'breast cancer in women'.

MBCT

An acronym for **mindfulness-based cognitive therapy**, a psychotherapeutic programme, based on mindfulness techniques, developed to prevent the recurrence of depression.

MBSR

An acronym for **mindfulness-based stress reduction**, a psychotherapeutical programme, based on mindfulness techniques, to help people in pain, or suffering from other conditions, such as anxiety and stress.

metastasis

The spread of cancer cells from the place where they were originally formed, or detected, to a location in another part of the body. Metastasis (plural, metastases) occurs when cancer cells detach themselves from the original tumour and travel through the blood or lymph system to form a new tumour in another organ or tissue of the body (adapted from the *National Cancer Institute Dictionary*).

microscopy

The examination of the aspects of the world invisible to, or undetectable by, the naked eye, with the help of a microscope. Microscopy is used to diagnose cancer and to identify which microbes are causing infection.

micturition

Urination, making water, or, more precisely, wanting to make water.

mindfulness

The psychological process of bringing one's attention to experiences occurring in the present moment (Wikipedia). Adam Dacey, the founder of Mindspace and former Buddhist monk, explained it as "living in the moment, a non-judgmental awareness of the present", as an antidote to anxiety and stress "brought about worrying about what might happen in the future". For critical comment, refer to Chapter 12.

mindfulness meditation

A psychological, or self-help therapy, based on mindfulness teaching, that aims to help a person change negative thoughts to more positive ones through meditation exercises(Macmillan).

MRSA

An acronym for **methicillin-resistant staphylococcus aureus**, a group of bacteria that are resistant to several antibiotics. Because

MRSA infections occur more frequently in hospital wards and nursing homes, the NHS has made it a priority to put in place hygiene measures to tackle MRSA in hospitals. Systematic measures to eliminate MRSA have been put in place on the New Cross Hospital site.

mucositis

Soreness, rawness and ulceration of the mouth, gums, or throat, one of the side effects of chemotherapy.

NHS

An acronym for the **National Health Service**, which is the publicly-funded national healthcare system in the United Kingdom, paid for in the main from taxation. It came into being on the 5th July 1948 under a Labour government committed to the ideal that good healthcare should be available to all, regardless of wealth. It was based on three principles: that it met the needs of everyone, that it was free at the point of delivery, and that it was based on clinical need, not on the ability to pay. Readers must judge for themselves whether these principles have been retained, or are being gradually eroded.

nausea

A feeling of sickness in the stomach, with an inclination to vomit.

neutropenia

The condition of having an abnormally low number of white blood cells, thus compromising the body's immune system and ability to fight disease. In my case, chemotherapy temporarily lowered my white blood cell count. **Neutropenic sepsis** is a potentially-life-threatening inflammatory response to bacterial or other infection brought about by a collapse in the neutrophil count caused by chemotherapy drugs.

neutrophils

A type of white blood cell which helps to fight infection by ingesting micro-organisms and releasing enzymes that kill them. Chemotherapy can weaken the immune system by lowering the number, or count, of white blood cells (an effect known as immuno-suppression). During my chemotherapy cycles, filgrastim injections were used to boost my white blood cell count.

nitrofurantoin

An antibiotic used to treat urinary tract infections.

Nivestim filgrastim

See filgrastim.

node negative cancer

Breast cancer where biopsy results show lymph nodes to be non-cancerous, in other words, when the breast cancer has not spread to the lymph nodes.

node positive cancer

Breast cancer which has spread to the lymph nodes.

normalisation

Business as usual – the maintenance of the habits and routines of everyday life.

nystatin

The active ingredient in **Nystan Oral Suspension** (brand name). Nystatin is an anti-fungal antibiotic used to prevent and treat fungal infections (thrush) of the mouth and throat,

oestrogen (US, estrogen)

A set of hormones that leads to the development and maintenance of the female characteristics of the body. Secreted chiefly by the ovaries and placenta, oestrogen hormones result in oestrus ('periods' of fertility), stimulate changes in the female reproductive organs during the oestrus cycle, and promote the development of female secondary sexual characteristics (Collins). Whereas testosterone is considered the male hormone, oestrogen and testosterone, are found in both sexes. Sexual distinctions are not qualitative differences, but arise from quantitative divergence in hormone concentrations and the differential expression of hormone receptors. In men, oestrogen is present in low concentrations in blood, but can be very high in semen (Pub Med, NCBI). Men's oestrogen levels increase with age, contributing to prostate problems, heart disease, and enlargement of the breasts. My breast cancer was oestrogen-receptor positive.

oestrogen-receptor positive breast cancer

Breast cancer that has developed in response to the hormone, oestrogen, where oestrogen, rather than progesterone, has led to the growth and spread of the cancer. Around 80 per cent of all breast cancer is oestrogen-reception positive, or 'ER-positive'. (See also ER-positive and ER-negative.

omeprazole

The medication, omeprazole is taken in capsule form to treat gastrinal reflux and peptic ulcers, the former caused in my case, by the chemotherapy drugs. Like lansoprazole, it is a proton pump inhibitor that reduces the levels of stomach acid.

oncology

The branch of medical science that deals with tumours and cancers, including the origin, development, diagnosis and treatment of malignant tissue growth. 'Onco' means 'mass', 'lump', or tumour, whereas 'logy' means 'study'. An **oncologist** is a medical practitioner who specialises in the diagnosis and treatment of cancers.

oncoplastic breast surgery

Breast surgery that removes breast cancer tissues, while retaining, or producing, a breast shape and appearance that resembles a normal breast. It combines the medical purpose of removing tumours and preventing the recurrence of cancer with the aesthetic cosmetic aim of preserving or improving the appearance of the breast.

ondansetron

A tablet used as an anti-emetic to prevent vomiting and nausea triggered by chemotherapy or radiotherapy, marketed under the brand name, Zofran.

orchiectomy

Orchiectomy, or castration, is the surgical removal of one or both testicles, a procedure that might be performed to reduce the body's androgen levels in order to treat the symptoms of breast cancer in men. (Androgens are the male hormones which the body may convert into oestrogens.)

palliative care

The active care of patients with advanced progressive diseases, who are often nearing the end of their lives. It frequently involves the management of pain and the provision of psychological and social support. 'Palliative' is also used in a broader sense to describe the care that is provided beyond clinical intervention.

peripheral neuropathy

Damage to the nerves which may affect sensation or movement. The symptoms of its onset are numbness and prickling or tingling in the hands (or feet), which can spread to the arms (or legs). Among its many causes are the side effects of chemotherapy drugs, referred to as **chemotherapy-induced peripheral neuropathy**.

phlebitis

Inflammation of a vein, often causing pain, redness of the skin, and swelling.

phlebotomy

The puncture and opening of a vein to draw off blood, often for a blood test. A phlebotomist is a person who draws venous blood for testing (or blood donation) by puncturing the vein. 'Phlebotomy' derives from the Greek: 'phlebo' meaning 'relating to a blood vessel' and 'tomia' meaning 'the cutting or severing of'.

physiotherapy

The treatment of injury, disease or malfunction by physical methods, usch as manipulation, massage, a routine of relevant exercises, or heat treatment. **Physiotherapists** are practitioners who help those affected by injury, illness, surgical procedures, and disability, to regain mobility and the full use of their limbs.

PICC line

An acronym for **peripherally-inserted central catheter**.

platelet

A cell fragment (without a nucleus) found in large numbers circulating in the blood stream. Platelets function by clumping or clotting together to stop bleeding from blood vessel injuries.

prostate

A walnut-sized gland surrounding the neck of the bladder in men which helps to make some of the fluid present in semen. The prostate is situated just in front of the rectum and can be detected and assessed by a rectal examination. An enlarged prostate means the prostate gland has grown bigger, which happens to most men in old age. Cancer of the prostate is the most common cancer in men.

PSA test

PSA is an acronym for the **prostate-specific antigen**. The prostate test is a blood test used to screen for prostate cancer by testing for an antigen or protein produced by cancerous and non-cancerous tissue in the prostate.

psychological and self-help therapies

Macmillan Cancer Care describes how psychological and self-help therapies are used to support cancer patients during and after their treatment, and mentions especially how support groups and self help groups provide an opportunity to share thoughts and feelings, and to learn how others have coped. Macmillan also lists other psychological therapies, such as mindfulness meditation, mindfulness-based cognitive therapy, and mindfulness-based stress reduction.

psychotherapy

Therapy used to treat emotional problems and mental health conditions. It involves talking to a trained therapist either on a one-to-one basis or in a group. It is the treatment of a behavioural disorder, a mental illness or any other condition by psychological means.

pyrexia

Raised body temperature above the normal range (37.5^0c and rising to 38.3^0c), a fever, or febrile condition.

radiographer

A person who specialises in the imaging of the human anatomy for the diagnosis and treatment of disease. A radiographer usually operates machines using radiation, especially x-rays, to take pictures of the inside of an organ/organism, or to treat a specific disease.

radiology

The science of dealing with x-rays and other high-energy radiation, and the use of that radiation for the diagnosis and treatment of disease. A **radiologist** is a person specialising in radiology, who uses x-rays for diagnosing and treating diseases.

radiotherapy

Radiotherapy is the use of x-rays, or other forms of radiation to treat disease, especially cancer. In radiotherapy, high-energy rays are used to destroy cancer cells and prevent them dividing and spreading. The rays are best used on well-defined cancers confined to a specific area of the body.

rectum

The rectum is the bottom end of the large intestine, terminating at the anus: the lowest section of the bowels or alimentary canal.

relaxation

The release of tension from muscles by physically lengthening the muscles and leading to a state of reduced stress and anxiety. (Jonas Mosby's *Dictionary of Complementary and Alternative Medicine*). **Relaxation therapy** is a form of treatment in which patients perform breathing and relaxation exercises and concentrate on pleasant situations.

saline solution

Saline solution or sodium chloride fluid is a mixture of sodium chloride and water and is used for a variety of purposes in medicine. It is used intravenously during chemotherapy to flush and hydrate before and between chemotherapy drugs. A saline flush is used to clean intravenous lines, such as a Hickman line, to prevent blood clotting.

secondaries

A common term for disease that has spread beyond the location of the primary disease to another part of the body, as in the metastisisation (see metastasis) of cancer.

Skene gland

Or **paraurethral gland** in women, is found in the area of the vulva, outside the vaginal wall and near the lower end of the urethra, and shares features with the prostate gland in men.

sentinel lymph node

The first lymph node in a row or cluster of nodes. It is likely to be the first organ to be reached by metastisising cells from a breast cancer tumour. If the sentinel node is free of cancer, it is assumed that the cancer has not spread beyond its original site.

septicaemia

Commonly referred to as blood poisoning, septicaemia is the invasion of the blood stream from a focal point of infection by microorganisms, such as bacteria, viruses or fungi, leading to acute illness of the whole body.

seroma

A gathering under the skin of serum fluid, consisting of blood plasma from injured cells – that may occur after surgery.

sonography

The use of reflected high-frequency sound waves to build up an image of a body organ. The image is known as a **sonogram**. A **sonographer** is a specialist in diagnostic medical sonography, who uses ultrasound to produce an image of an organ.

sphygmomanometer

Using abbreviated to 'sphyg', a sphygmomanometer is an instrument for measuring blood pressure, usually consisting of an inflatable rubber cuff which tightens around the arm to record systolic and diastolic blood pressure.

steroids

Different types of chemical substances that are produced in the body, or artificial forms of those substances that are used as medications. Examples include oestrogen and testosterone, and the anti-inflammatory dexamethasone.

subcutaneous

Situated, used or introduced under the skin, as in the case of a subcutaneous injection.

Sudocrem

A medicated cream used to treat nappy rash, eczema, bedsores, acne and chilblains. Ingredients include a water-repellent base of oil and wax, emollients, antibacterial and antifungal agents and a mild anaesthetic. Originally manufactured by a Dublin pharmacist, the current brand name still reflects Dubliners' colloquial pronunciation of 'soothing cream'.

surgical stockings

These are elasticated compression stockings, a form of hosiery worn to prevent the development of venous (vein) disorders, such as, oedema, phlebitis and thrombosis.

sutures

Stitches that are inserted to hold together the edges of a wound, or close up a surgical incision.

tamoxifen

A selective oestrogen-receptor modulator of the triphenylethylene group that is used to treat and prevent the recurrence of breast cancer in both women and men. It is usually taken by mouth on a daily basis for five years after other adjuvant therapies for breast cancer. It is sold under the brand name, Nolvadex.

tamsulosin

A drug used to treat urinary retention, benign prostatic hyperplasia, and to help in the passage of kidney stones. It works by relaxing bladder neck muscles, thus making it easier to urinate.

therapy

A widely-used term deriving from the Greek word, *therapeíã*, meaning 'treatment', as in chemotherapy, psychotherapy, radiotherapy, hormone therapy, complementary therapy, etc.

thorax

The part of the body between the neck and the diaphragm, commonly called the chest, including the content encased by the ribs, especially the heart and lungs.

thrombo-phlebitis

Inflammation of a vein (phlebitis) relating to the presence of a blood clot (thrombus). Symptoms include pain to the affected area, redness to the skin, and swelling. In my case, the thrombo-phlebitis was located in my arm which, at one stage, I was unable to straighten. It was caused by the insertion into the vein of an intravenous needle and catheter and the injection through them of chemotherapy drugs.

trimethoprim

An antibiotic used mainly to treat urinary tract infections.

urea and electrolytes

The most commonly requested biochemistry tests, providing information about a person's health, such as the levels of sodium and potassium in the body, the functioning of the kidneys, and renal disease. (*Nursing Times*, 24.01.2014).

urology

The branch of medicine concerned with the function and disorders of the urinary system. A **urologist** is a doctor who specialises in the treatment of the urinary system.

visualisation or **guided imagery**

A psychotherapeutic technique aimed at altering mental imagery to bring about beneficial change to thought patterns and behaviour, thus reducing symptoms of pain, anxiety and stress.

Xailin Fresh

A brand name for eye drops containing carmellose sodium which are used to treat red, sore or itchy eyes.

ZeroAQS emollient cream

A cream containing macrogol cetastearylether, cetostearyl, alcohol, chlorocresol, white soft paraffin, liquid paraffin, and purified water. ZeroAQS is an emollient (having the property of softening and soothing the skin) and a cleanser. It is used to treat and soothe skin affected by the radiation administered during radiotherapy.

Directory of persons

This is a directory of the names of family members, friends, surgeons, physicians, nurses and therapists who, in the course of my breast cancer, comforted, cared for, supported, or treated me, and whose first names and surnames appear in this book. Persons involved in the course of my treatment at the hospital or GP surgery are referred to by pseudonyms in order to accommodate an expressed preference for privacy. An unaltered name is signalled by the use of Roman script, a pseudonym by Italic.

Abbassi, Dr Salma

Dr Salma Abbassi was the doctor who discussed my test results with me on the 15th May 2018, when I was a patient on the Acute Medical Unit at New Cross Hospital.

Agrasen, Dr

Following my urinary problems, I made an appointment on the 25th September 2017 at the Castlecroft Medical Centre, where I saw *Dr Agrasen*, a GP, who suggested my complaint was likely to be a consequence of the anaesthetic I had been given, and prescribed the antibiotic, trimethoprim, for a urinary infection.

Ahmed, Dr Tasleema

A GP at the Castlecroft Medical Practice, *Dr Tasleema Ahmed* examined the lump in my breast on the 9th August 2017, and arranged an appointment for me on the 23rd August, with the breast cancer consultant at New Cross Hospital.

Bianchi, Dr Monica

Dr Monica Bianchi is a GP at the Castlecroft Medical Practice, who, on the 14th May 2018, recognised the potentially serious nature of my condition and directed me to go immediately to the New Cross Hospital Emergency Department.

Bilson, Councillor Peter

Peter Bilson is deputy leader of Wolverhampton City Council and cabinet member for city assets and housing.

Bowker, Staff Nurse Christine

Staff Nurse Christine Bowker conducted my discharge interview from the Appleby Suite, after the operation for the insertion of my Hickman line on the 8th March 2018.

Brock, Student Nurse Michelle

Student Nurse Michelle Brock, from the University of Wolverhampton, on placement at the Appleby Suite, comforted and supported me, following my operation for the insertion of a Hickman line on the 8th March 2018.

Catterall, Nurse Margery

Nurse Margery Catterall, a member of the New Cross Hospital Breast Cancer Nursing Team, gave practical advice and support and checked my seroma (for example, on the 28th November and 6th December 2017).

Channar, Nurse Saiju

Nurse Saiju Channar helped take blood samples from me on the Durnall Oncology Day Care Unit on the 14th June 2018.

Chevannes, Lloyd

Lloyd is my brother-in-law, who lives in Sutton Coldfield, with wife, Bernadette. He and Bernadette came to visit me at home and have regularly asked after my health.

Chevannes, Professor Mel

Mel has been my wife for 42 years and is the mother of my three children, Toussaint, Spartaca and Robeson. Since my breast cancer diagnosis, she has served as my primary carer, accompanying me to hospital appointments, making sure I took my medicines on time, administering my injections at home, and keeping me fed and clean. Trained as a nurse, midwife and health visitor, with a former career in higher education as a professor of nursing, she has been in a position to offer me both the practical and intellectual support and advice that has made it possible to write this book.

Chevannes-Osborne, Caio Darwin

Caio is Toussaint Chevannes-Osborne and Luc Osborne's son, and Frank and Mel's grandson, who on a number of occasions came with his mother and father to stay when I was undergoing my treatment for breast cancer. Caio was born on the 27th July 2017, at the time that my breast cancer first came to light, Caio's arrival coming to symbolise rebirth, rejuvenation and the triumph of life over disease, despair and death.

Chevannes-Osborne, Toussaint

Toussaint is one of Frank and Mel's daughters, who lives in London with husband, Luc, and their baby boy, Caio, one of Frank and Mel's grandsons. Toussaint, Luc and Caio visited me on numerous occasions while I was undergoing treatment for breast cancer.

Chevannes-Reeves, Spartaca

Spartaca is one of Frank and Mel's daughters, who lives in Nairobi Kenya with husband, Patrick. She called us on the 10th February 2018, to tell us the heartening news that she was expecting a baby. She communicates on a regular basis, via Facetime, with Mel and me to inquire about my health.

Coburn, Nurse Samantha

Nurse Samantha Coburn, who has worked as an oncology nurse for fifteen years, conducted my line care on the Durnall Oncology Day Care Unit on the 21st March and 11th May 2018.

Cornwallis, Columbine

Columbine Cornwallis is a hospital counsellor and member of the Cancer Psychology and Counselling Service, who led a session of the visualisation and relaxation group for cancer patients (newly diagnosed and in active treatment), which I attended on the 27th April 2018.

Curtis, Helen (née Lewis)

Helen is my second cousin who telephoned me on Wednesday 22nd May 2018 to inform Mel and me of the death of her mother, Joy Etteridge (née Wiggins), (my late father's cousin).

Dasent, Margaret

Margaret is a longstanding family friend, who used to baby-sit our children, and now works as a nurse in General Practice. She visited and telephoned regularly to inquire after my health.

Davis, Councillor Norman, and wife, Mary

Norman Davis OBE was a friend and political colleague of Mel, when she served on Wolverhampton City Council. He recognised me from his trolley bed as he was wheeled towards the Deanesly Oncology Centre on the 22nd January 2018. Mel attended his funeral at St Leonard's Church in Bilston on the 1st May 2018. Norman was leader of Wolverhampton's Labour Group and leader of the council from1973 to 1984, and from 1986 to 2002.

Dean, Nurse Heather

Nurse Heather Dean conducted my line care and took blood samples from me on the Durnall Oncology Day Care Unit on the 24th and 31st May 2018.

Denktash, Sister Neshele

Sister Neshele Denktash performed my Hickman line care on the 15th May 2018, when I was a patient on the Acute Medical Unit at New Cross Hospital.

Dharma, Aaron

Aaron Dharma is the founder of *Mindspan* and tutor to the mindfulness eight-week beginner course (commencing on the 18th April 2018) that I attended at the Newman Centre, Tettenhall, Wolverhampton. A former Buddhist monk, *Aaron* has over 20 years of experience practising and teaching mindfulness meditation.

Dobson, Nurse Donna

Nurse Donna Dobson, a member of the New Cross Hospital Breast Cancer Nursing Team, gave practical advice and support after my breast cancer operations and drained my seroma (for example, on the 31st October and 7th November 2017).

Eden, Dean

Dean Eden is a ward assistant on the Durnall Oncology Day Care Unit, who cheerfully offered to make tea for Mel and me, every time we went on the ward for line care.

Edmunds, Sister Natalie

Sister Natalie Edmunds was New Cross Hospital's lead palliative care nurse who conducted an assessment meeting with me, accompanied by Mel, on the 27th December 2017, prior to the start of my chemotherapy course. Afterwards, we met her working on the Durnall Oncology Day Care Unit, where she performed my fifth line care on the 6th April and, sixth line care on the 13th April 2018, prior to her retirement from work on the 30th April 2018.

Finucane, Patrick

Patrick is my secondary-school friend of 56-years standing. On learning of my cancer, he made arrangements to travel from Kent to Wolverhampton, especially to visit me, staying with us from the 19th to the 21st February 2018. During his stay, we scoped out a post-treatment celebration holiday for September in Western Ireland.

Frankel, Dr Anna

Dr Anna Frankel is a long-standing friend and former colleague who, on learning of my breast cancer, inquired after my health on a regular basis and assisted me in developing the theory and practice of industrial history therapy, on the 13th February 2018, when we met at the Birmingham Jewellery Quarter, and on the 26th April 2018, when we visited the Black Country Living Museum.

Gill, Dr Chetpal

Dr Chetpal Gill is a GP from Bradley. Mel and I have known him for many years through mutual friends. We encountered Dr Gill and his wife at the Durnall Oncology Day Care Unit on the 21st March 2018.

Grigoryev, Dr Grozdan

Dr Grozdan Grigoryev is a consultant oncologist at New Cross Hospital. He met with me and Mel on the 27th November 2017, when he proposed successive courses of adjuvant chemotherapy, radiotherapy, and hormone therapy, to prevent the recurrence of my breast cancer. Together with *Dr Gupta*, he reviewed my first cycle of chemotherapy on the 22nd January 2018, and continued to monitor my progress throughout my treatment..

Gupta, Dr Hetu Charitha

Dr Hetu Charitha Gupta is a specialist registrar in oncology working with *Dr Grigoryev*, a consultant oncologist, at New Cross Hospital. Following our initial meeting with *Dr Grigoryev* and *Dr Gupta* on the 27th November

2017, *Dr Gupta* conducted reviews of my treatment and progress on the 5th March, the 26th March, and the 16th April 2018.

Harrington, Peter

Peter Harrington is an advanced practitioner of radiotherapy and a lymphoedema therapist, working in the Directorate of Oncology and Clinical Haematology at New Cross Hospital. He gave Mel and me advice on radiography, radiotherapy and lymphoedema prevention on the 10th May 2018.

Hart, Nurse Eleanor

Nurse Eleanor Hart, Acute Oncology Specialist Nurse, gave me information, advice and help when I was a patient in the Acute Medical Unit at New Cross Hospital on the 15th May 2018.

Hepworth, Amber

Amber Hepworth was one of the clerical officers for the Durnall Oncology Day Unit. Her friendly and helpful demeanour contributed greatly to the welfare of cancer patients.

Higgins, Nurse Sandra

Nurse Sandra Higgins conducted my line care on the Durnall Oncology Day Care Unit on the 7th June 2018.

Hii, Dr

Dr Hii was the doctor in charge on the Acute Medical Unit at New Cross Hospital, when I was admitted in the early morning hours of Tuesday 15th May 2018.

Holmes, Professor Diana

Di and her husband, Nick Cheesewright, are longstanding friends. Di is a professor of French at the University of Leeds and works, in particular, on women writers, and gender in literature and film. She had breast cancer herself in 2002 and remembers how supportive Mel was then. She has read earlier drafts of *Breast Cancer Man* and supplied critical advice, for which I am most grateful..

Holyoak, Sister Jemima

Sister Jemima Holyoak administered the first session of my chemotherapy on the 3rd January 2018 at the Snowdrop Millennium Suite, and the third cycle on the 14th February 2018. *Jemima* also telephoned on a number of occasions to update me on neutrophils readings.

Hopkins, Nurse Elspeth

Nurse Elspeth Hopkins was the nurse in attendance at my meeting with *Dr Gupta* on the 5th March 2018. She took us to the Snowdrop Suite to seek the chemotherapy nurses' opinion on the suitability of my veins for chemotherapy injections, following my thrombo-phlebitis,.

Hurd, Professor Geoff

Geoff Hurd and his wife, Stella, are longstanding friends. Before his retirement, Geoff was deputy vice-chancellor at the University of Wolverhampton, at the same time that Mel served as the Dean of the School of Health. On learning of my cancer, Geoff telephoned the house and spoke with Mel about my health and offered to help in any way possible. Geoff took me out for a series of therapeutic coffee mornings: on the 4th and 24th April, etc., and has supplied critical advice on earlier drafts of *Breast Cancer Man,* for which I am most grateful.

Hurst, Nurse Lindsay

Nurse Lindsay Hurst was the practice nurse at the Castlecroft Medical Practice who, on the 21st June 2018, took out the stitches from my chest following the procedure to remove my Hickman line.

Iqbal, Dr Rukhsana

On the 28th September 2017, while suffering from urinary problems, I visited the New Cross Walk-in Clinic and saw *Dr Rukhsana Iqbal*, who tested my urine and prescribed the antibiotic, nitrofurantoin.

Jevons, Sister Carys

Sister Carys Jevons leads the New Cross Hospital Breast Cancer Nursing Team. She was present when *Mr Venkatramanan* diagnosed my breast cancer and briefed us afterwards about what happened next, presenting me with a copy of Macmillan's *Understanding Breast cancer in Men*. After my mastectomy and lymph node clearance, *Sister Jevons* regularly drained the seroma I developed under the breast tissue.

Kowalczyk, Krystyna

Krystyna Kowalczyk is a senior therapy radiographer in the New Cross Directorate of Oncology and Clinical Haematology. With colleagues, she administered my radiotherapy on numerous occasions during the period of my treatment from 4th June to the 22nd June 2018.

Lawrence, Councillor Roger

Roger Lawrence is leader of Wolverhampton City Council and chair of the cabinet, with responsibility for corporate strategy. He is also chair of the Health and Wellbeing Board.

Lewis, Frank

Frank Lewis is the son of our old friend, Essie Lewis. We met Frank and his wife, Tina, at the Deanesly Oncology Unit on the 16th April 2018.

Lopez, Gem and Philip

Gem and Philip Lopez, who live in Tettenhall like us, are close friends of ours and we have been on holiday together. In recent years, Philip has helped me greatly in computer applications, preparing manuscripts for publication, including that for *Breast Cancer Man*. Gem, like me, is a trustee of Wolverhampton Citizens Advice and took me to board meetings during my treatment.

Mainwaring, Sister Cassia

Sister Cassia Mainwaring is sister-in-charge of the chemotherapy unit at the Royal Wolverhampton Hospital Trust's Cannock hospital. She administered my fourth session of chemotherapy (the first of docetaxel) at the Snowdrop Millennium Suite on the 14th March 2018.

Major, Bob

Bob is a long-standing friend of Frank and Mel, who lives in Harlech, north-central Wales. While Mel and I retain regular telephone contact with him, we were unable to deal with him face-to-face during my cancer treatment because of his persistent shingles.

Maryniuk, Dr Maksym

Dr Maksym Maryniuk is a registrar in oncology at New Cross Hospital. He examined and treated me on the Durnall Oncology Day Care Unit on the 27th February and again on the 21st March 2018, when he prescribed me omeprazole capsules.

McGrath, Senior Nurse Mary

Senior Nurse Mary McGrath is the manager of the Snowdrop Millennium Suite at New Cross Hospital.

McLean, Staff Nurse Michelle

Staff Nurse Michelle McLean administered the second session of my chemotherapy on the 29th January 2018 at the Snowdrop Millennium Suite, as well as the sixth and final session on the 30th April 2018. She also took blood samples from me on the Durnall Oncology Day Care Unit on the 14th June 2018.

Montagu, Elsie

Elsie Montagu is the phlebotomy team leader at the Deanesly Oncology Outpatients Department, New Cross Hospital, who took my blood samples on the 12th February 2018.

Narayani, Dr Haripriya

Dr Haripriya Narayani was a registrar in attendance at the Durnall Oncology Unit, who examined my Hickman line on the 17th May 2018, and removed it under local anaesthetic on the 15th June 2018..

Osborne, Luc

Luc is our son-in-law, married to Toussaint, our daughter, and the father of baby Caio Darwin. Luc visited me on a number of occasions during my breast cancer treatment to give me practical help and emotional support.

Oyawale, Dr Bidemi

Following the development of sores between my buttocks, I made an emergency appointment to see *Dr Bidemi Oyawale*, a GP at the

Castlecroft Medical Practice. She examined the area and wrote a prescription for Fucibet cream.

Parkinson, Philippa (Pip), née Reeves

Pip is one of my three sisters, who resides in Arley, north Warwickshire, with husband, John. Pip regularly inquired after my health and the progress of my treatment, giving me sensible advice.

Puttock, Nurse Rosie

Nurse Rosie Puttock took blood samples, changed my dressing, and undertook my line care at the Durnall Oncology Day Care Unit on the 12th March 2018.

Qian, Dr Yu Yan

Dr Yu Yan Qian examined my right arm on the 23rd February 2018 at Durnall Oncology Day Care Unit, and referred me for an ultrasound scan and further blood samples, which subsequently revealed I was suffering from thrombo-phlebitis.

Raja, Dr Tahir

Dr Tahir Raja is a registrar on oncology working with *Dr Grigoryev*, a consultant oncologist at New Cross Hospital. On behalf of *Dr Grigoryev*, *Dr Raja* conducted a review of my chemotherapy on the 1st February 2018, prior to the third cycle, and diagnosed my thrombo-phlebitis on the 23rd February 2018, prescribing flucloxallin, hydrocortisone cream and filgrastim injections.

Raza, Waliyah

Waliyah Raza was a therapy radiographer in the Deanesly radiotherapy department who helped prepare me for my radiotherapy course.

Reeves, Dr Francis (Frank)

Author of this book, I am Frank Reeves, the 72-year-old man (now 73), identified forever in NHS records as 'Francis Reeves' (additionally confirmed by my date of birth and address). I am married to Mel Chevannes, with whom I have three children, who themselves have given us grandchildren. *Breast Cancer Man* is an account of my diagnosis, operations, and treatment for breast cancer at New Cross Hospital, an NHS hospital in the West Midlands.

Reeves, Genevieve (Vieve)

Genevieve is Robeson and Tasha Reeves' daughter, and Frank and Mel's granddaughter. She was brought on a number of occasions to visit me, her grandfather, during my treatment for breast cancer, thus giving me renewed inspiration for living.

Reeves, Margaret (Maggie)

Maggie is one of my three sisters, who resides in Southwell, with husband, Barrie. She gave me a book at Christmas 2017, which distracted me from the injections of my first session of chemotherapy on the 3rd January. Maggie has assiduously inquired after my progress and provided me with all the love and support that a brother could reasonably expect at such times.

Reeves, Maximus (Maxi)

Maximus is Robeson and Tasha Reeves' son, and Frank and Mel's grandson. He was brought on a number of occasions to visit me, his grandfather, during my treatment for breast cancer, thus giving me renewed inspiration for living.

Reeves, Robeson

Robeson is our son, married to Tasha, and father of Maximus and Genevieve, two of our grandchildren. During my breast cancer treatment, he phoned me regularly to ask after me, and drove from London to Wolverhampton to visit me on many occasions, cooking me cordon-bleu meals to rekindle my post-chemo sense of taste.

Reeves, Tasha (née Harvey)

Tasha is our daughter-in-law, married to Robeson, our son, and mother of Maximus and Genevieve, two of our grandchildren. During my breast cancer treatment, Tasha showed me great love and affection, including making me real ginger tea, and made sure she brought our grandchildren to visit on a regular basis.

Ridley, Charles

Charles Ridley is a clinical psychologist working with the Cancer and Renal Psychology Service at New Cross Hospital. On the 11th May 2018, he led a session of the visualisation and relaxation group.

Roberts, Bartholomew

Bartholomew Roberts is chair of the Royal Wolverhampton NHS Trust, with ten years experience as a non-executive director.

Rose, David and Clare

David and Clair are our next-door neighbours at 55 Woodthorne Road and are clinical psychologists by profession.

Rush, Rosanne

A phlebotomist at the Deanesly Centre, *Rosanne Rush* took blood samples from me on 5th March 2018.

Samuel, Dr Guthrie

On the 8th March 2018 at New Cross Hospital's Appleby Suite, *Dr Guthrie Samuel* operated on my chest under local anaesthetic to insert a Hickman line, or central venous catheter (CVC).

Seagrove, Nurse Shelley

Nurse Shelley Seagrove conducted my fourth line care at the Durnall Oncology Day Care Unit on the 28th March 2018, and was friendly and pleasant when I visited Durnall again on the 4th May.

Shakeshaft, Dr

Dr Shakeshaft was the lead GP at the Castlecroft Medical Practice, to whom official correspondence about patients was generally addressed.

Shastri, Mr Tajim

Mr Tajim Shastri is a consultant in oncoplastic breast surgery and general surgery at New Cross Hospital. His picture appears along with that of *Mr Venkatramanan* in the Wolverhampton and District Breast Cancer Action group's recent recruitment leaflet.

Shergill, Mr Anil

Mr Anil Shergill is a consultant sonographer at New Cross Hospital's Imaging Department, who on the 23rd February 2018, diagnosed me as having thrombo-phlebitis.

Shome Mr Hiyan

Mr Hiyan Shome is a consultant urologist surgeon at New Cross Hospital, who examined my prostate gland and discussed my post-operative urinary symptoms at the urology outpatients' department on the 1st February 2018.

Singh, Dev and Marie

Dev and Marie are our next-door neighbours at 51 Woodthorne Road. Dev works as a consultant diabetician at New Cross Hospital and Marie is an advanced nurse practitioner in Brewood.

Spittle, Lucan

Lucan is a boiler engineer, partner to Emma, the daughter of Gem and Philip Lopez. He came to our assistance on the 2nd February 2018, when our boiler broke down, and refused to be paid for his work!

Summer, Nurse Dionne

Nurse Dionne Summer was a New Cross Hospital Emergency Department triage nurse who admitted me with suspected neutropenic sepsis on the 14th May 2018, and later administered antibiotics and Hartmann's solution through my Hickman line.

Townsend, Angela (Annie), née Moane, adopted Reeves

Annie is one of my three sisters, who resides in Ripple with husband, Pete. Annie constantly inquired after my health and the progress of my treatment and came to visit me on Sunday the 21st January 2018.

Trainer, Nurse Janice

Nurse Janice Trainer flushed my line and took blood samples on the 27th April 2018 at the Durnall Oncology Day Care Unit.

Venkatramanan, Mr Suri

Mr Suri Venkatramanan is a consultant oncoplastic breast surgeon at New Cross Hospital who specialises in the management of breast conditions, breast cancer, and breast reconstruction. I was referred to his outpatient clinic on the 23rd August 2017 when, after a biopsy of the lump in my left breast, he diagnosed me on the 29th August 2017 to have breast cancer.

Mr Venkatramanan performed my mastectomy and sentinel node biopsy on the 22nd September 2017, the biopsy result on the 10th October making it necessary for him to undertake a lymph gland clearance operation on the 20th October 2017. I was pleased to learn that *Mr Venkatramanan* is the West Midlands breast screening quality assurance surgeon responsible for ensuring all breast surgeons screening breast cancer patients in the West Midlands adhere to the highest standards.

Walsgrove, Derek

Derek Walsgrove is a friend and former colleague of mine from Bilston College. We recognised one another on the Deanesly Millennium Suite on the 14th February 2018 when he was accompanying his partner to an oncology appointment.

Warmington, Staff Nurse Liza

Staff Nurse Liza Warmington works at the Durnall Oncology Day Care Unit, New Cross Hospital. She took blood samples from me and administered my line care on the 23rd February, 9th March, 20th April, 4th May, and 17th May 2018.

Wilson, Staff Nurse Jean

Staff Nurse Jean Wilson conducted my admission procedure to the New Cross Hospital Appleby Suite on the 8th March 2018, prior to an operation to insert a Hickman line in my chest. She comforted me beforehand with a very-welcome bear hug.

Subject index

bubbles in drip tube, alarm, 165.

cancer: & age, 338; & Darwinian principles, 161; & depression, 327-328; diagnosis, research to speed it up, 160; & outlook on life, 336-344; selective perception of c news, 78, 337; & travel, 334-336; & work, 329-331.

car parking charges at hospital, see New Cross Hospital, Wolverhampton.

Castlecroft Medical Practice, Wolverhampton, 4, 25, 245-246, 288, 305.

central line, see Hickman line.

chemotherapy, 36, 37-38, 41, 187, 310-312; alternatives, 82; coping with, 182; cycles of, (1) 47-62, (2) 63-86, (3) 94-109, (4) 128-147, (5) 163-180, (6) 218-244; sessions of, (1) 47-49, (2) 63-65, (3) 94-96, (4) 129-131, (5) 164-165, (6) 218-220.

Citizens Advice, Wolverhampton, 73, 137, 157, 317.

Compton Hospice change of name, 168.

cramp attacks, 134, 135, 141, 145, 170, 225, 227, 230.

CT scans, 36.

Davis, Norman, friend and former councillor: funeral, 221; patient at New Cross, 60-61.

DCIS (ductal carcinoma in situ), 28.

deaths of relatives and friends, their depressing effect, 162, 163, 164, 223.

sonography, 15.

sphygmomanometer, 219.

tamoxifen, 36, 37-38, 174, 283-289; benefits, 283-284; preferable to castration, 284; side effects, 284-286; supply, 288.

taste, loss of, 168, 172, 173, 230, 231, 232.

therapy, 182-215; complementary, 197, 204, 331; earfulness, 215; holiday t, 199; industrial history/roots t, 188-191; meditation, 204-205; mindfulness, 205-215; nature of t, 194-195, 196; psychological ts, 204, 331-332; relief through t, 203-204; visualisation and relaxation, 191-194, 233.

thrombo-phlebitis, 105, 107, 108, 109, 111-126.

urology: interlude, 87-92.

vaccination, chemotherapy's effect on, 62, 334.

vulnerability, feelings of, 76, 78, 79-81, 85, 157.

Windrush: government's hostile environment, 180; W and NHS joint 70 years celebration in Manchester, 271, 276.

Wolverhampton Royal Hospital Trust, 4, 291, 294, 313.

Wolverhampton Wanderers, emotional uplift at their promotion to Premiership, 177.

How to obtain copies of *Breast Cancer Man*

Breast Cancer Man has been written with the aim of informing those newly diagnosed with breast cancer about the treatment they are likely to be given, and the possible physical, mental and social impact it may have on them, in the hope that they will be better prepared for the subsequent course of events, for example, the surgical interventions and/or adjuvant therapies. Newly-diagnosed breast cancer patients can obtain free single copies of the first edition of *Breast Cancer Man* by emailing blueroofbooks@yahoo.com, or by writing to Blue Roof Books, 53 Woodthorne Road, Tettenhall, Wolverhampton WV6 8TU. Please supply your name, and postal address and provide a reason for your interest, for example, you have been diagnosed with breast cancer, or are employed in the NHS. Other customers will be charged a subsidised standard RRP of £10 (inclusive of postage and packing). Appreciative readers are encouraged as a quid pro quo to make a donation to Supporter Donations, Macmillan Cancer Support, FREEPOST LON15851, 89 Albert Embankment, London SE1 7UQ.

Copies of *Breast Cancer Man* are also available on Amazon.